SELF ASSESSMENT IN RADIOLOGY

Cardio-Thoracic Imaging

Michael B Rubens
MB, BS, DMRD, FRCR

*Consultant Radiologist at the London Chest Hospital
and the National Heart Hospital, and Honorary
Senior Lecturer at the Heart & Lung Institute,
University of London*

Wolfe Medical Publications Ltd

Copyright © Michael B Rubens, 1989
First published in 1989 by Wolfe Medical
Publications Ltd
Printed by W. S. Cowell Ltd,
Ipswich, England
ISBN 0 7234 0906 4

All rights reserved. No reproduction, copy or transmission of this publication may be made without written permission.

No part of this publication may be reproduced, copied or transmitted save with written permission or in accordance with the provisions of the Copyright Act 1956 (as amended), or under the terms of any licence permitting limited copying issued by the Copyright Licensing Agency, 33-34 Alfred Place, London, WC1E, 7DP.

Any person who does any unauthorised act in relation to this publication may be liable to criminal prosecution and civil claims for damages.

A CIP catalogue record for this book is available from the British Library.

This book is one title in a series of radiology self-assessment question and answer books. For a full list of other titles in the series, plus details of all our medical and surgical atlases, please write to Wolfe Medical Publications Ltd, Brook House, 2-16 Torrington Place, London WC1E 7LT.

Some other subjects of titles in the series:
Ear, nose and throat radiology
Gastrointestinal radiology
Mammography
Paediatric radiology
Neuroradiology
Nuclear medicine
Urological radiology

Preface

This book is one in a series entitled *Self Assessment in Radiology & Imaging*. A decade and a half ago such a series would have been entitled simply *Self Assessment in Radiology*. The modalities that necessitate the addition of *Imaging* to the series title—radio-nuclide imaging (RN), ultrasonography (US), computed tomography (CT) and magnetic resonance imaging (MRI)—have all been developed since then, and are now an essential part of our diagnostic armamentarium. Nevertheless, the chest radiograph (CXR) remains the most frequently performed single radiographic or imaging procedure. The CXR is often the initial investigation in a patient with known or suspected systemic disease. Moreover, countless CXRs are performed routinely on patients entering hospital for almost any reason, or for immigration purposes, or for pre-employment or insurance medical examinations. The wisdom of performing these routine CXRs is debatable, but the fact is that they are done and someone has to interpret the films. All too often this is not a formally trained radiologist.

This book is aimed at anyone who looks at CXRs. As in earlier books in the series, it comprises a sequence of cases presented in a question-and-answer format. In many instances the CXR is supported by some other imaging modality. Most common thoracic abnormalities are represented, and the book may also be used as an atlas by referring to the diagnostic index.

In order to encourage an orderly approach to analysis of the CXR the cases are arranged, more or less, into abnormalities of the chest wall, diaphragm (and upper abdomen), pleura, lung, heart and mediastinum.

Q1

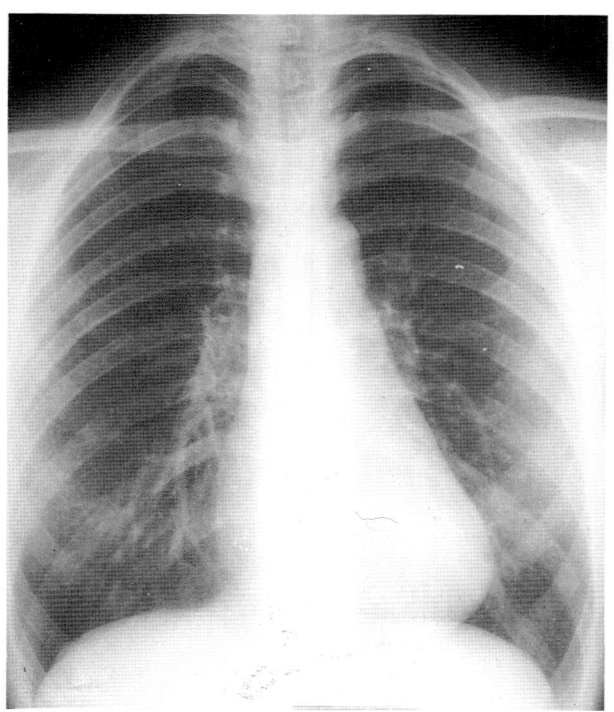 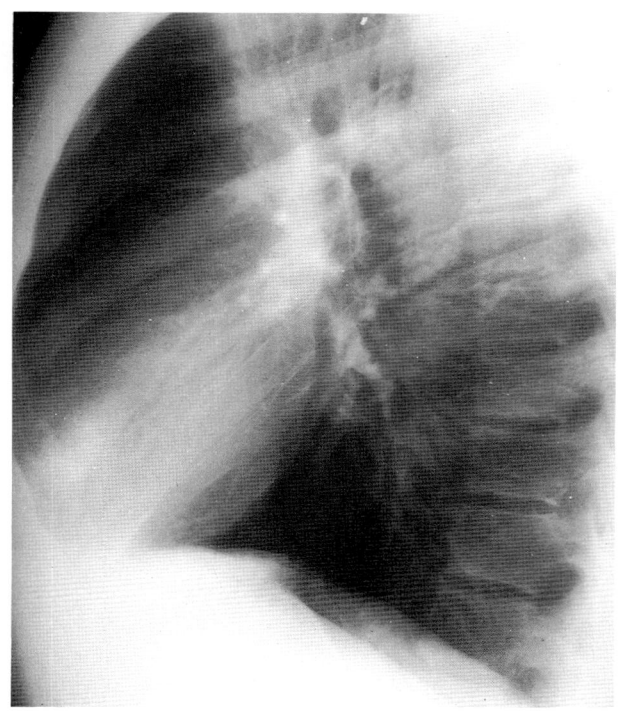

A 42-year-old man presented with a normal PA and lateral CXR.

- What does PA mean, and how does the appearance differ from an AP film?

- On the PA film, what structures form:
  a) The right cardiovascular silhouette?
  b) The left cardiovascular silhouette?

- On the lateral film what structures form:
  a) The anterior cardiac silhouette?
  b) The posterior cardiac silhouette?

A1

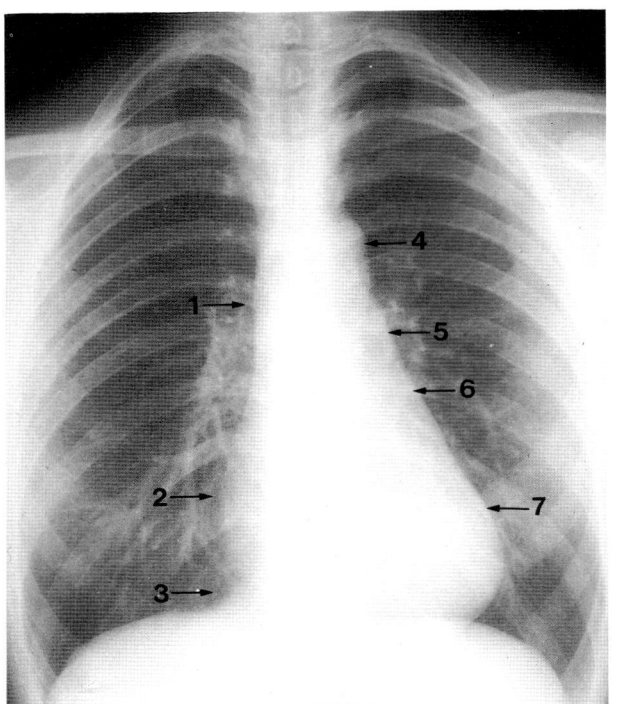
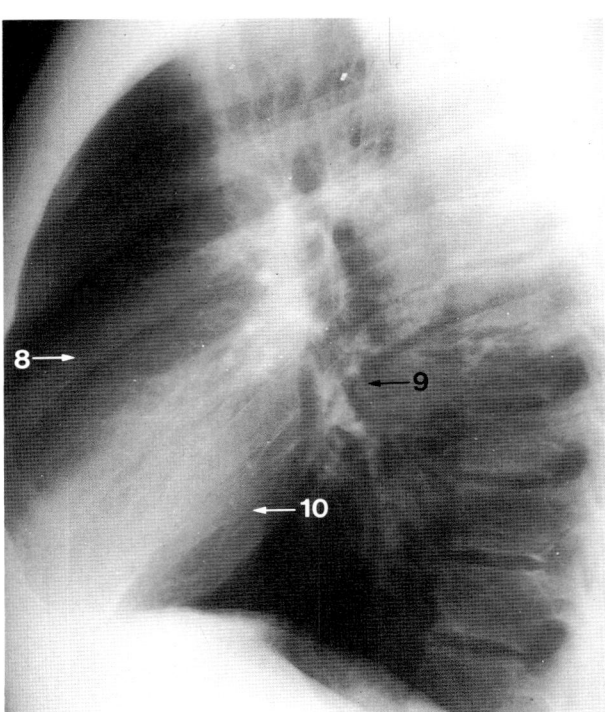

PA means postero-anterior, and refers to the direction of the x-ray beam through the patient. The patient is positioned with his anterior chest wall against the film and his back to the x-ray tube. For an AP CXR, the patient's back is against the film, and the heart, which is an anterior structure, is further from the film, and is therefore magnified.

The right cardiovascular silhouette comprises the superior vena cava (1), the right atrium (2), and the inferior vena cava (3). The structures forming the left cardiovascular silhouette are the aortic knuckle (4), the pulmonary trunk (5), the left atrial appendage (6), and the left ventricle (7). The anterior cardiac silhouette is formed by the right ventricle (8). The posterior cardiac silhouette comprises the left atrium and pulmonary veins (9) and the left ventricle (10).

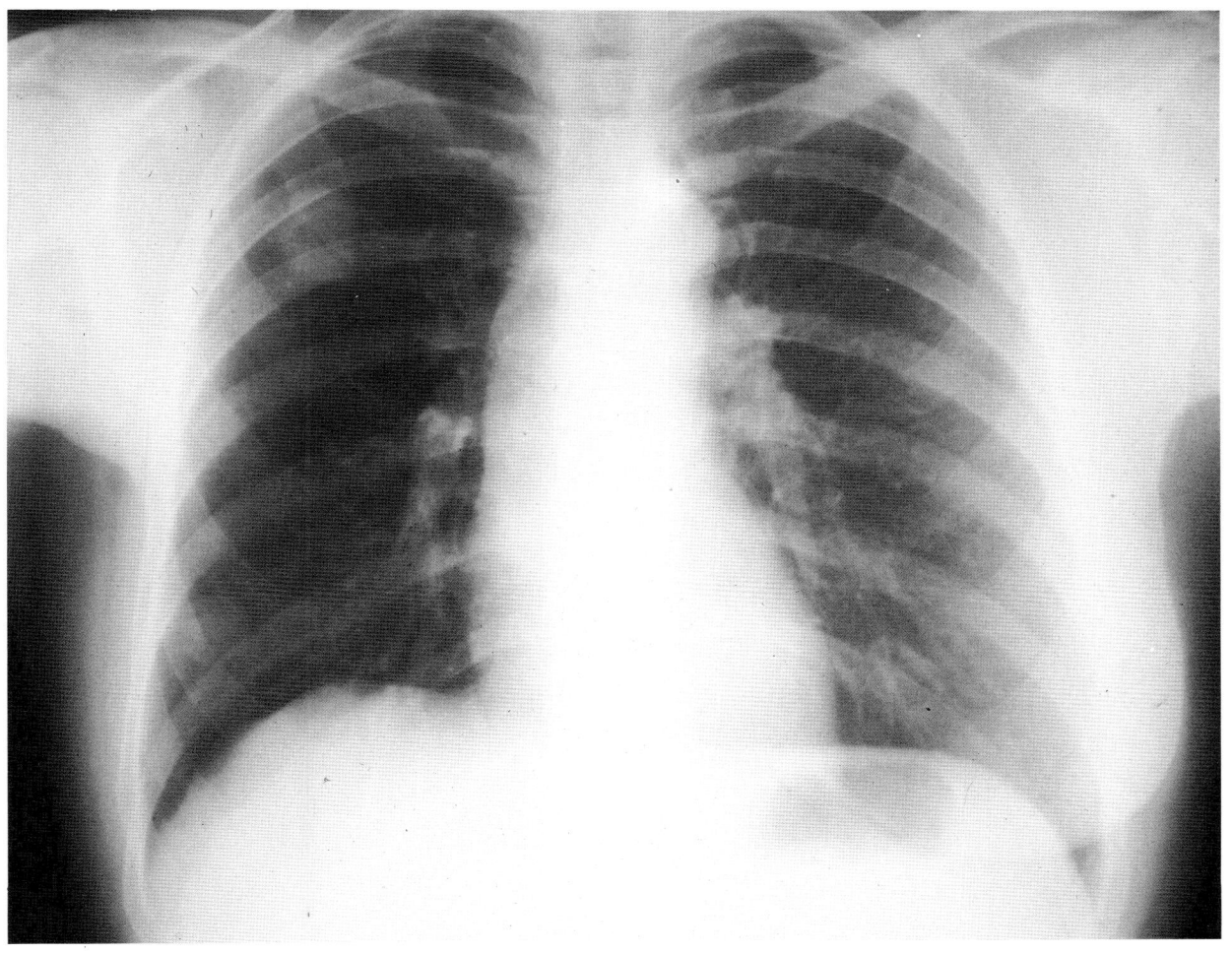

A 45-year-old woman presented with right-sided chest discomfort. Three years previously she underwent surgery.

- Comment on the relative density of the lungs.
- What was the operation?
- What is the diagnosis?

A2

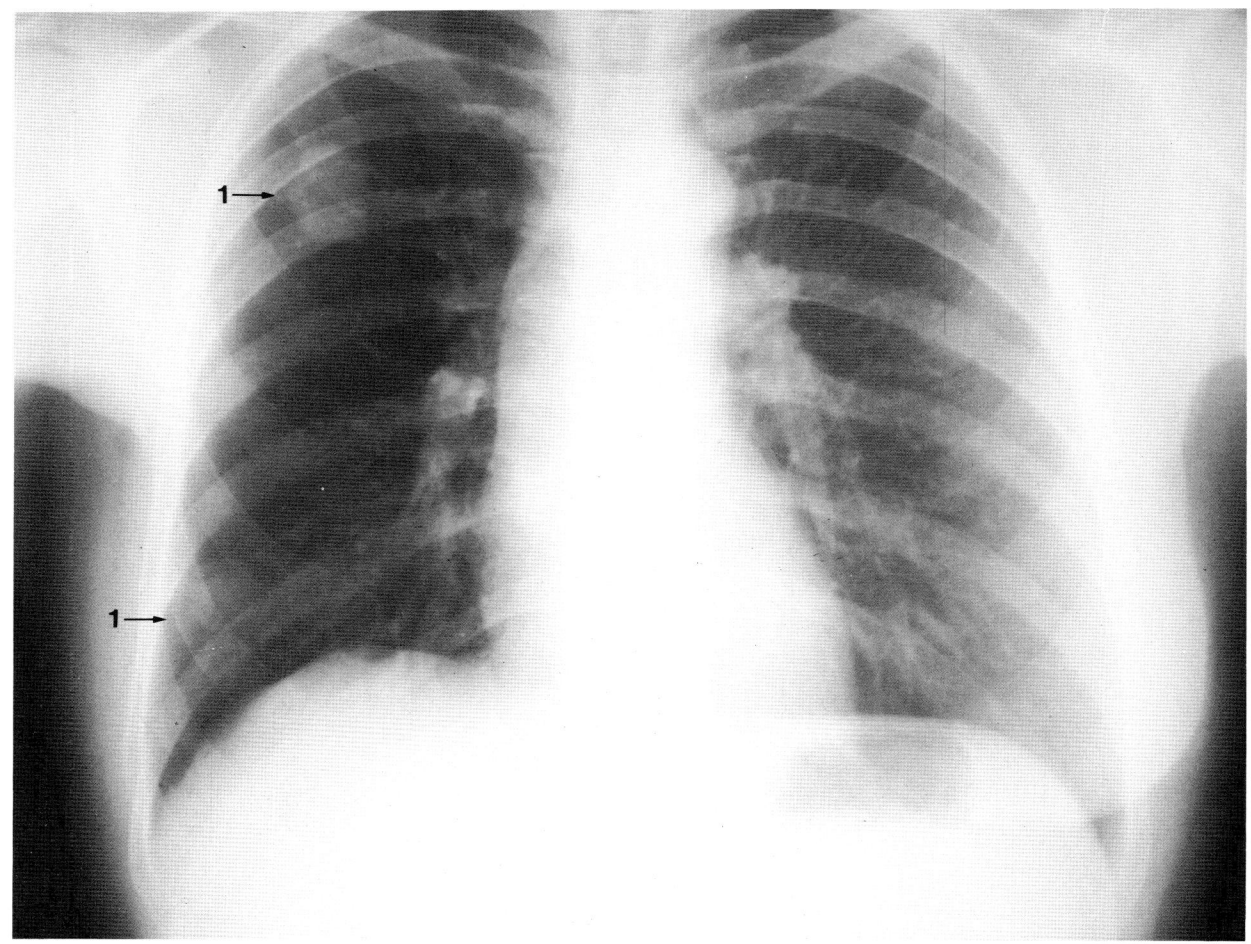

The right lung is hypertransradiant. The left breast is visible, but not the right. In addition, two opacities (1) are visible in the right lung. The patient has had a right mastectomy. The diagnosis is pulmonary metastases from carcinoma of the breast.

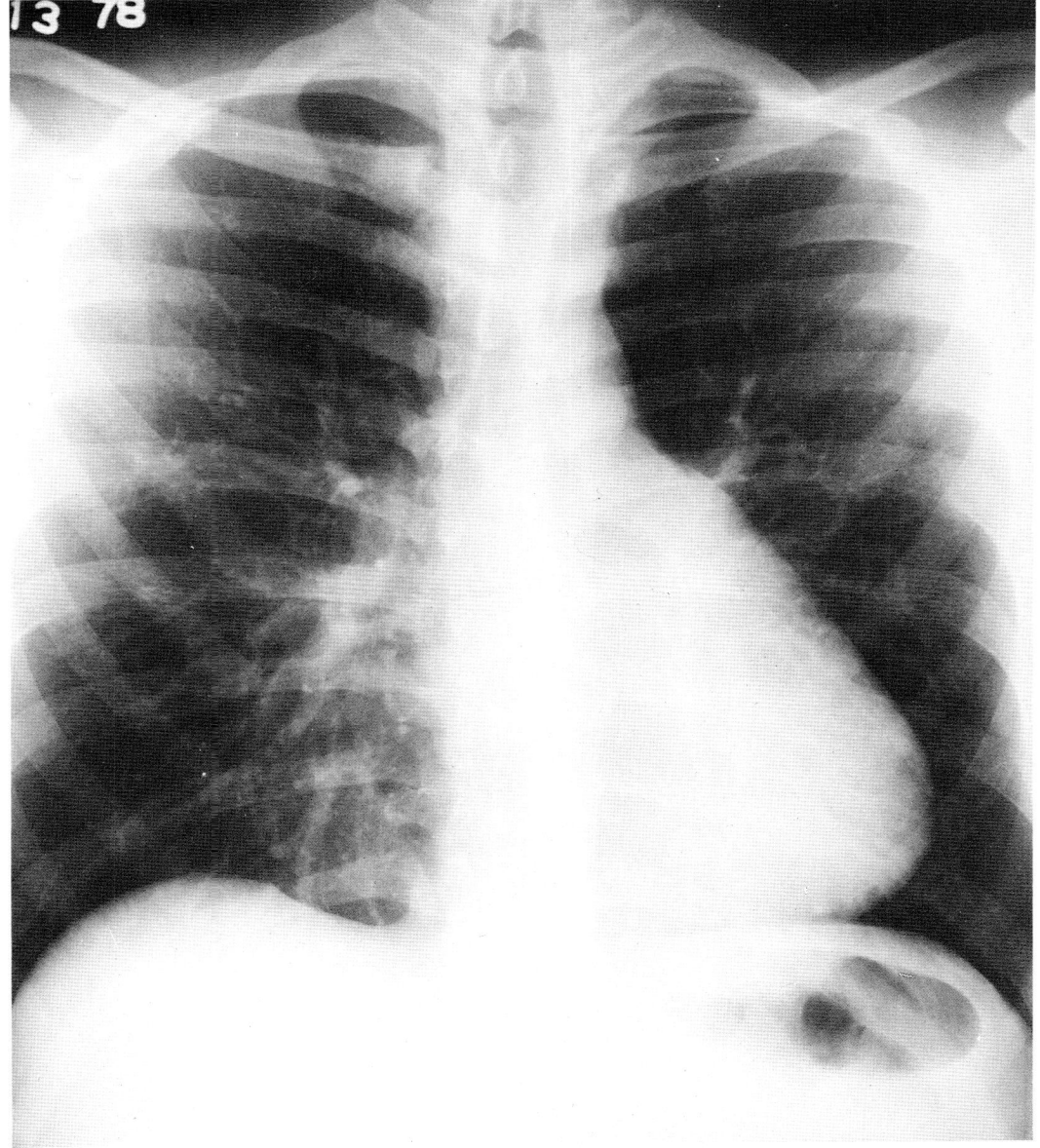

This CXR was taken during a routine medical examination. The patient is a fit 36-year-old man.

- Comment on the position and shape of the heart.
- Comment on the appearance of the ribs.
- What did clinical examination of the chest show?

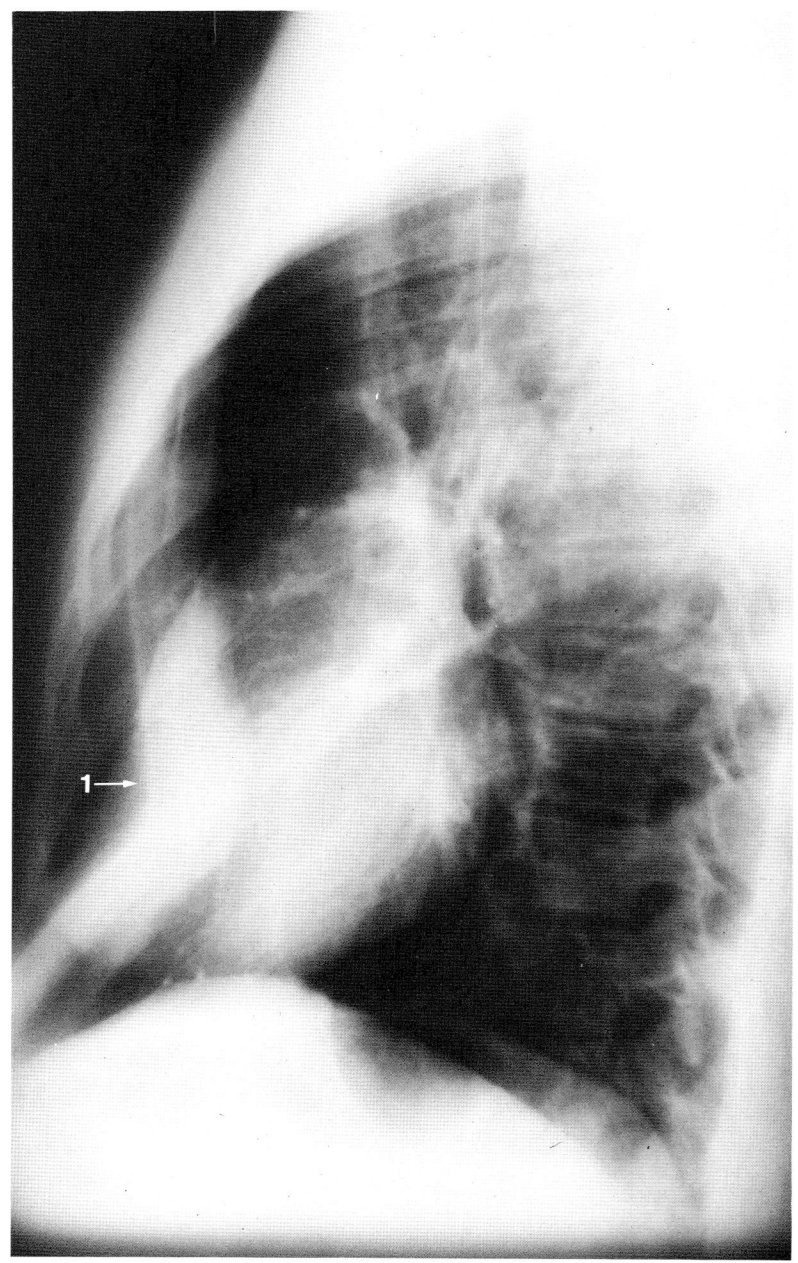

The heart is displaced to the left, and the left heart border is straighter than usual. Compared with normal, the ribs slope upward posteriorly and are more steeply inclined anteriorly. The patient has a depressed sternum (pectus excavatum). This is well demonstrated on the lateral film: the depressed sternum (1) is displacing the heart posteriorly.

Q4

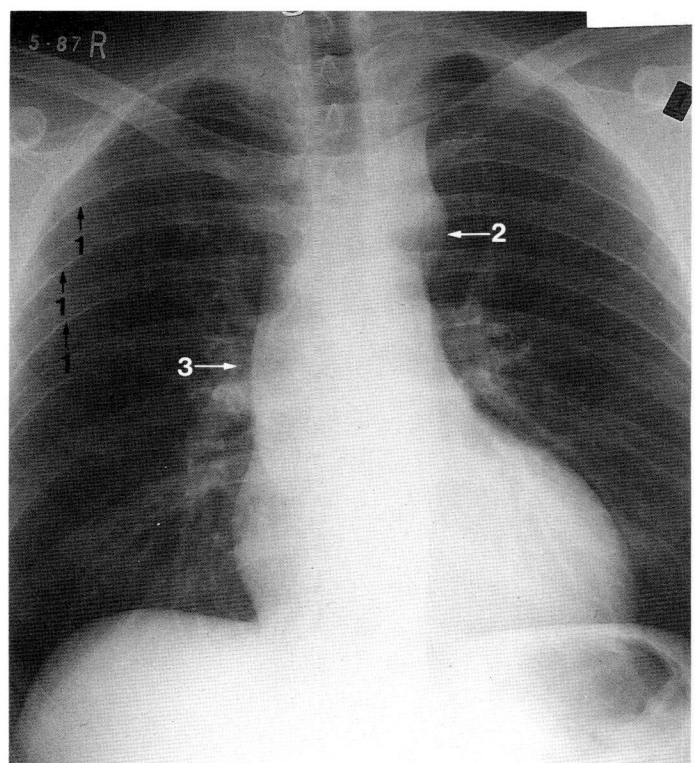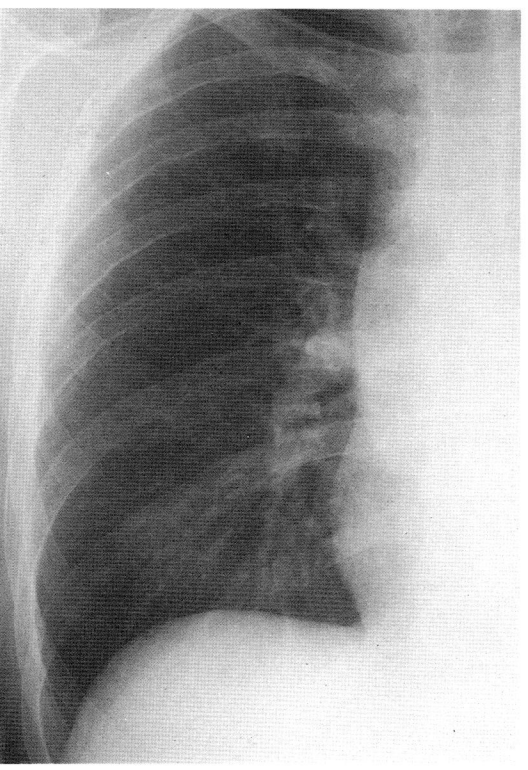

A 26-year-old man presented with headaches. On clinical examination the blood pressure was elevated and an ejection systolic murmur was heard.

- What is the diagnosis?
- Comment on the ribs (1).
- Comment on the aortic knuckle (2).
- Why is the ascending aorta (3) prominent?

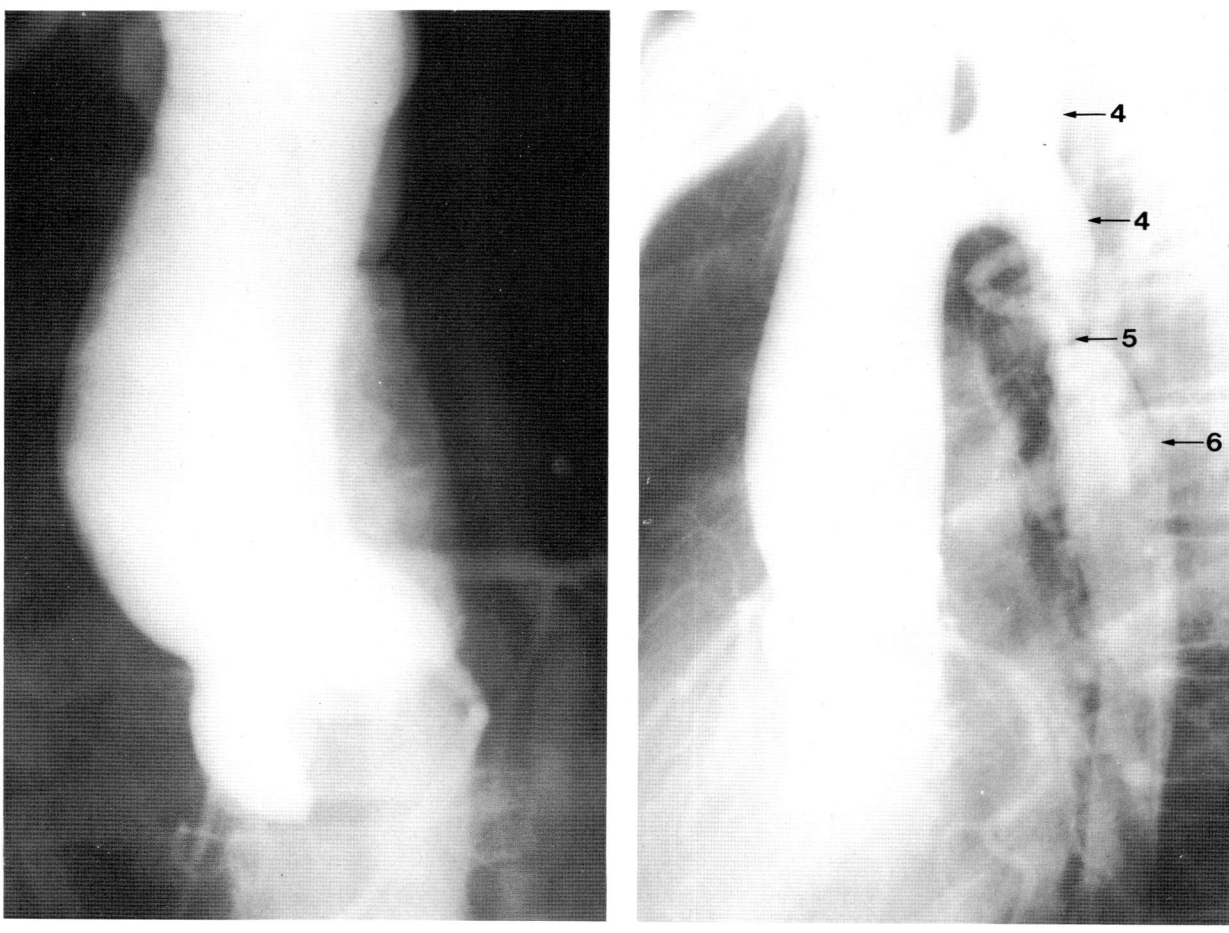

The diagnosis is coarctation of the aorta. There is rib notching, which is caused by dilatation and tortuosity of the intercostal arteries. The aortic knuckle shows an abnormal double density. Aortography shows that this is produced by aorta and dilated left subclavian artery (4) proximal to the coarctation (5), and post-stenotic dilatation of the aorta (6) distal to it.

In addition, there is a stenosed bicuspid aortic valve with post-stenotic dilatation of the ascending aorta. Up to 80 per cent of cases of coarctation of the aorta have a congenitally abnormal aortic valve.

Q5

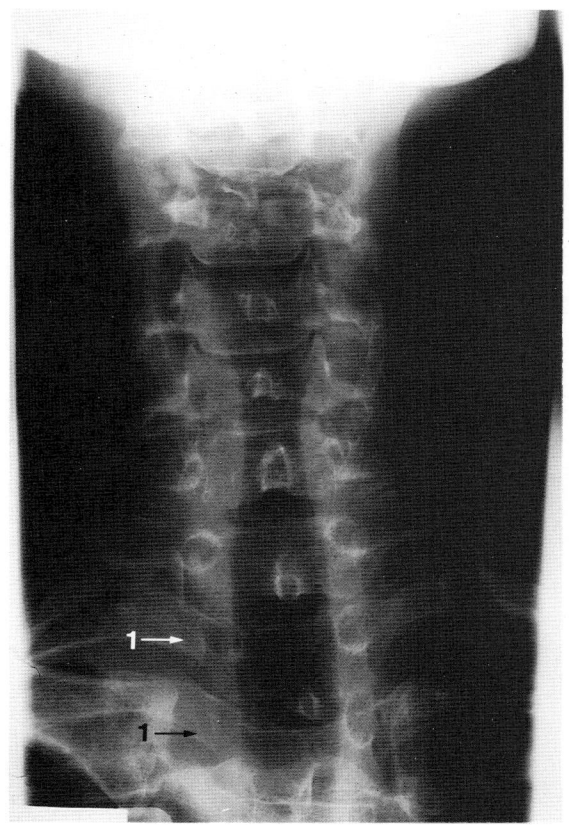
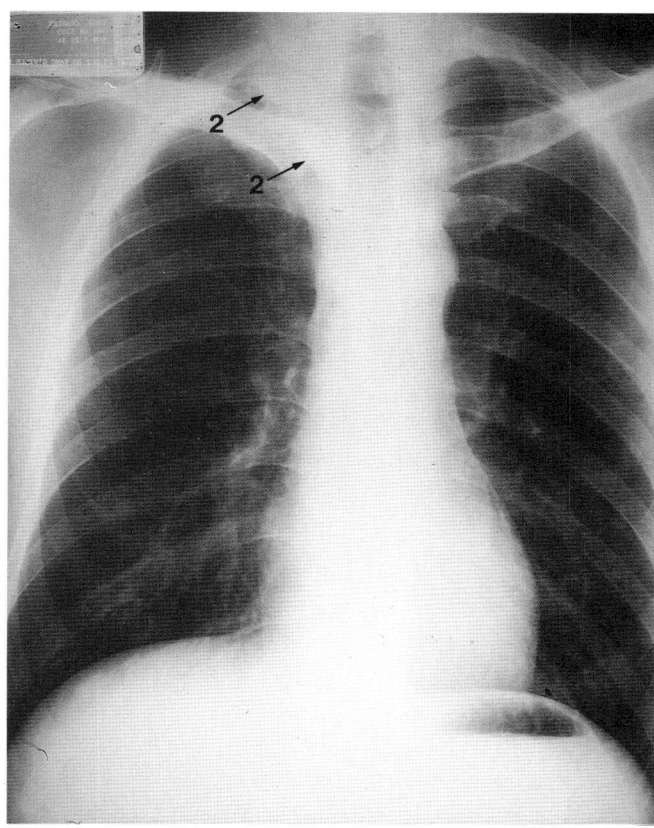

A 46-year-old man presented with pain in the neck and right arm.

- What bony abnormality (1) is seen in the cervical spine?
- Describe the abnormality (2) seen on both films at the right apex.
- What is the diagnosis?
- What investigations would you do next?

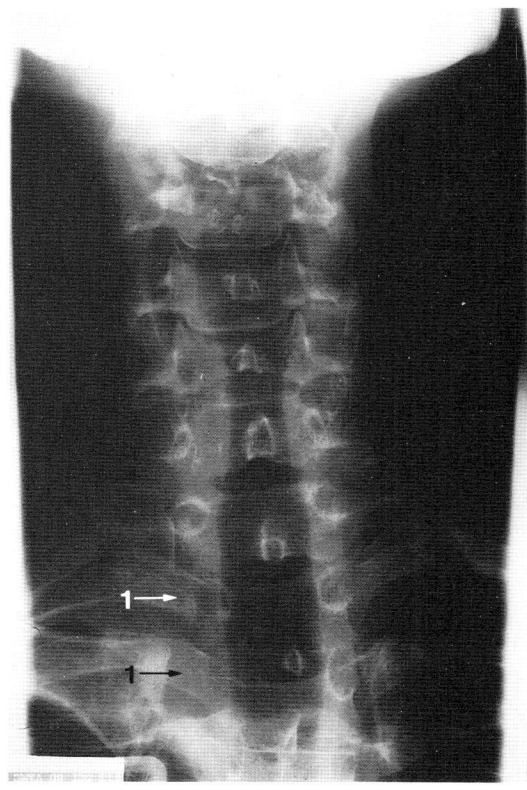
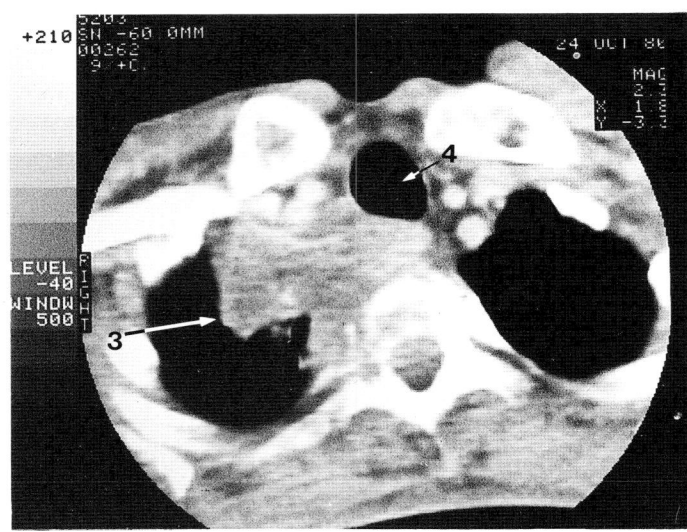

The right pedicles of T-2 and T-3 are destroyed. Extensive pleural shadowing is present at the right apex. The left apex is clear. The diagnosis is a Pancoast tumour.

Sputum examination for malignant cells should be undertaken. A bronchoscopy is likely to be negative with such a peripheral lesion, but might provide good material for cytological examination. The CT scan demonstrates the extent of the right apical mass (3) extending between trachea (4) and spine, and also shows invasion of the vertebral body. Percutaneous needle biopsy provided a tissue diagnosis of anaplastic large cell carcinoma of the bronchus.

Q6

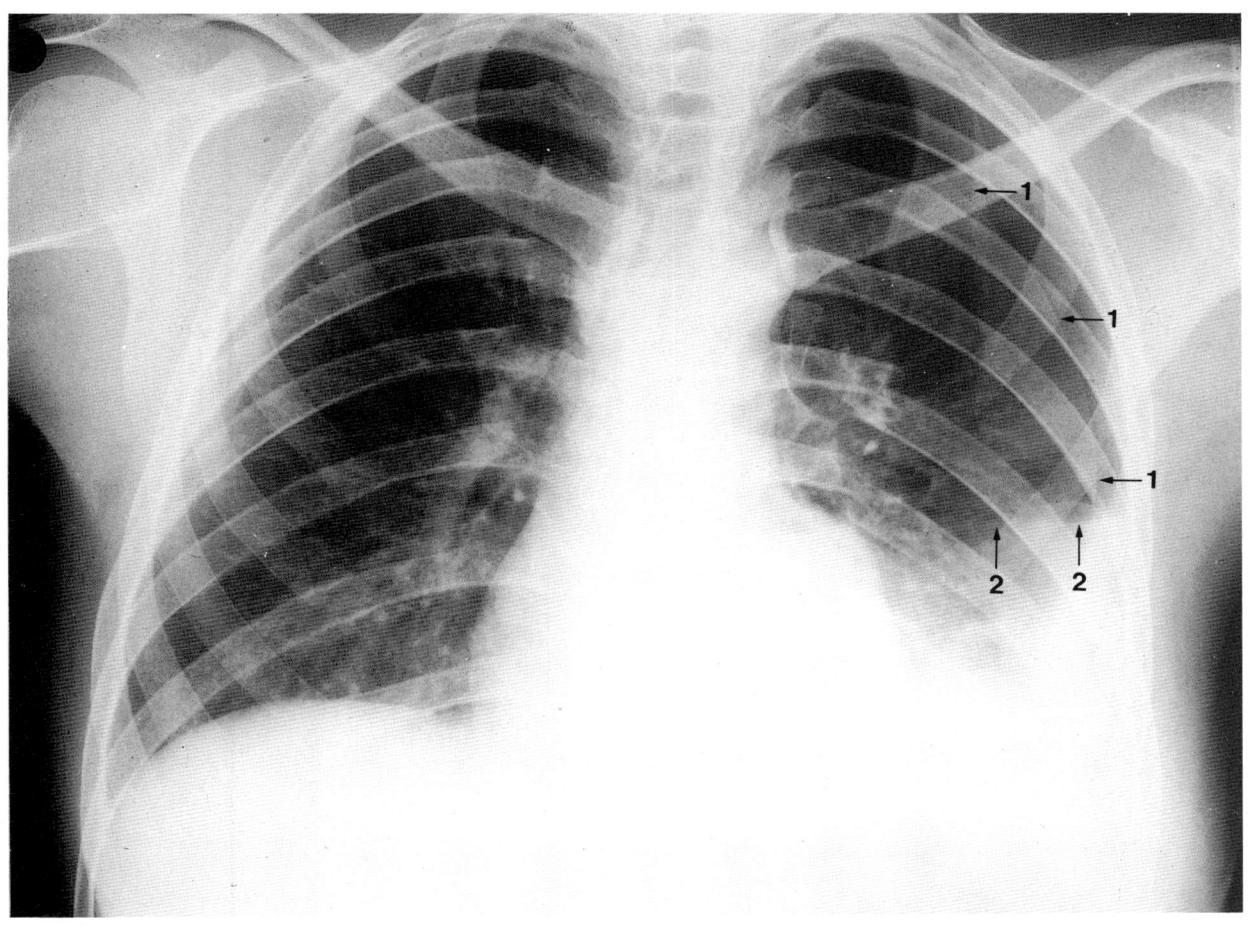

A 42-year-old female was involved in a car crash.

- What chest injuries has she sustained?
- What structure is indicated by (1)?
- What is the line indicated by (2)?

A6

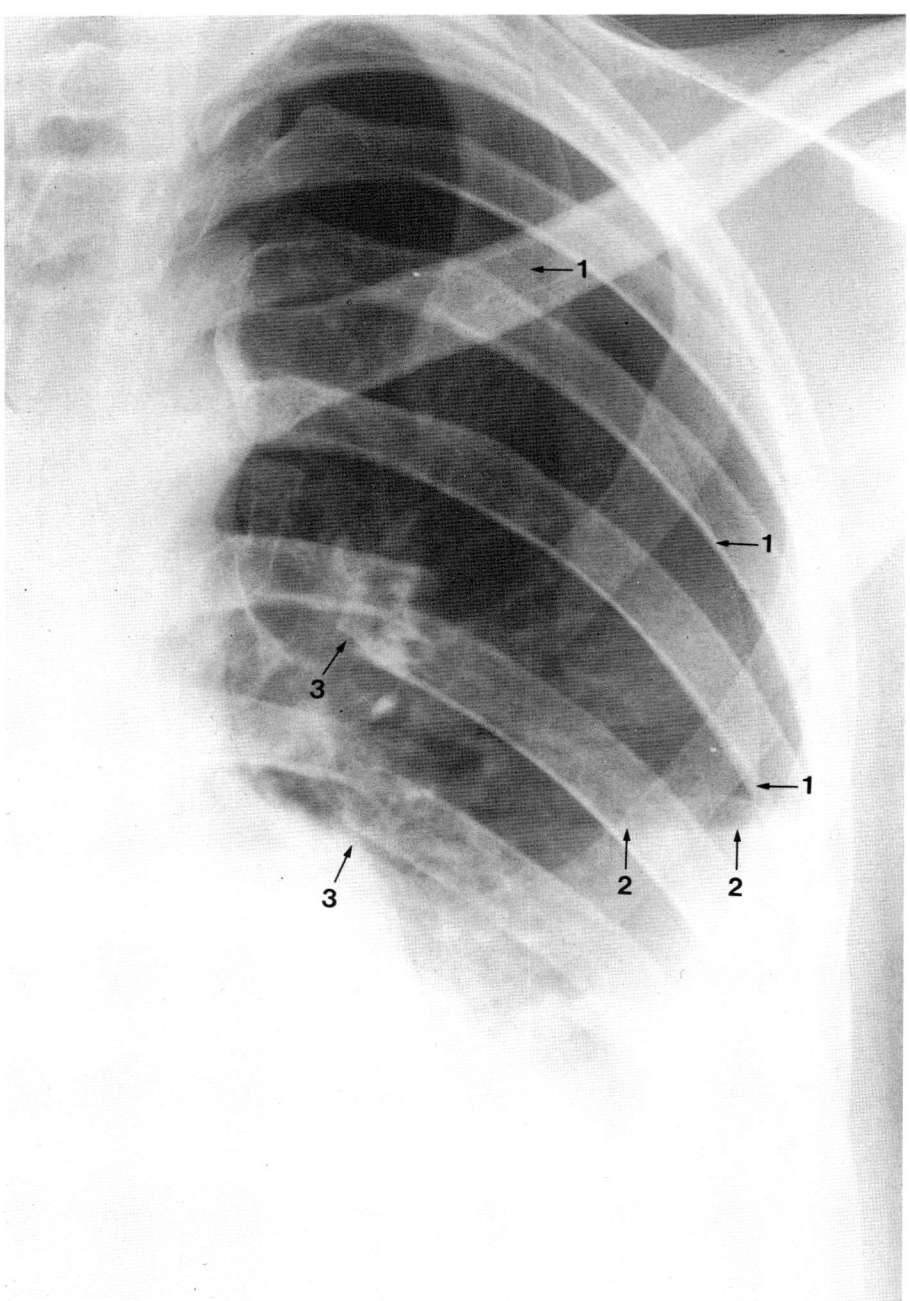

She has fractures of the left seventh and eighth ribs (3), complicated by a hydropneumothorax. (1) = the edge of the partially collapsed left lung. (2) = a fluid level in the pleura, which in this case is due to blood.

Q7

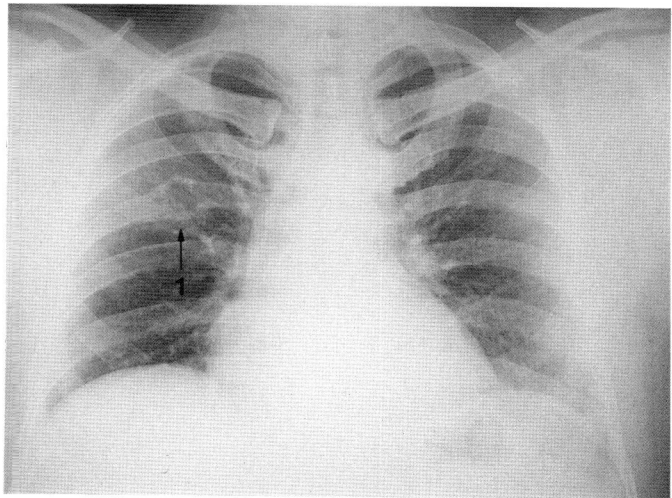

A 55-year-old asymptomatic man was x-rayed on arrival in the United Kingdom as an immigrant. An expanding, lucent lesion was noted in the right sixth rib (1).

- What is the differential diagnosis?

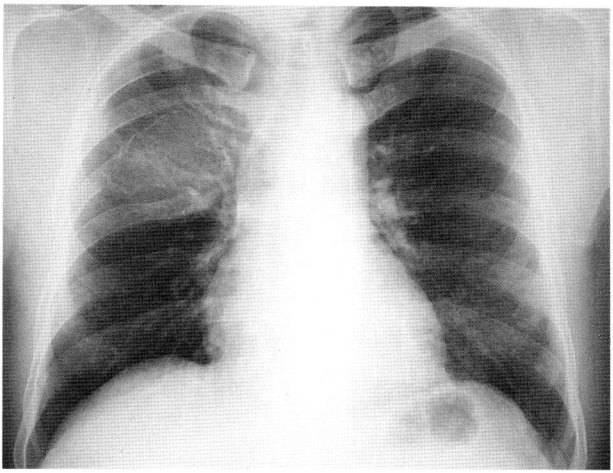

He did not wish to be investigated further at that time. However, he presented two years later complaining of right-sided chest pain. A firm mass was now palpable in the thyroid gland.

- How has the CXR changed?
- What is the likely diagnosis?

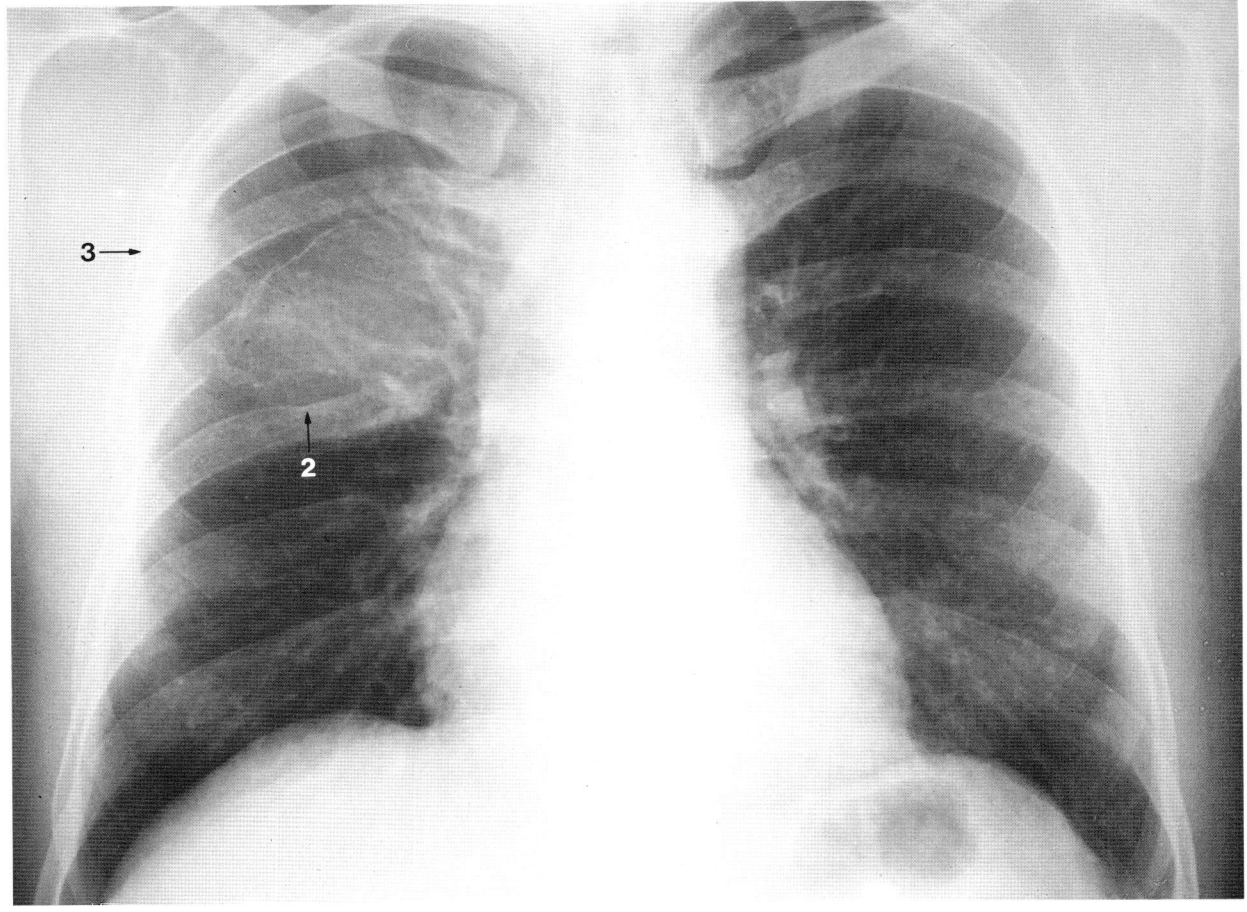

Fibrous dysplasia, chondroma, plasmacytoma or metastasis were considered most likely. Brown tumour of hyperparathyroidism and osteomyelitis were considered less likely, as were primary bone tumours.

Two years later, the lesion in the right sixth rib has expanded and destroyed the rib further, and caused pressure erosion on the superior aspect of the seventh rib (2). There is also a new lesion in the fourth rib (3). The diagnosis was metastatic thyroid carcinoma.

Skeletal metastases are rarely expansile, except from renal and thyroid tumours.

Q8

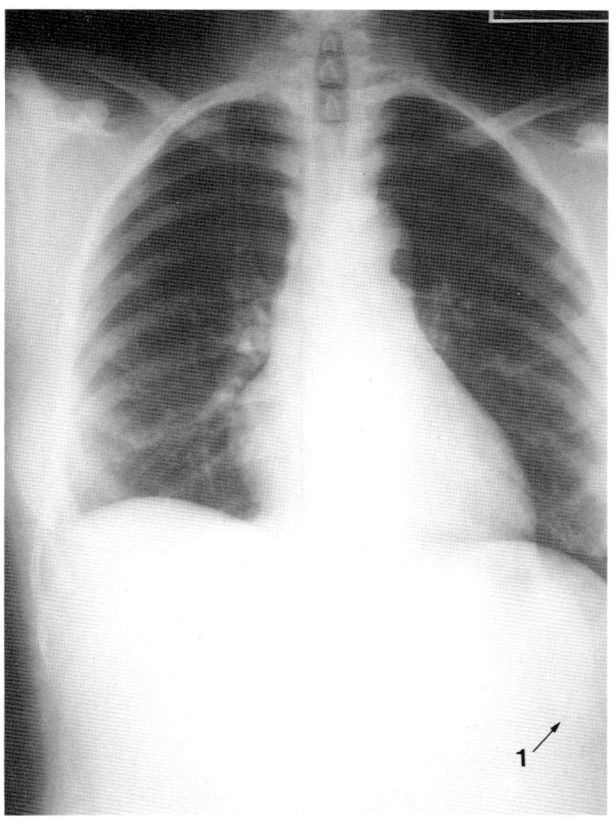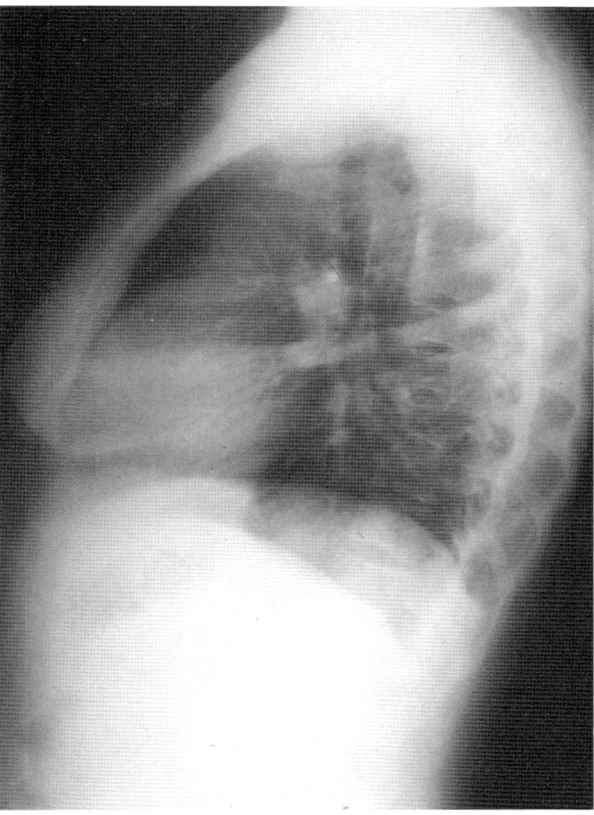

A 35-year-old black female presented with repeated episodes of skeletal and abdominal pain.

- Comment on the density of the bones, especially the ribs.
- What are the commoner causes of widespread bony sclerosis?

Now examine the spine on the lateral film.

- What is the diagnosis of this case?
- What is structure (1)?

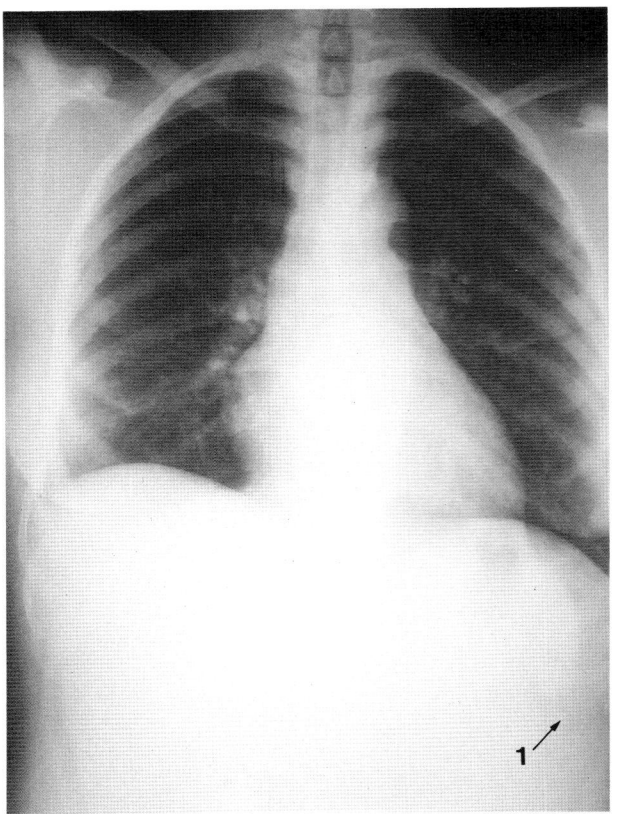 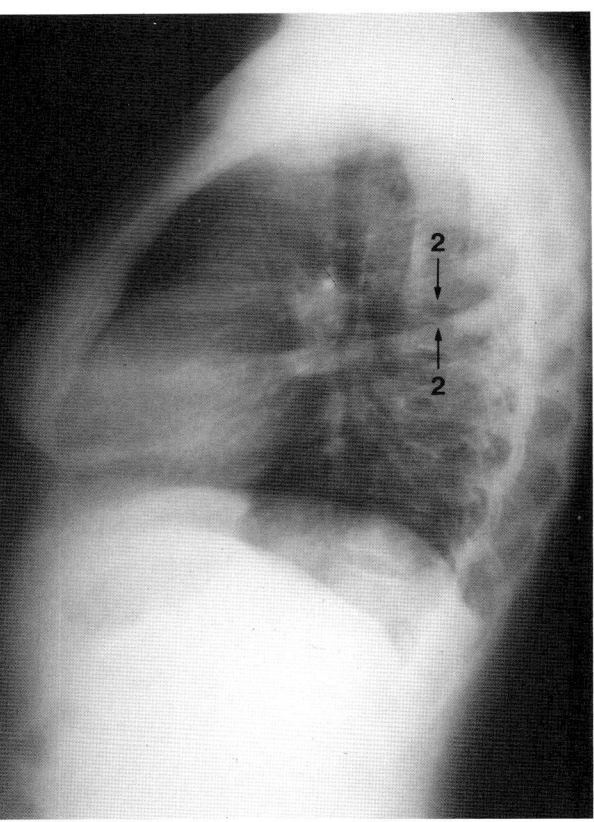

The bones are diffusely sclerotic. The commoner causes of widespread bony sclerosis are osteoblastic metastases, myelofibrosis, Paget's Disease, and sickle cell disease. In this case the diagnosis is sickle cell disease. The vertebral end plates are depressed (2) secondary to metaphyseal infarction. Similarly the widespread bony sclerosis is due to ischaemic osteonecrosis. (1) = the spleen. It is small and calcified due to multiple episodes of infarction.

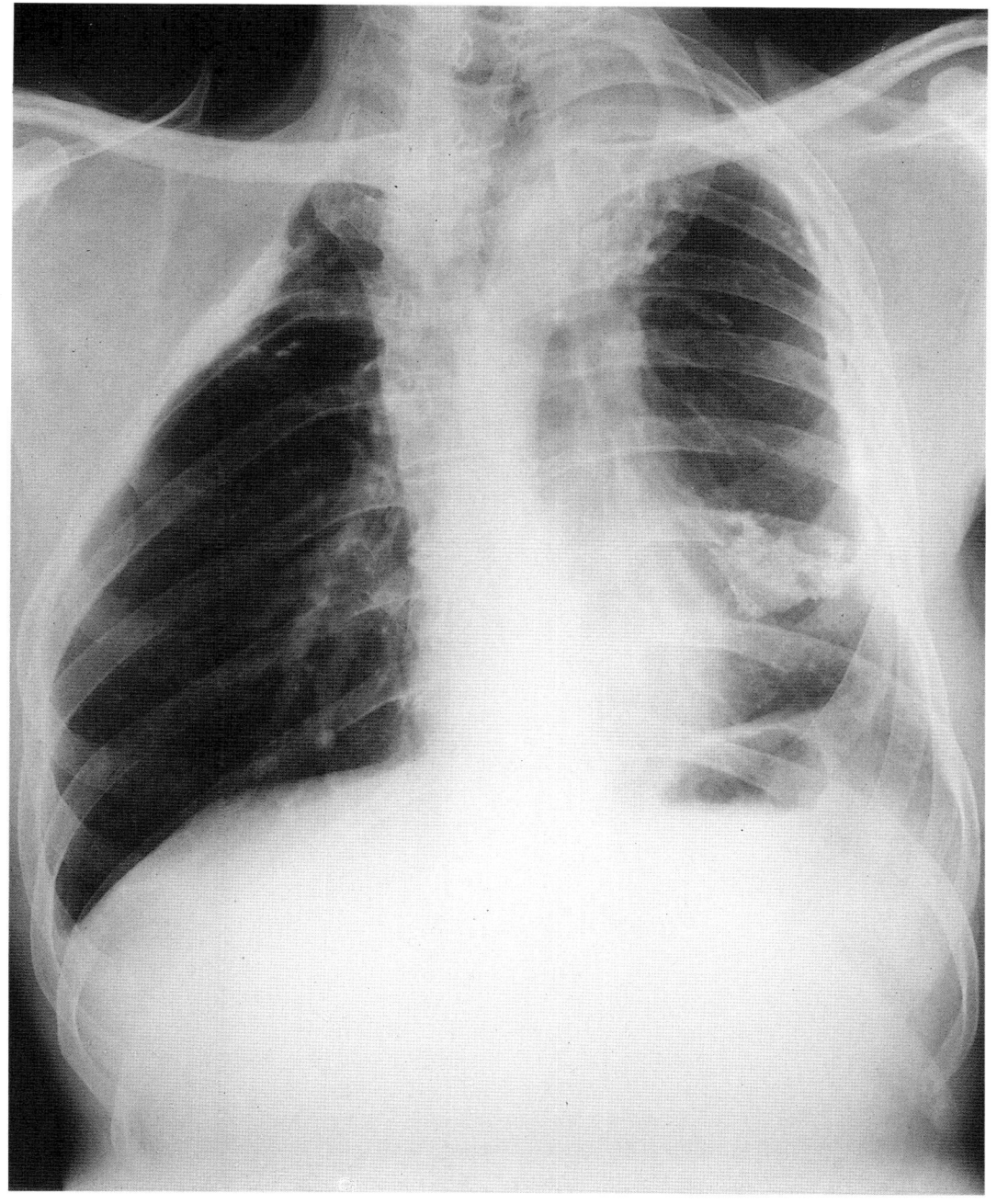

A 75-year-old man presented with a past history of right upper lobe pulmonary tuberculosis.

- How was he treated previously?
- Was his disease confined to the right upper lobe?

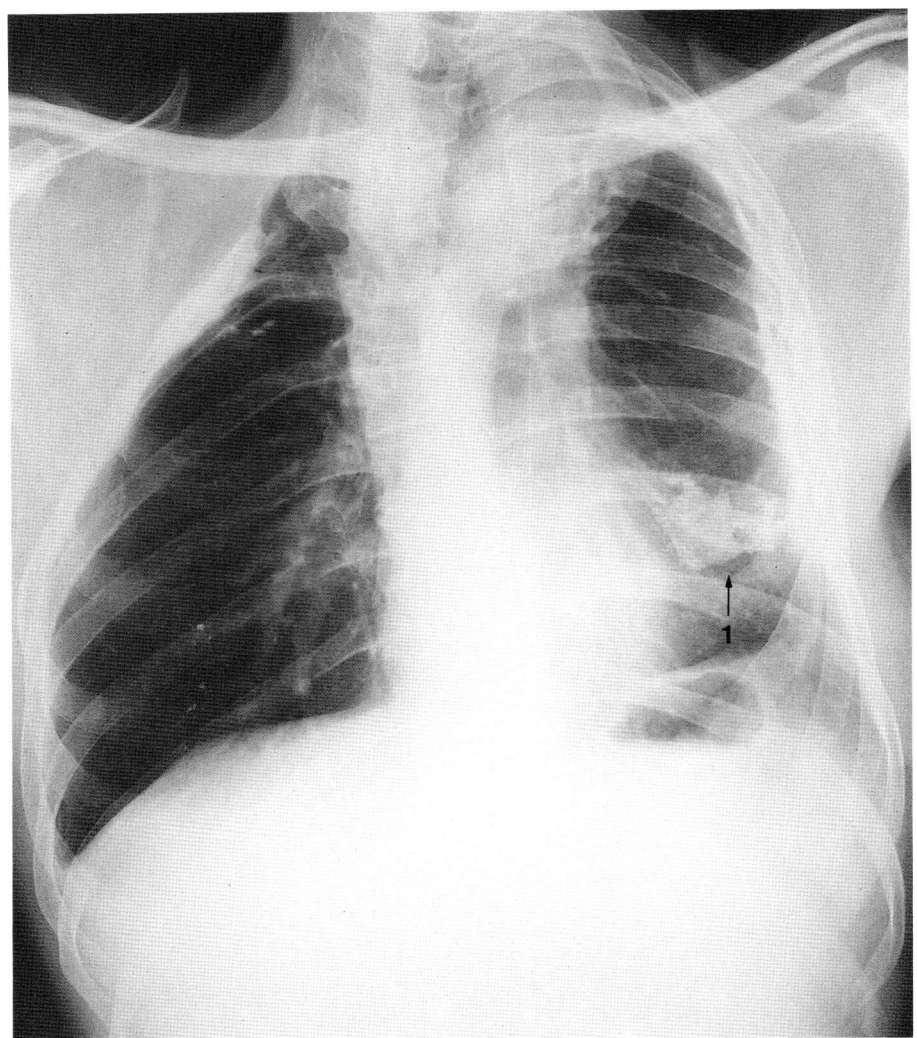

He had previously undergone thoracoplasty. The right first to fifth ribs have been removed to produce collapse of the infected upper lobe. Prior to the availability of the anti-tuberculous chemotherapy, collapse therapy of the infected lung was commonly practised. Other methods included artificial pneumothorax and insertion of various inert materials, such as lucite balls. There are still many patients alive today whose CXRs show the sequelae of such procedures.

The disease was not confined to the right upper lobe. Left upper zone fibrosis and calcified nodules indicate previous left upper lobe infection, and left pleural calcification (1) was caused by pleural infection.

Q10

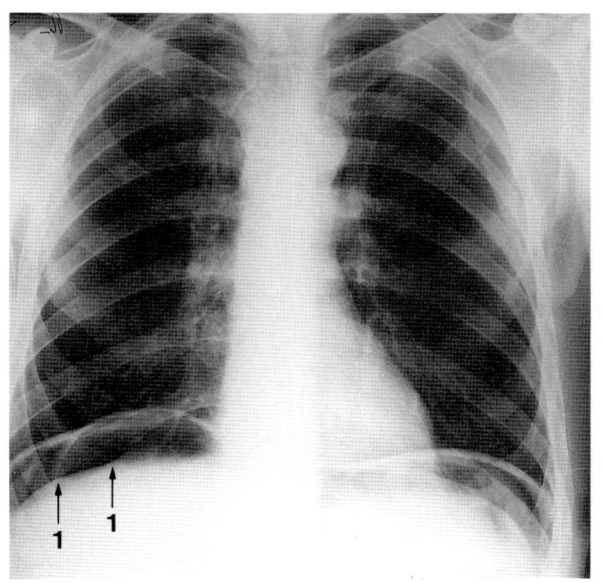
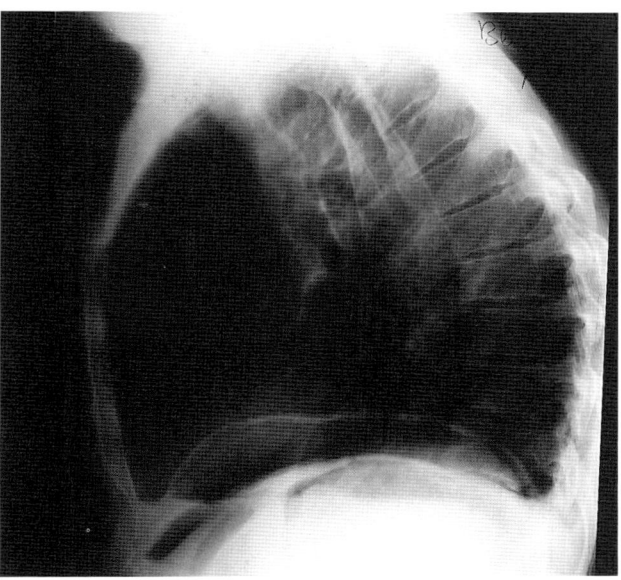

A 57-year-old man presented with sudden, severe abdominal pain.

- What is structure (1) and why is it visible?
- What is the diagnosis?

A10

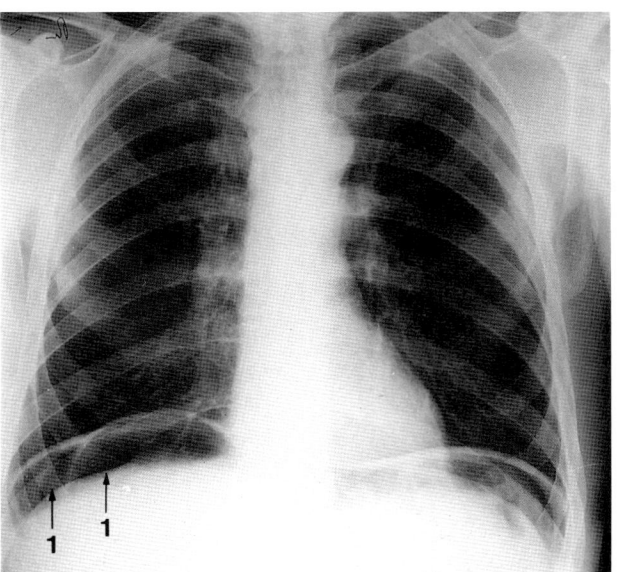 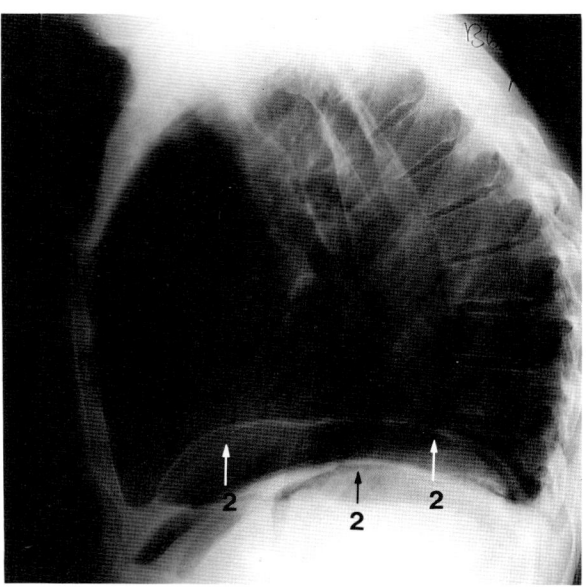

(1) = the superior surface of the liver. It is visible because there is free air between the liver and diaphragm. Similarly, the inferior surface of the diaphragm is visible (2). The diagnosis is pneumoperitoneum. At surgery a perforated peptic ulcer was found.

Q11

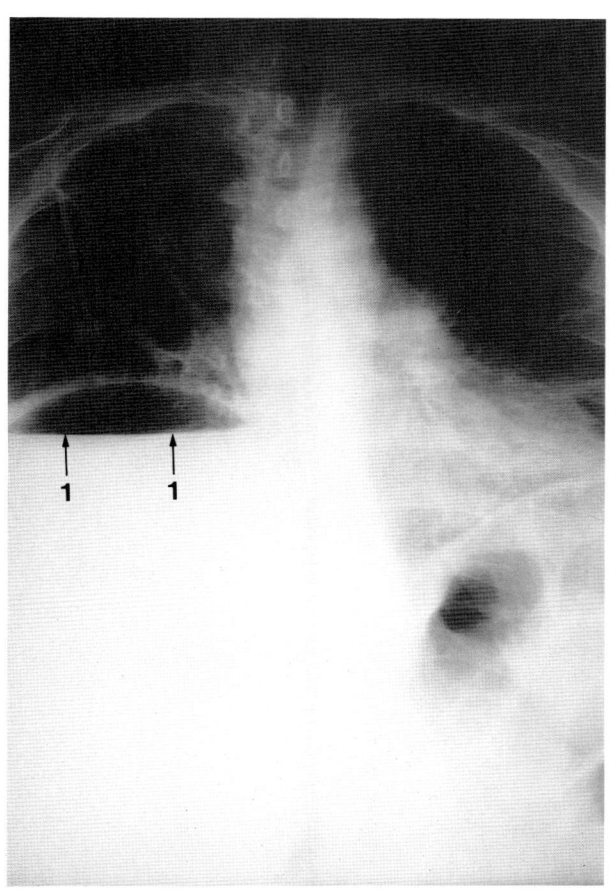
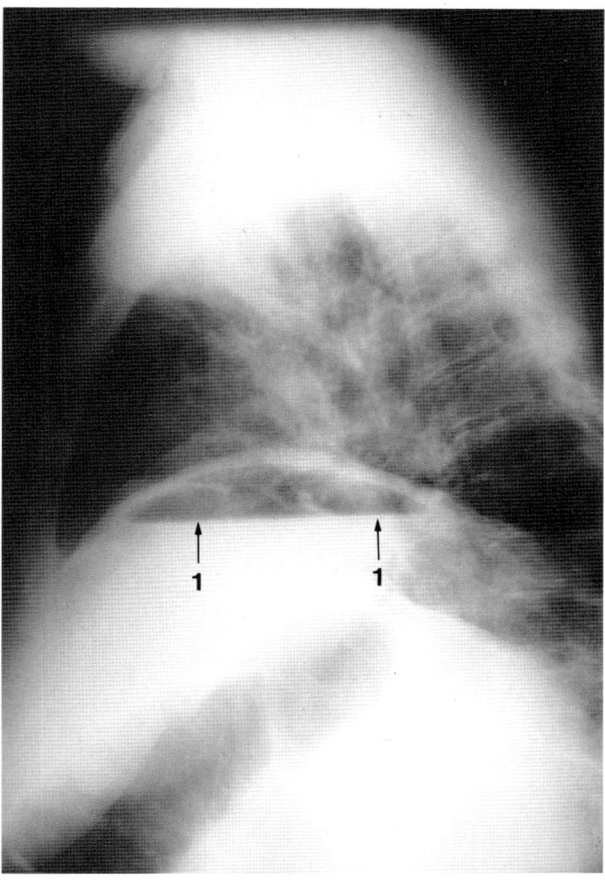

A 40-year-old woman presented with abdominal pain, fever and absent bowel sounds.

- Where is this fluid level (1) and what is its significance?

- Compare the level and width of the right hemi-diaphragm with that in case 10. What are the differences?

- What is the diagnosis?

A11

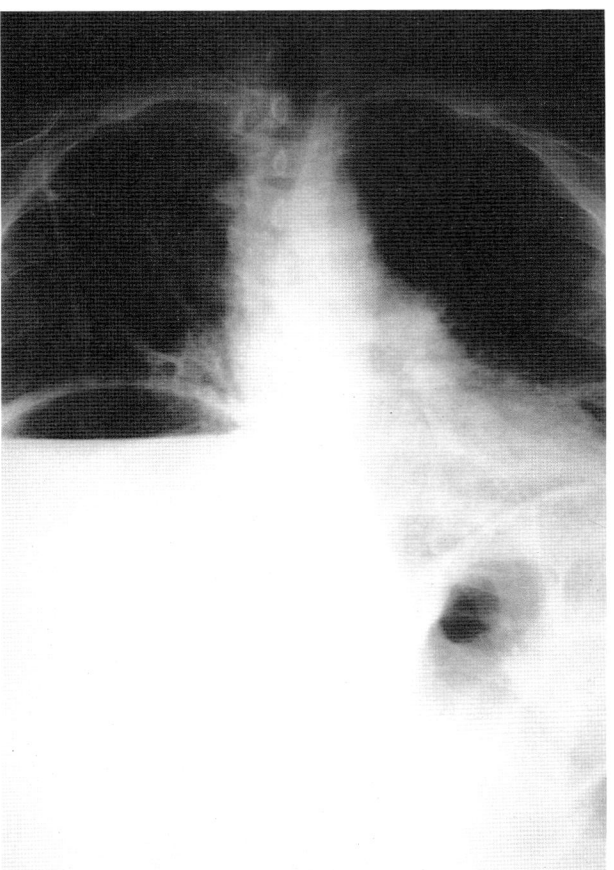
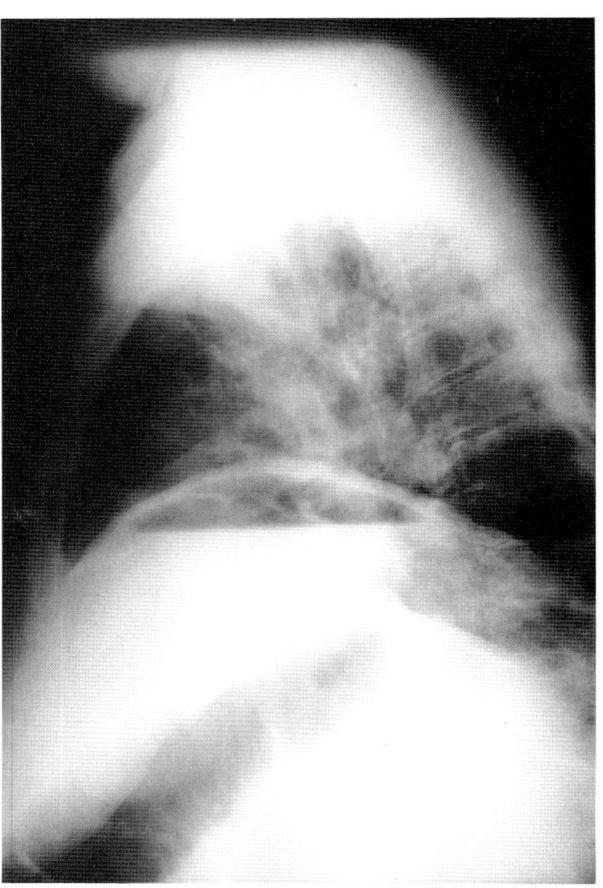

The fluid level is in the right subphrenic space. The combination of both fluid and gas suggests a subphrenic abscess. The right hemi-diaphragm is elevated. It appears thickened because there is a pleural effusion above it. The diagnosis is subphrenic abscess. This may be a complication of laparotomy. However, when it develops spontaneously it is usually due to perforation of a viscus. This patient had a perforated appendix.

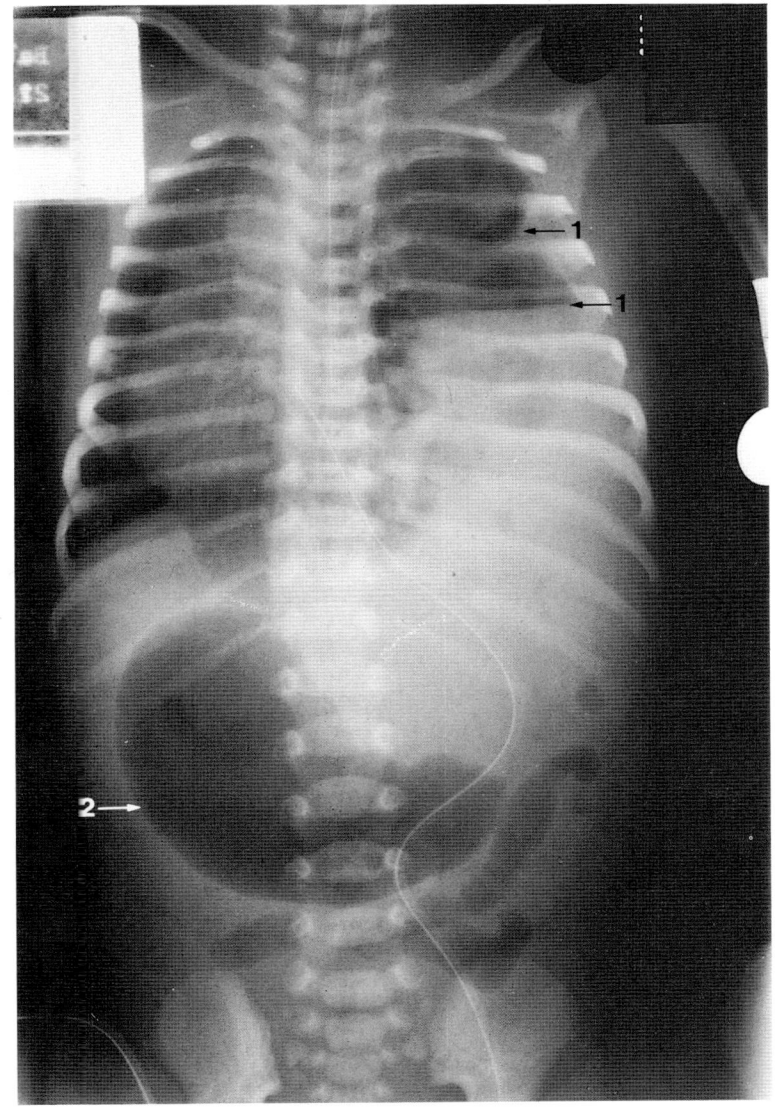

A 2-day-old child presented with cyanosis and hypoxia.

- Comment on the position of the mediastinum.
- The lower half of the left hemithorax is opaque, and areas of lucency (1) are also seen in the left hemithorax. What is causing this appearance?
- What is structure (2)?
- What is the probable diagnosis, and what further test would you do?

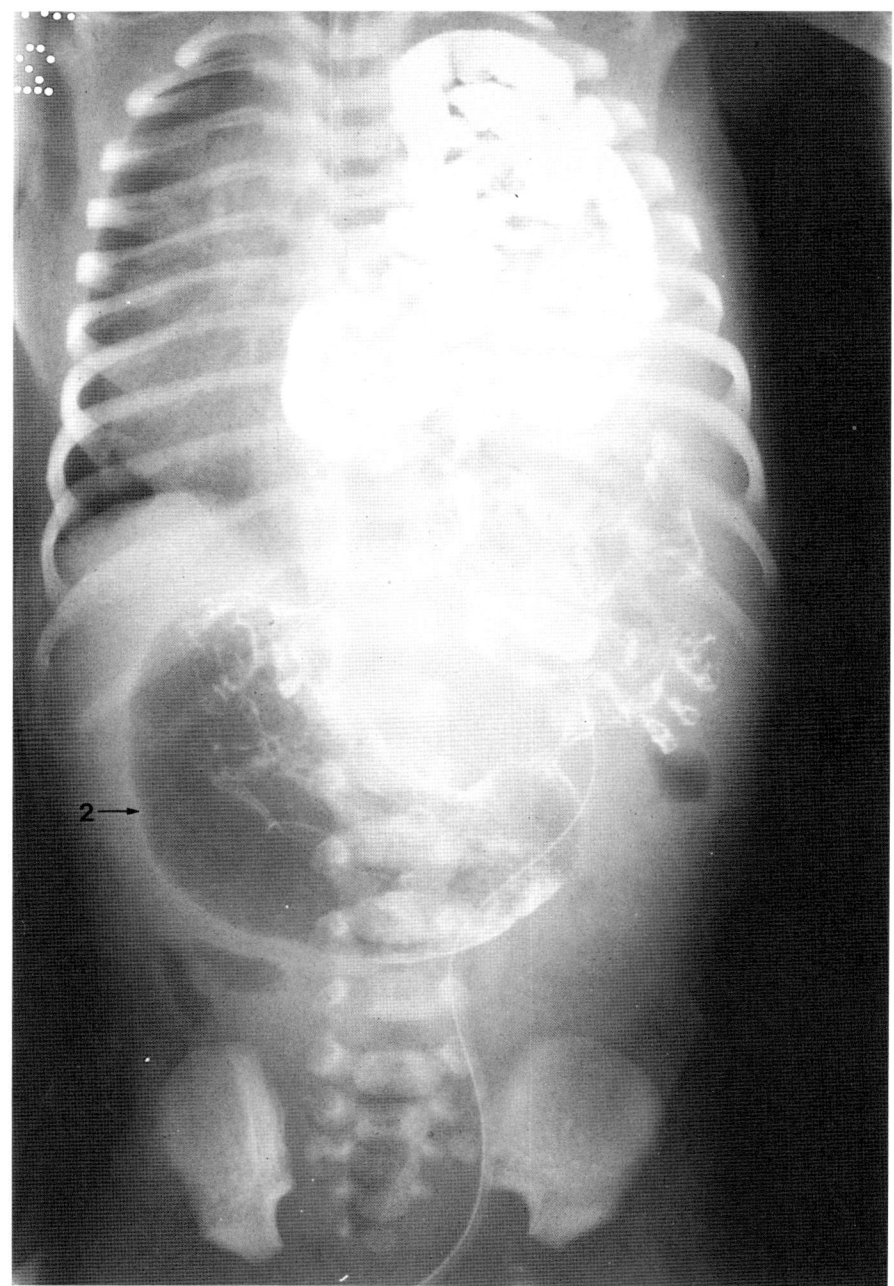

The mediastinum is pushed to the right. Multiple loops of bowel are present in the left hemithorax. (2) = the stomach. It is dilated. Barium meal and follow-through are indicated. This confirms that the left hemithorax is occupied by multiple loops of small bowel due to a congenital diaphragmatic hernia.

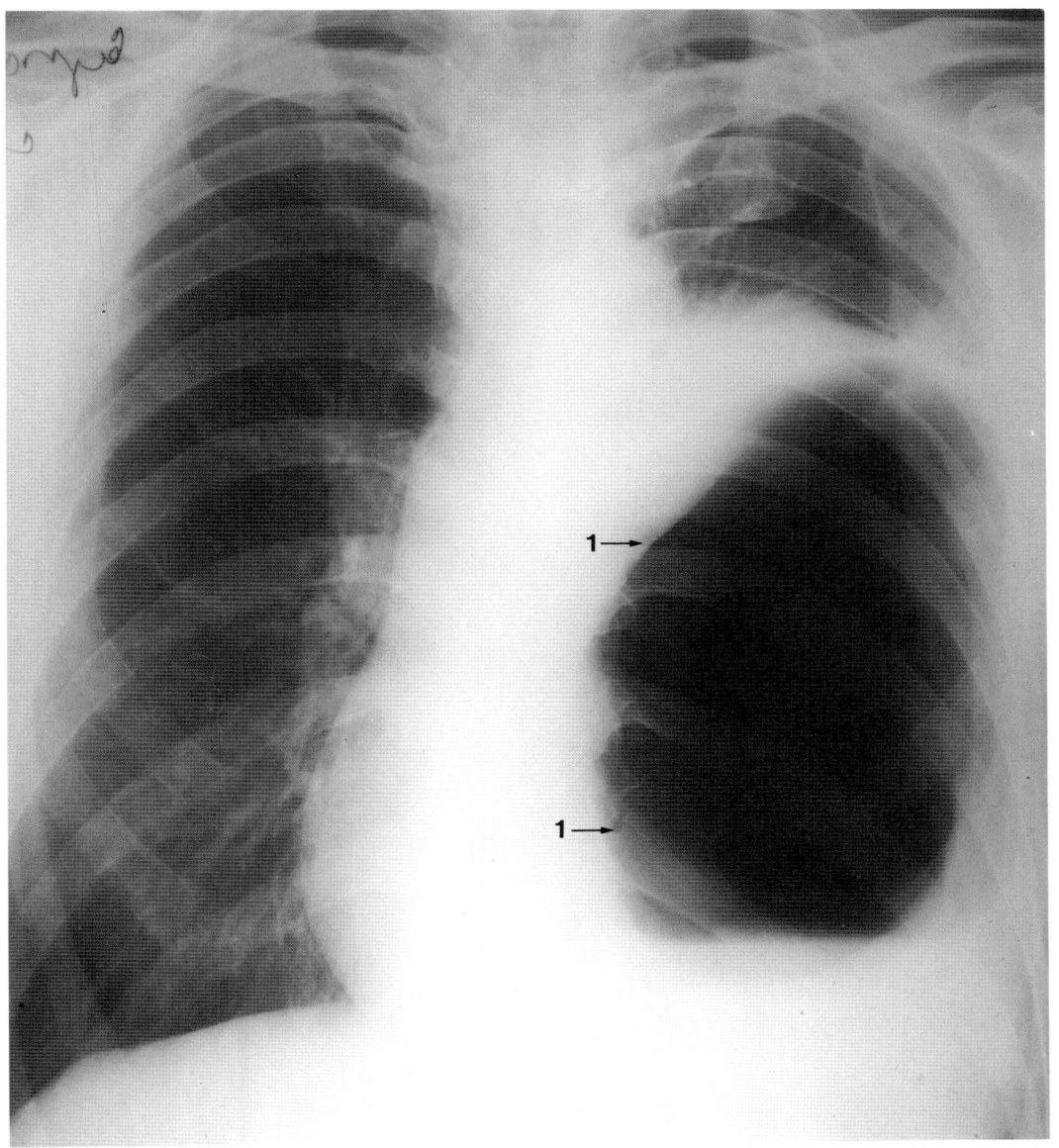

A 58-year-old man presented with a seven-day history of vomiting. On examination a succussion splash was heard over the left chest. Eleven years earlier he sustained broken legs and pelvis after falling from a building.

- What is the gas filled structure (1) in the left hemithorax?
- What is the diagnosis?
- What test would confirm it?

A13

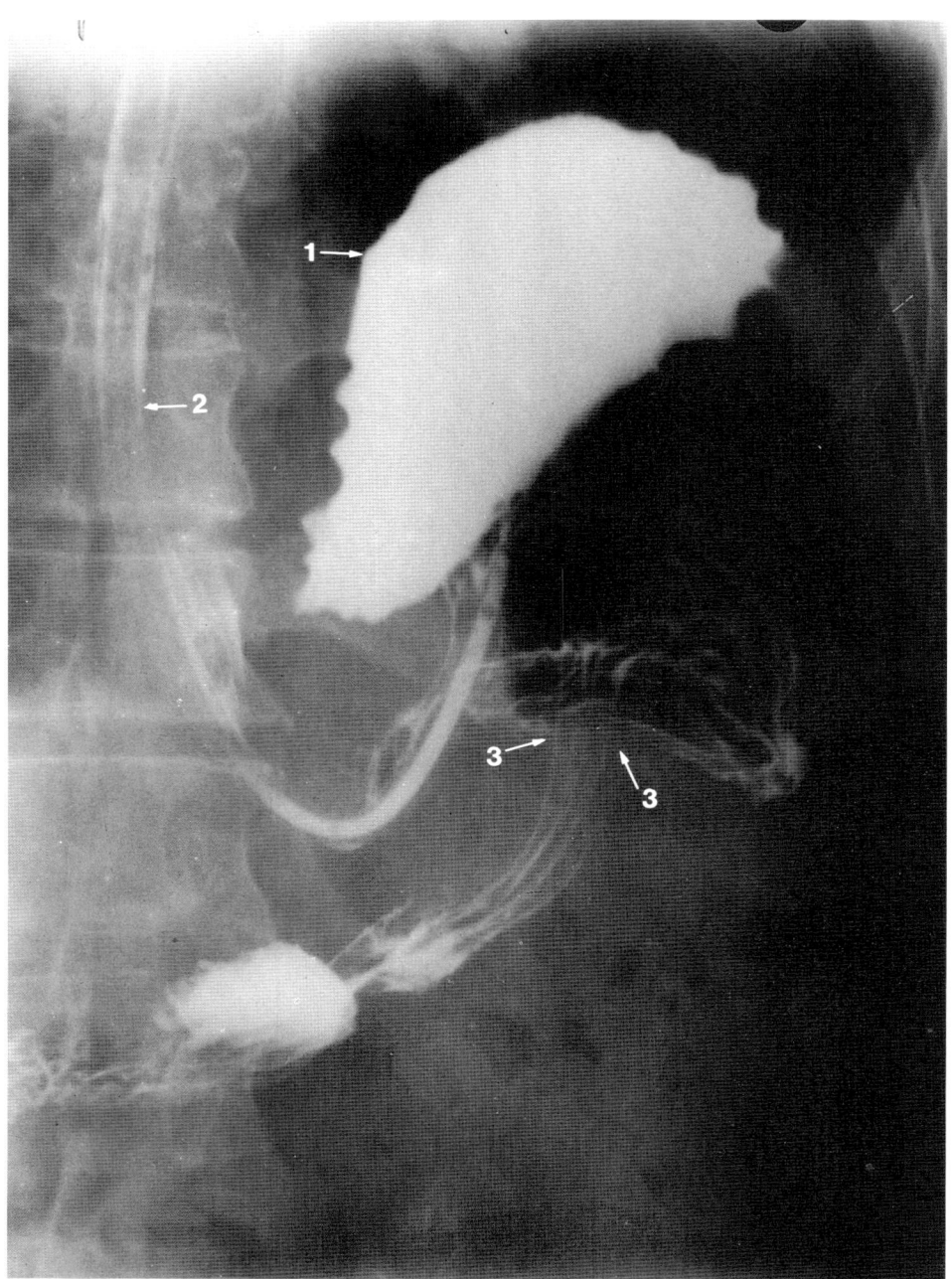

(1) = the stomach. The diagnosis is rupture of the left hemi-diaphragm. A barium study would confirm it. Barium has been passed down a Ryle's tube (2) which has been used to decompress the stomach. At surgery the stomach was found to have herniated through a 5 cm rent in the diaphragm; this can be seen on the barium study (3).

Q14

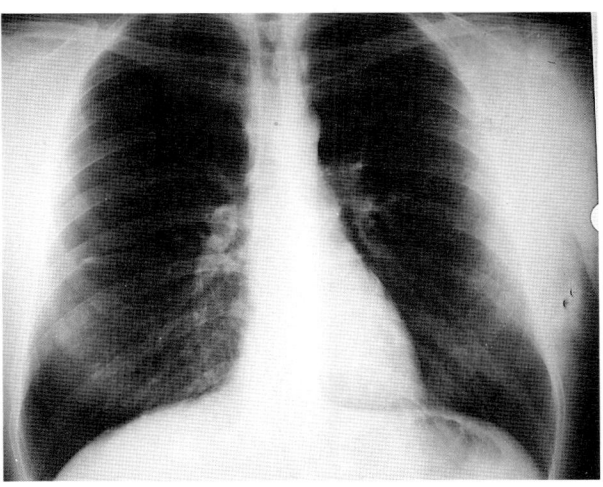 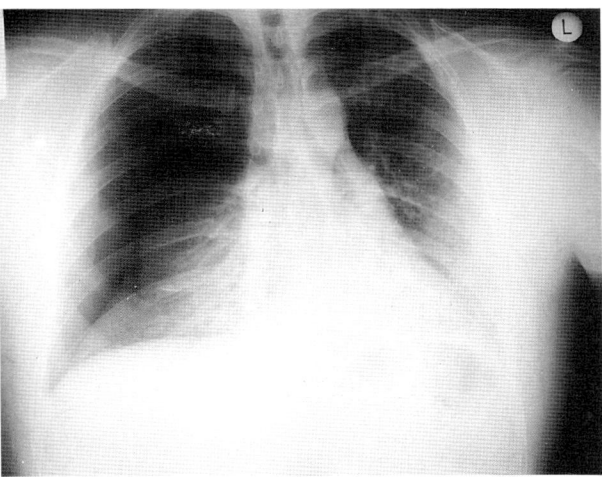

A 27-year-old man presented with sudden onset of right-sided chest pain, worse on respiration, and associated with breathlessness.

- Two CXRs were taken when the patient presented. Why?
- What is the diagnosis, and what is the probable cause?

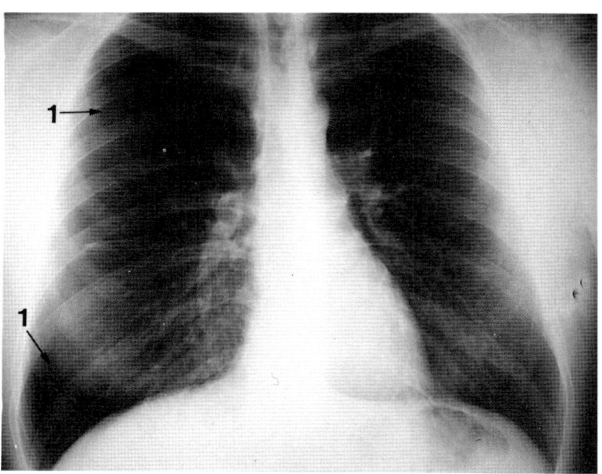 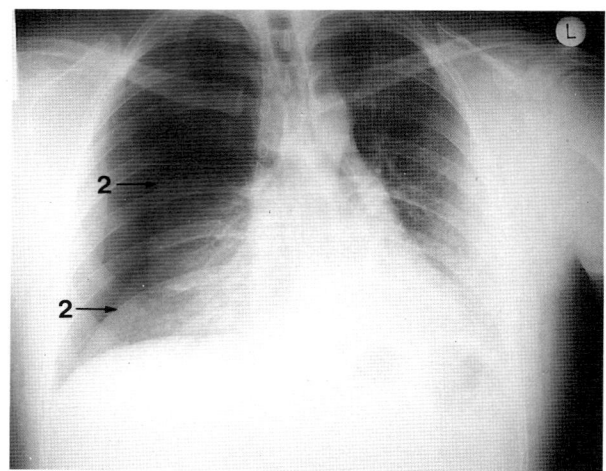

The first film is in full inspiration, and the second is in full expiration. The clinical presentation suggests a pneumothorax. A small pneumothorax may be difficult to see on full inspiration. In this case the lung edge (1) is just visible. However, on expiration the lung volume diminishes but the amount of intrapleural air is unchanged, making the lung edge easily visible (2).

The diagnosis is spontaneous pneumothorax. In young men this is usually due to rupture of an apical sub-pleural bleb.

Q15

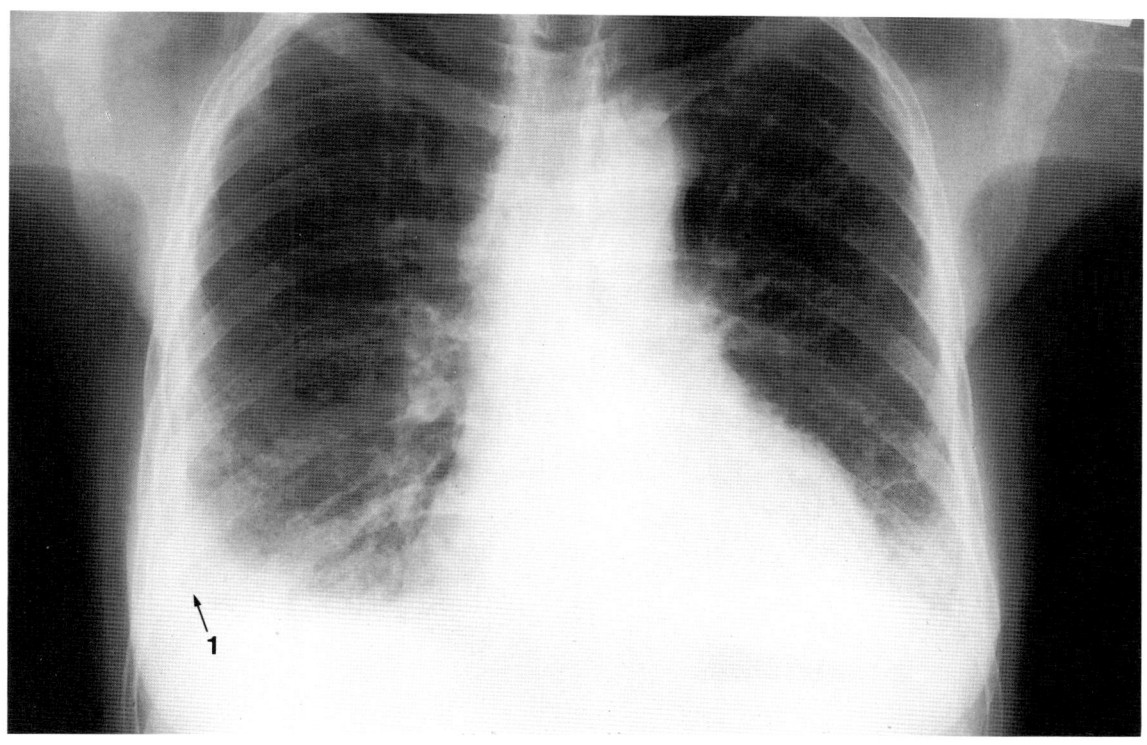

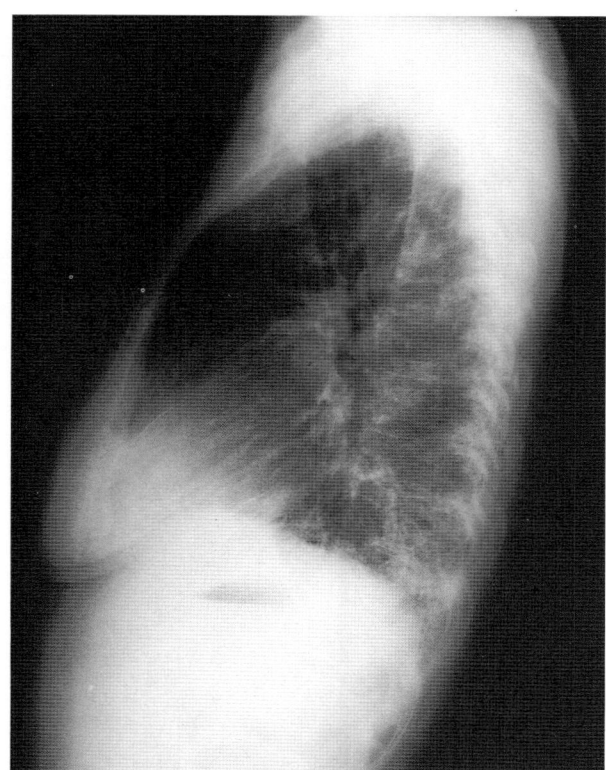

A 60-year-old woman presented with joint pains and mild dyspnoea. On physical examination crackles were heard at both bases, and soft tissue swelling was present around several of the joints of both hands.

- What is causing the shadowing (1) at the right base?
- What are the commoner causes of this abnormality?
- Is the lung parenchyma normal?
- What is the diagnosis?

A15

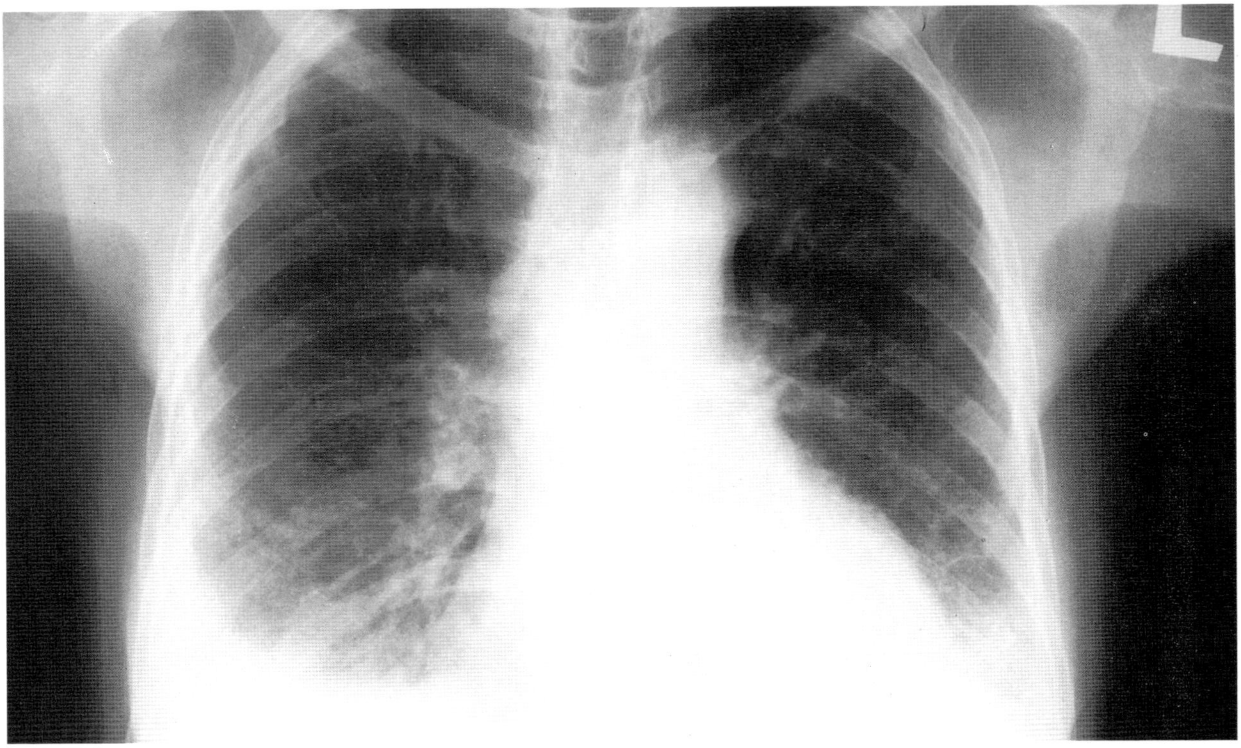

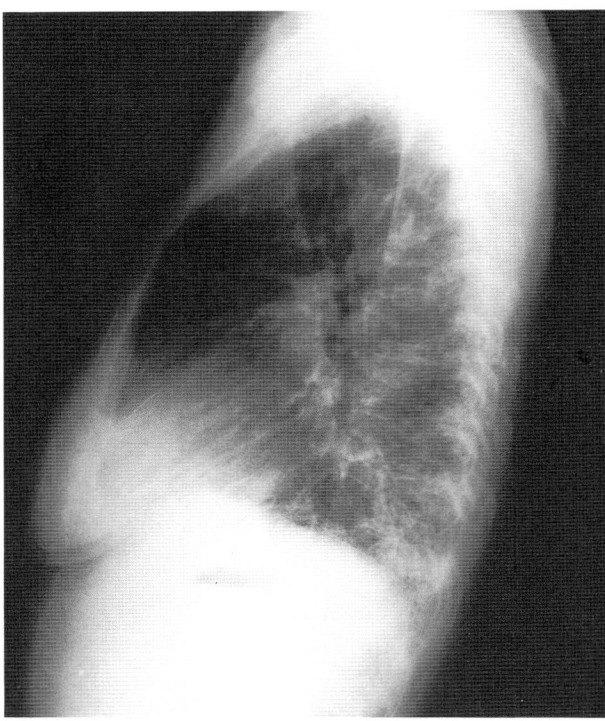

The shadowing is caused by a pleural effusion. A smaller effusion is present at the left base. The commoner causes of pleural effusion are pneumonia, heart failure, lung cancer, pleural metastases, pulmonary infarction, lymphoma and connective tissue disorders. The lung parenchyma is not normal. Reticulo-nodular shadowing is present in both lower zones; it is particularly well seen on the lateral film. This appearance indicates interstitial lung disease. The diagnosis is rheumatoid disease.

Q16

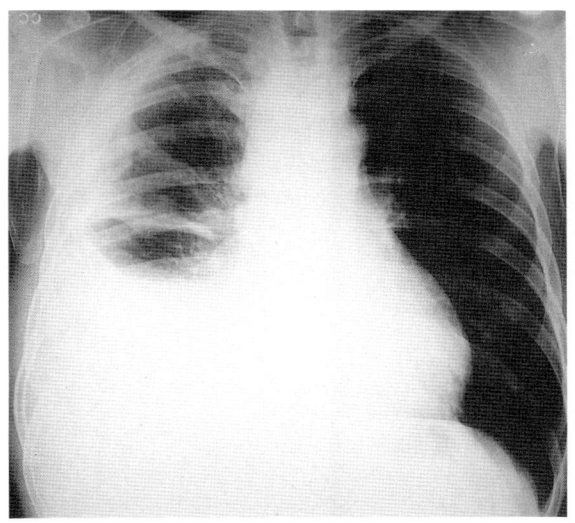
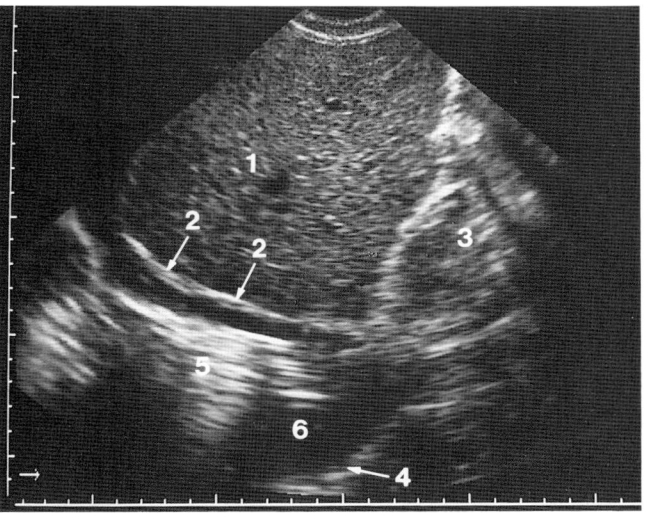
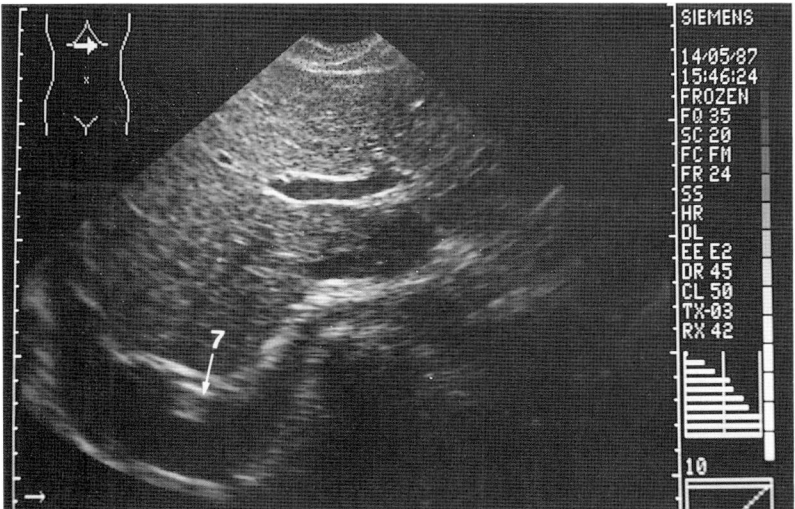

A 50-year-old man presented with a non-productive cough and dyspnoea.

- What does the CXR show?

An ultrasound examination of the upper abdomen and right side of the chest was performed.

- On the longitudinal scan of the right upper quadrant of the abdomen, name the numbered normal structures (1-4).
- What are (5) and (6)?
- What is the abnormality (7) indicated on the transverse scan?
- What further investigation would you do?

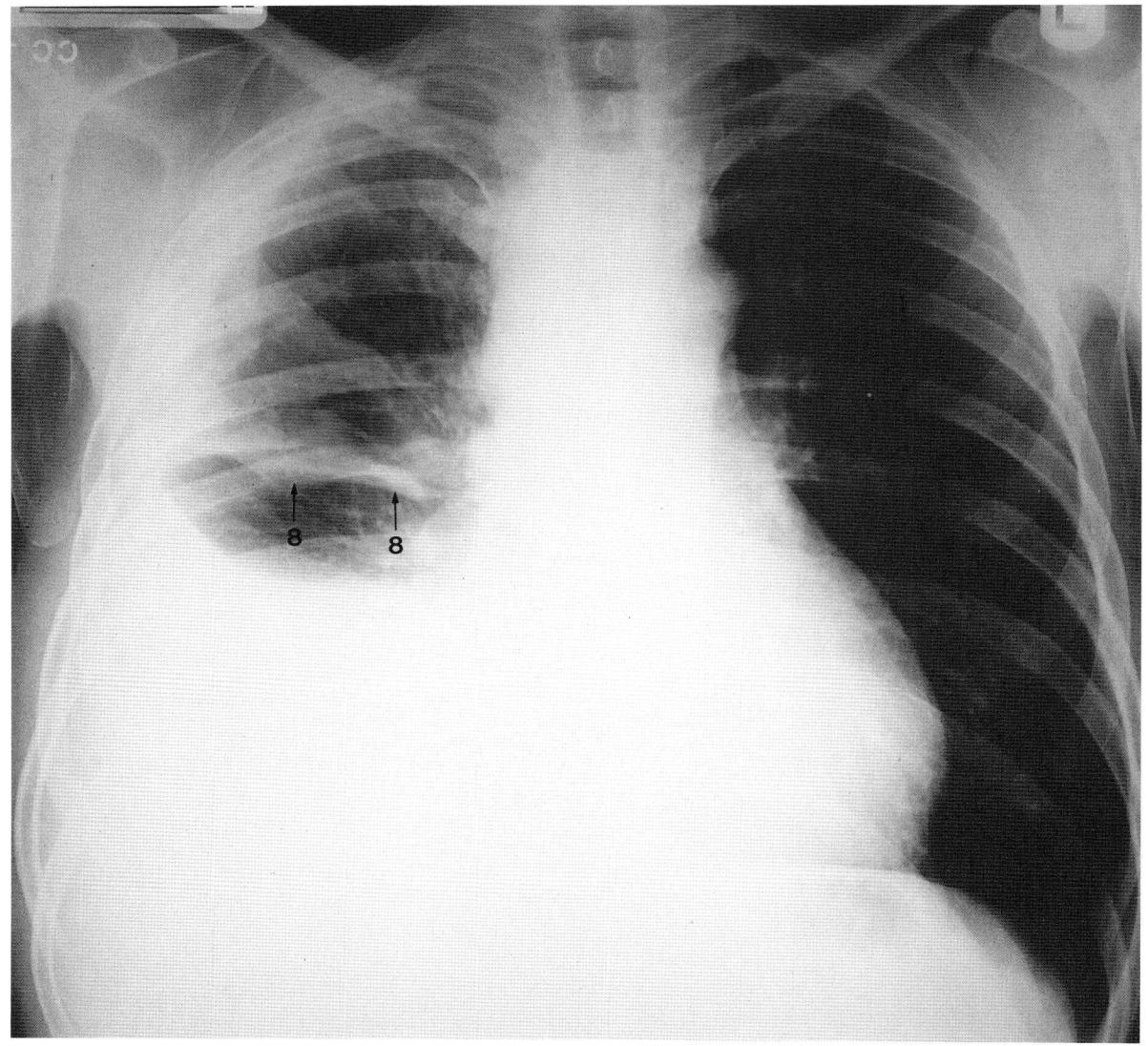

The CXR shows a large pleural effusion extending into the horizontal fissure (8).

(1) = liver; (2) = right hemi-diaphragm; (3) = upper pole of right kidney; (4) = posterior chest wall. (5) = right lower lobe; (6) = pleural effusion. (7) = pleural mass.

Pleural fluid was aspirated for bacteriology and cytological examination, but no organisms or malignant cells were found. Since the pleural mass was so close to the liver it was biopsied via a thoracoscope rather than with ultrasound guidance. The biopsy showed adenocarcinoma. The primary tumour was not discovered.

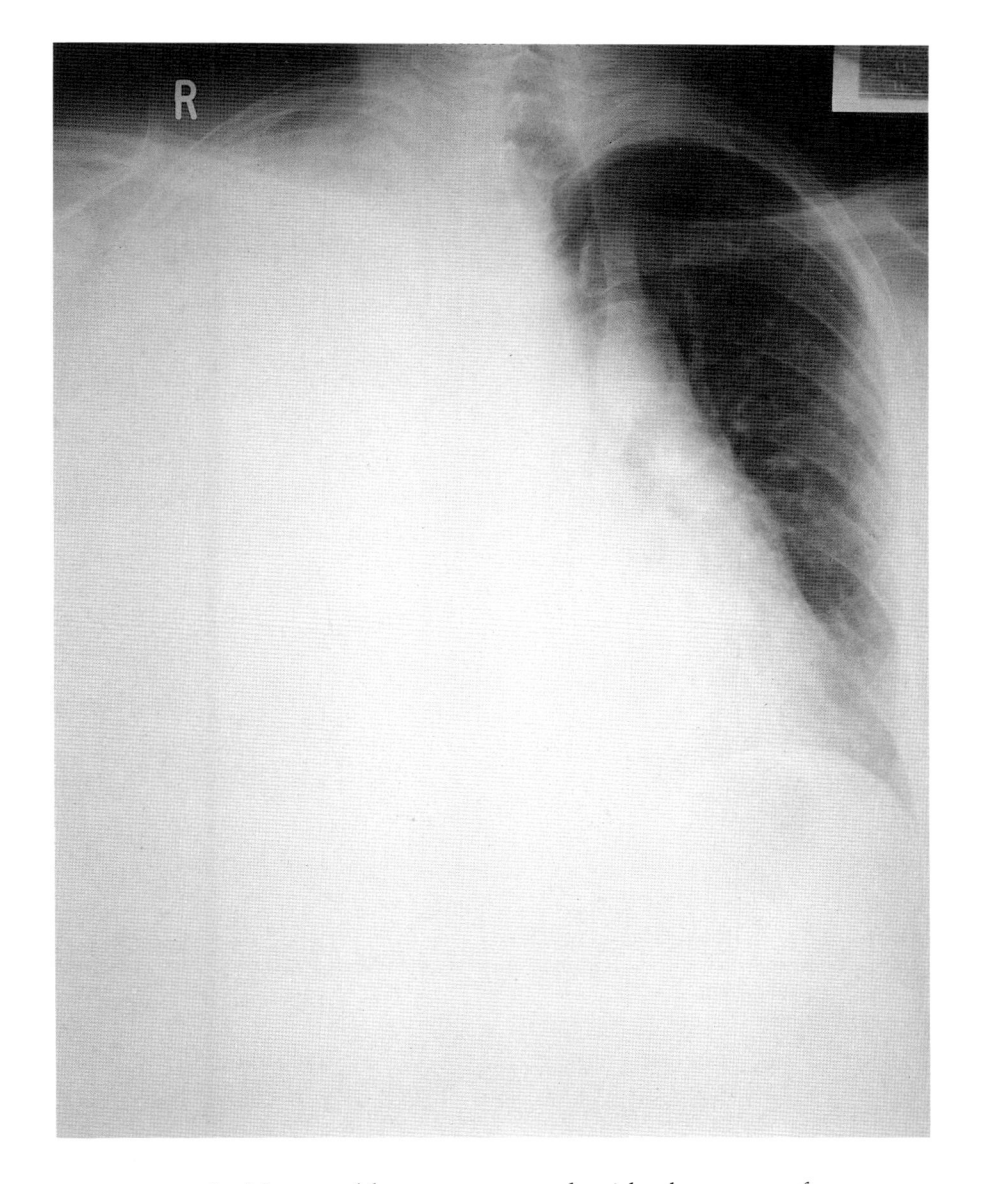

A 46-year-old man presented with shortness of breath and opacification of the right hemithorax. Complete opacification of a hemithorax may be due to:

a) Complete collapse of a lung (or pneumonectomy),
b) Complete consolidation of a lung, or
c) Large pleural effusion.

- What is the cause in this case, and why?
- How would you prove it?

A17

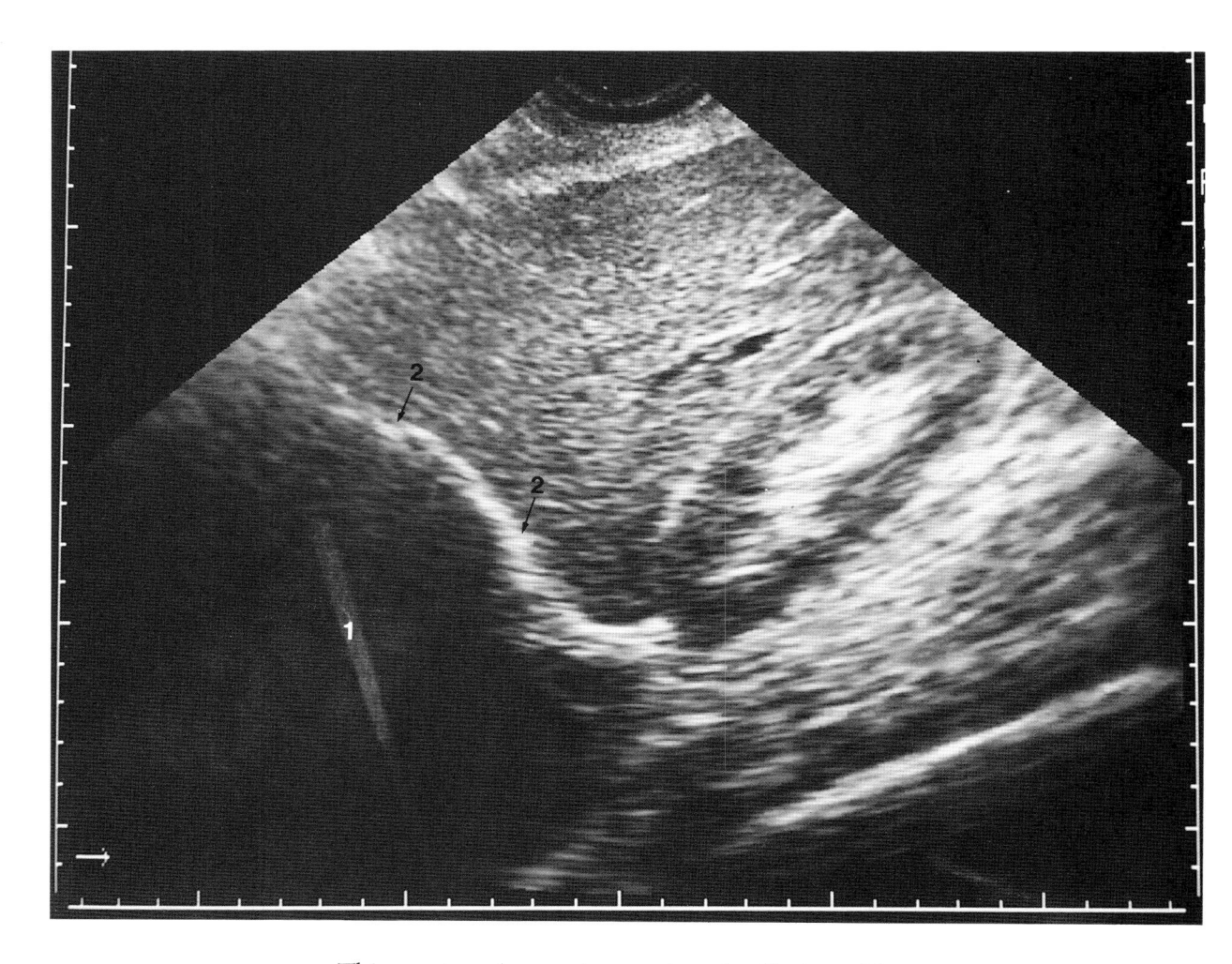

This patient has a large pleural effusion. The mediastinum is pushed away from the opaque side, indicating that the abnormality is space-occupying. Note the deviated trachea. Consolidated lung is usually similar in volume to normal lung, and in complete collapse of a lung the mediastinum is pulled toward the abnormal side. The presence of a large pleural effusion could be proved by an ultrasound scan. The longitudinal scan clearly shows a large echo-free effusion (1) above the right hemi-diaphragm (2).

Q18

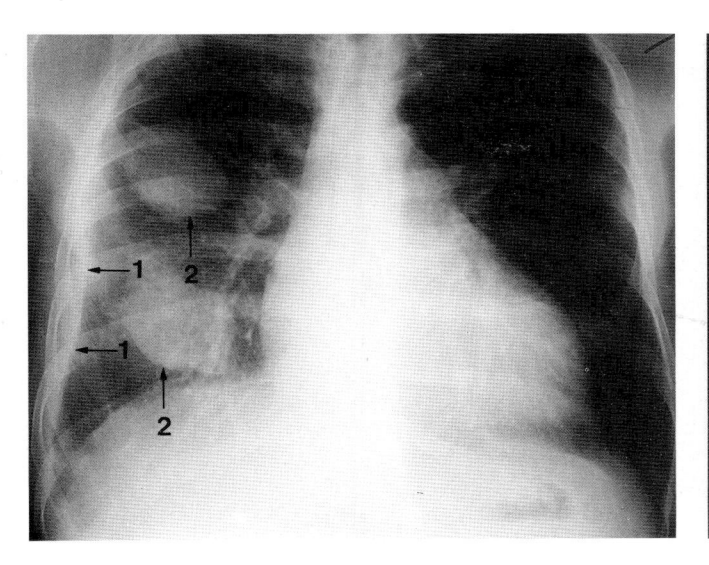

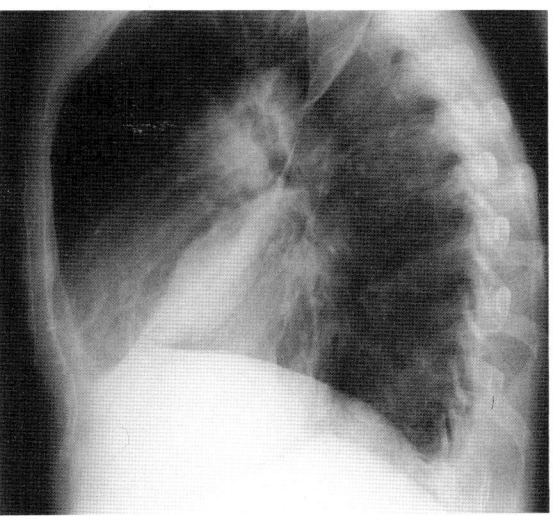

A 52-year-old man presented with heart failure due to congestive cardiomyopathy.

- What is the shadowing (1) in the periphery of the right mid and lower zones?
- What are the round densities (2) in the right upper and lower zones? What is their anatomic location?

A18

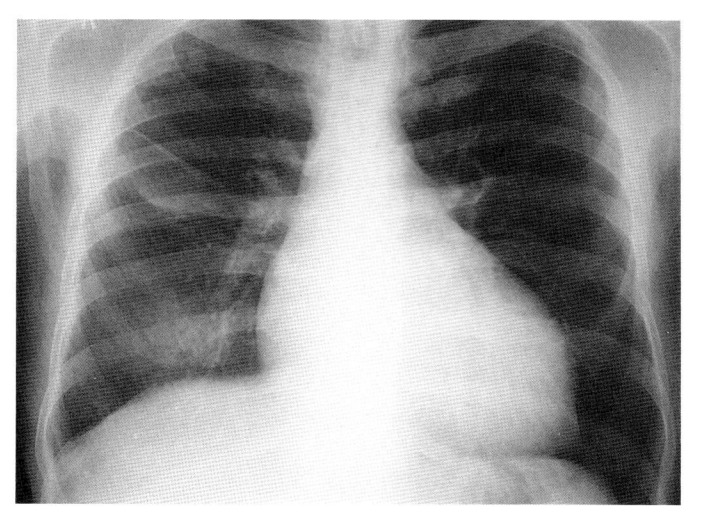

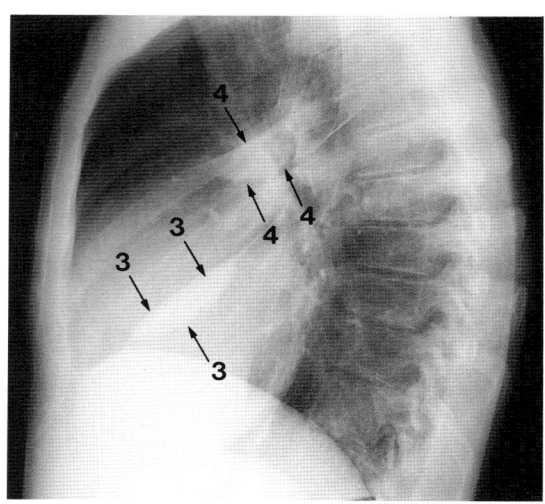

The CXRs on this page were taken three weeks later. The shadowing in the periphery of the right mid and lower zones was a lamellar pleural effusion which has now resolved. The round densities in the right upper and lower zones are encysted pleural effusions, located in the oblique (3) and horizontal (4) fissures.

Q19

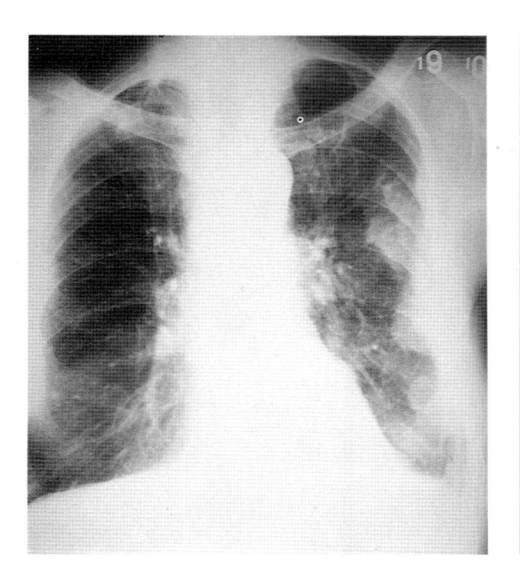

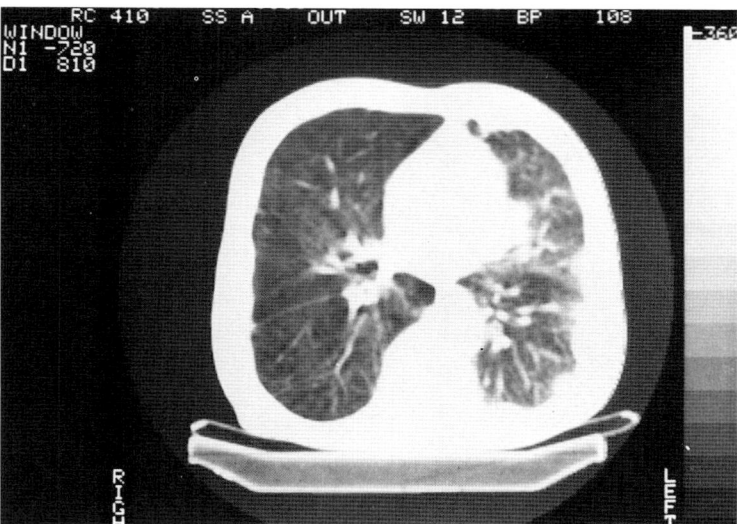

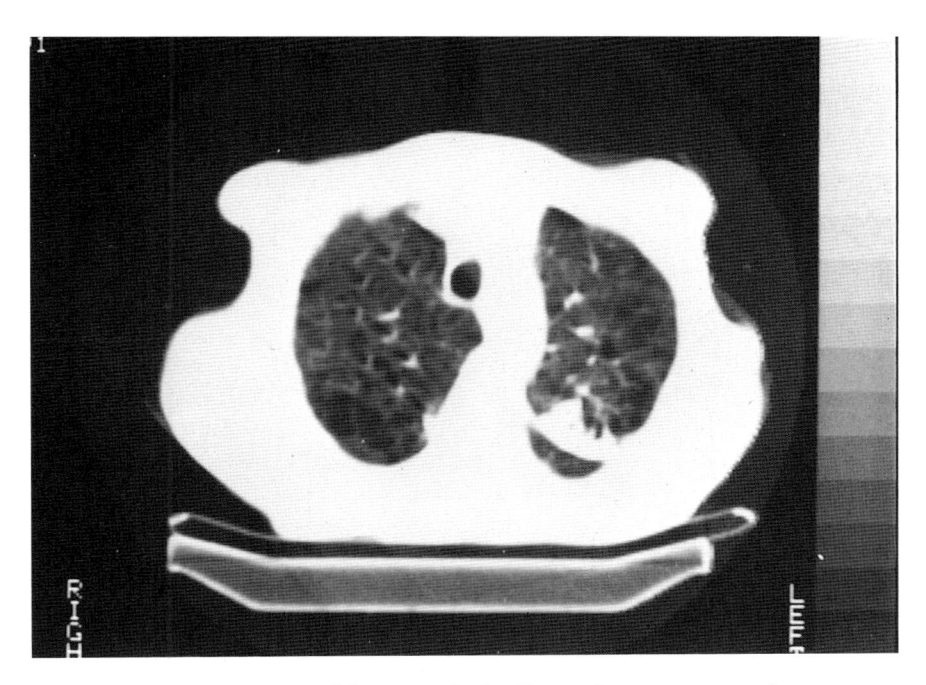

A 71-year-old retired boilermaker presented with left-sided chest pain.

- What abnormality does the CXR show?
- What additional information is shown on the CT scans?
- What is the probable diagnosis?
- What investigation would you do next?

A19

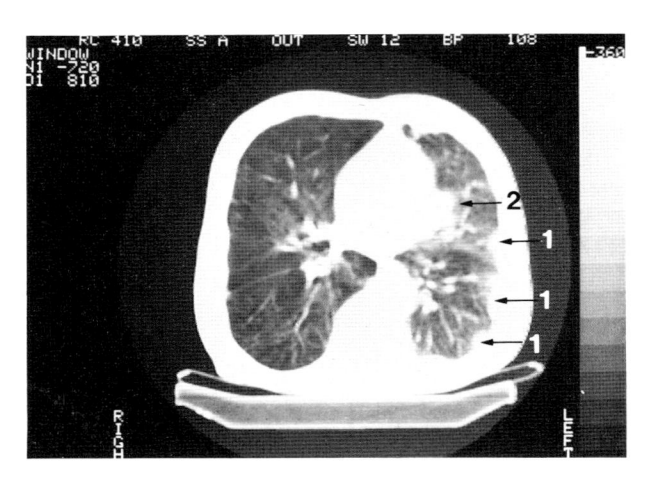

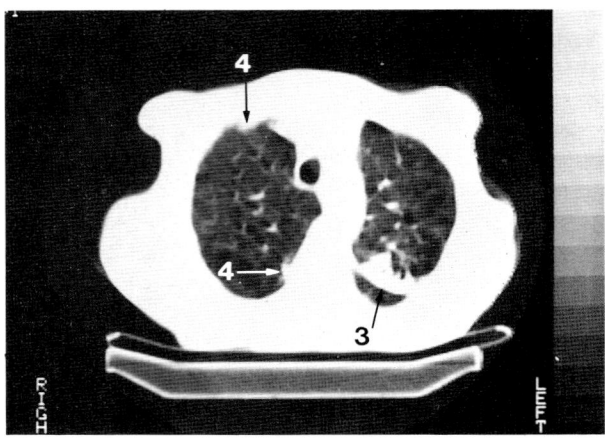

The CXR shows lobulated pleural densities surrounding the left lung. The CT scans also show that:

a) The volume of the left lung is reduced.
b) In addition to peripheral pleural masses (1), nodules are present adjacent to the mediastinum (2).
c) Pleural masses extend into the interlobar fissure (3).
d) Pleural plaques (4) are present in the right hemithorax.

The presence of bilateral pleural plaques is very suggestive of asbestos exposure, and the extensive pleural disease on the left almost certainly indicates malignant change. Percutaneous needle biopsy of the pleura provided a tissue diagnosis of malignant mesothelioma.

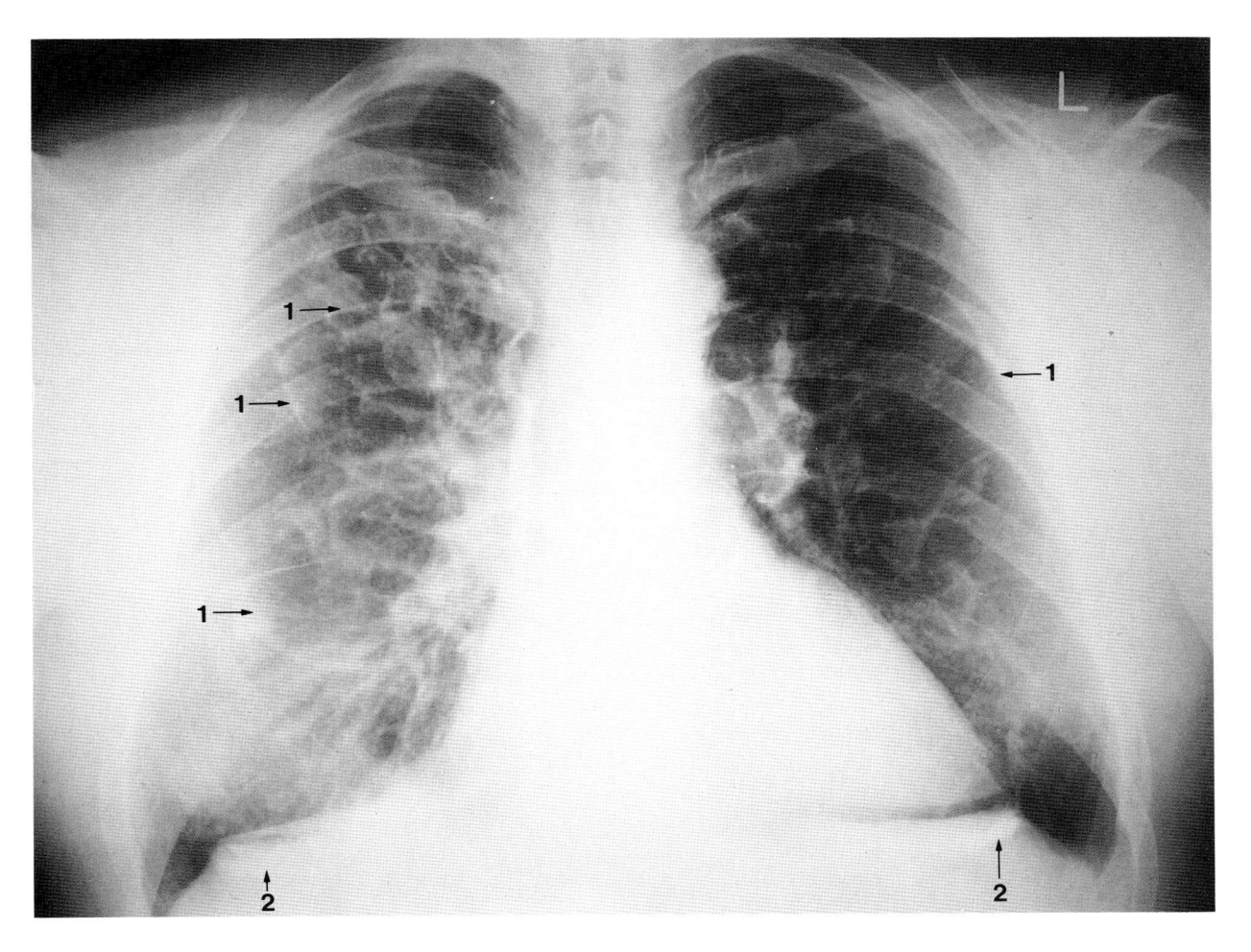

A 65-year-old man was asymptomatic, but had a history of asbestos exposure.

- Multiple calcified densities are seen in the periphery of the lungs (1) and over the diaphragm (2). Where are they located and how can they best be demonstrated?
- Is there evidence of asbestosis on this CXR?

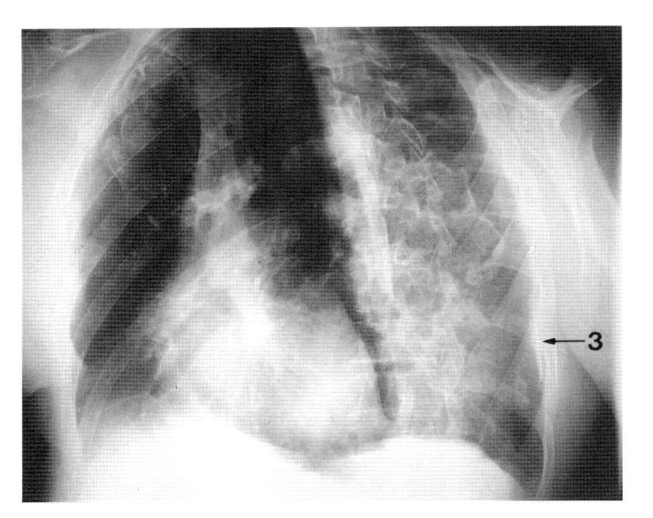

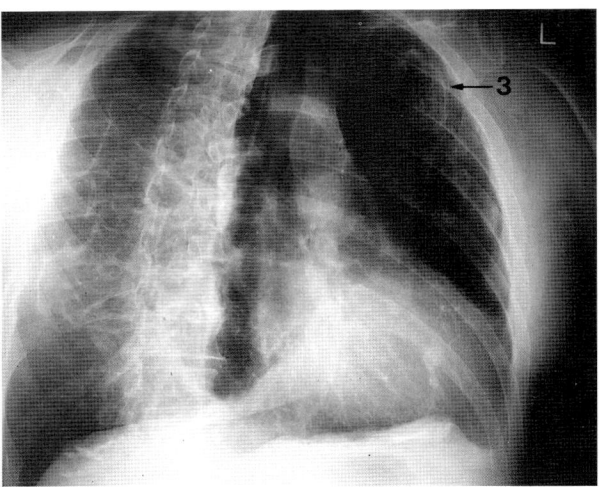

The calcified pleural plaques of asbestos exposure are typically located in the parietal pleura. Oblique films, preferably aided by fluoroscopy, may demonstrate plaques (3) not easily seen on a frontal CXR. CT is even more sensitive. There is no evidence of asbestosis. Asbestosis implies pulmonary fibrosis due to asbestos exposure. This patient's films show only pleural abnormalities.

Q21

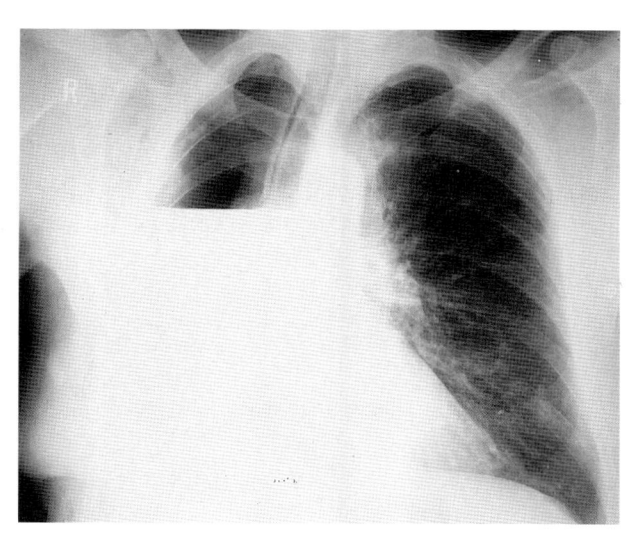

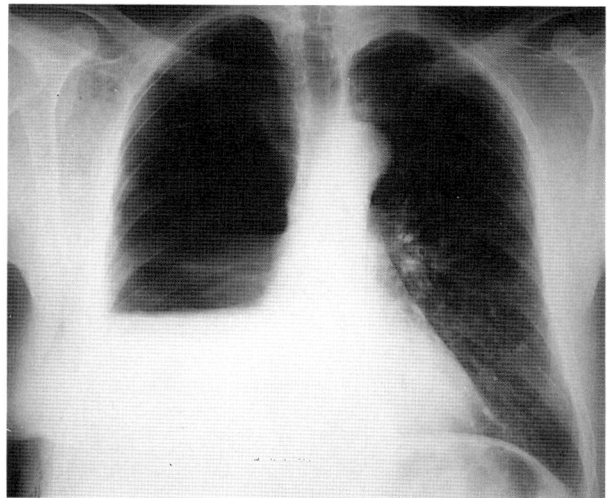

A 65-year-old man with carcinoma of the bronchus was treated by right pneumonectomy. The first CXR was taken 12 days postoperatively. Two days later the patient suffered a severe bout of coughing during which a large amount of brown fluid was expectorated. The second CXR was taken after this episode.

- Following pneumonectomy, what normally happens to the space previously occupied by the removed lung?
- What complication occurred between these two CXRs?
- What investigation should be done next?

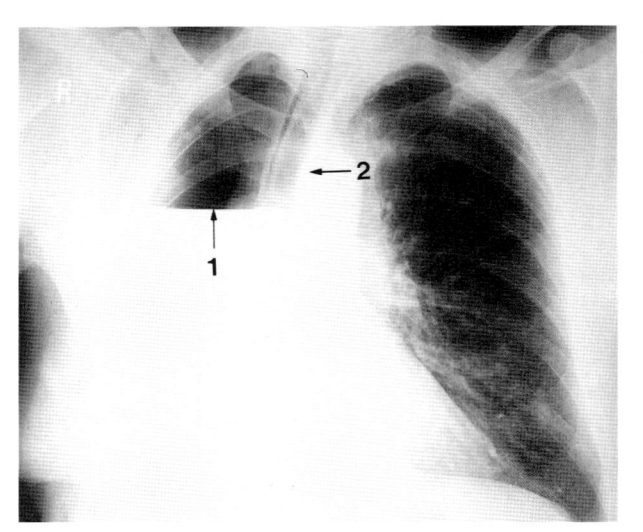

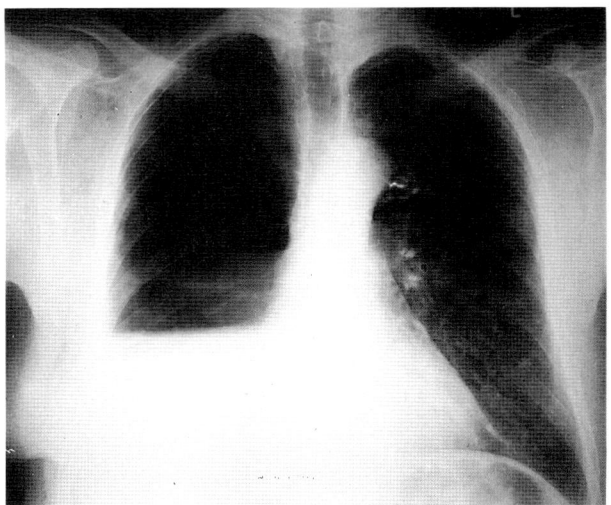

After pneumonectomy, the space gradually obliterates by accumulation of fluid (1) and shift of the mediastinum. Note the deviation of the trachea (2). Between the CXRs a bronchopleural fistula occurred. This resulted in expectoration of much of the fluid in the pneumonectomy space so that the fluid level has fallen, and air replacing the fluid has allowed the mediastinum to return to the mid line. Bronchoscopy confirmed the diagnosis, which was due to a broken ligature.

Q22

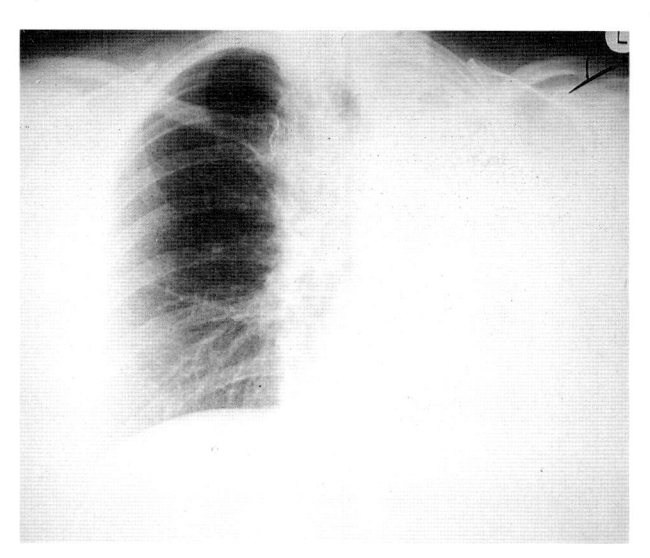

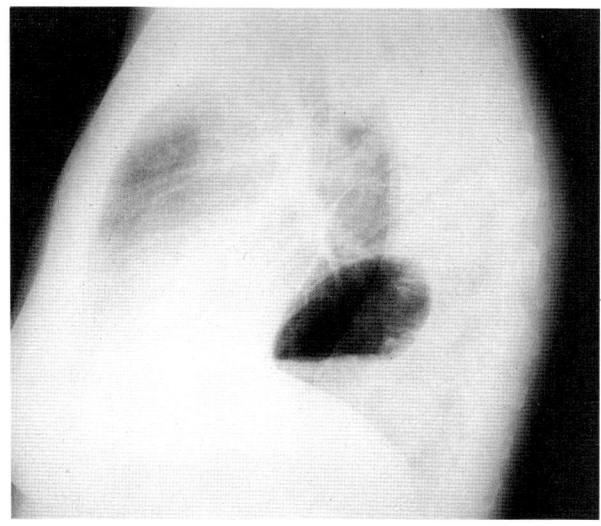

A 65-year-old woman presented with shortness of breath and haemoptysis. The CXR shows opacification of the left hemithorax.

- Comment on the position of the mediastinum and the left hemi-diaphragm.
- Is this appearance due to a large pleural effusion, or collapse or consolidation of the left lung?
- What did bronchoscopy reveal?

A22

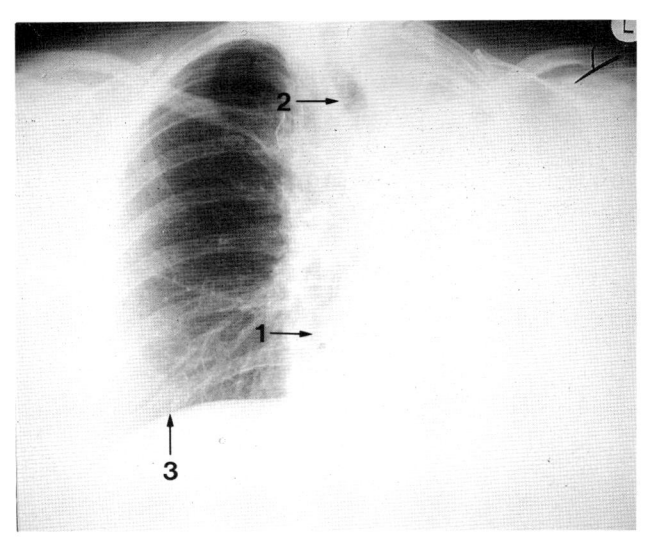

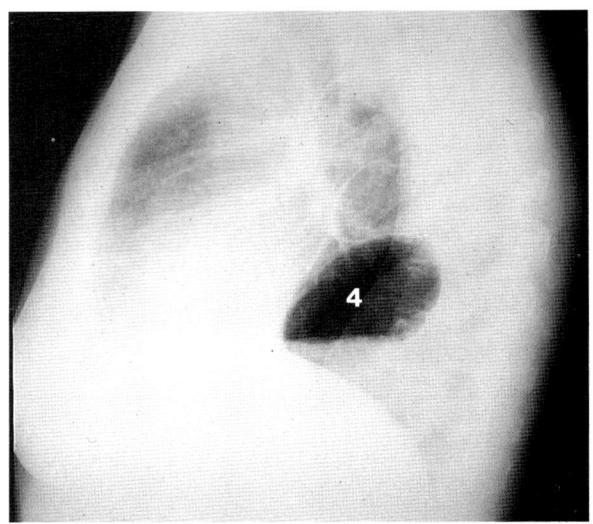

The heart (1) and the trachea (2) have been pulled to the left. The right hemi-diaphragm (3) is seen in its normal position. The left hemi-diaphragm is not visible since there is no aerated lung above it. However, the air-filled gastric fundus (4) is clearly higher than usual, indicating that the left hemi-diaphragm must also be elevated. Opacification of the left hemithorax is due to collapse of the left lung. Bronchoscopy revealed that the left main bronchus was obstructed by a carcinoma.

Q23

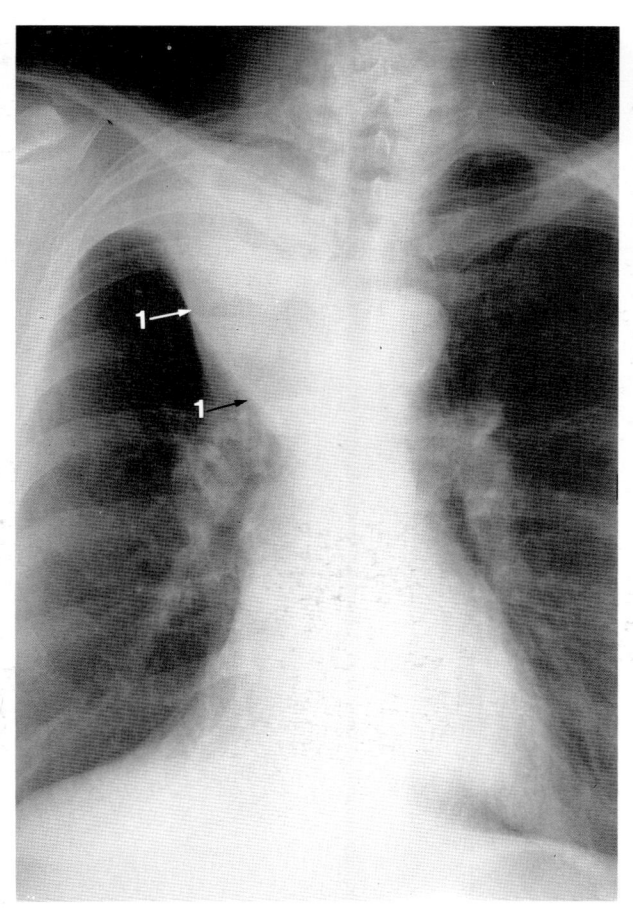

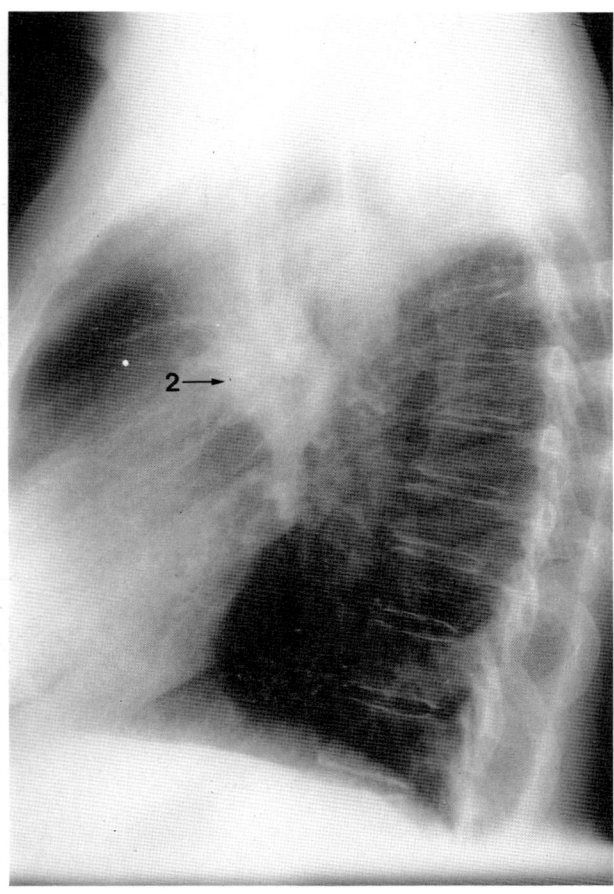

A 50-year-old man presented with a chronic cough and recent haemoptysis.

- What is this structure (1)? Comment on its position.
- What is the density in the right upper zone?
- What is this density (2)?
- What is the diagnosis?

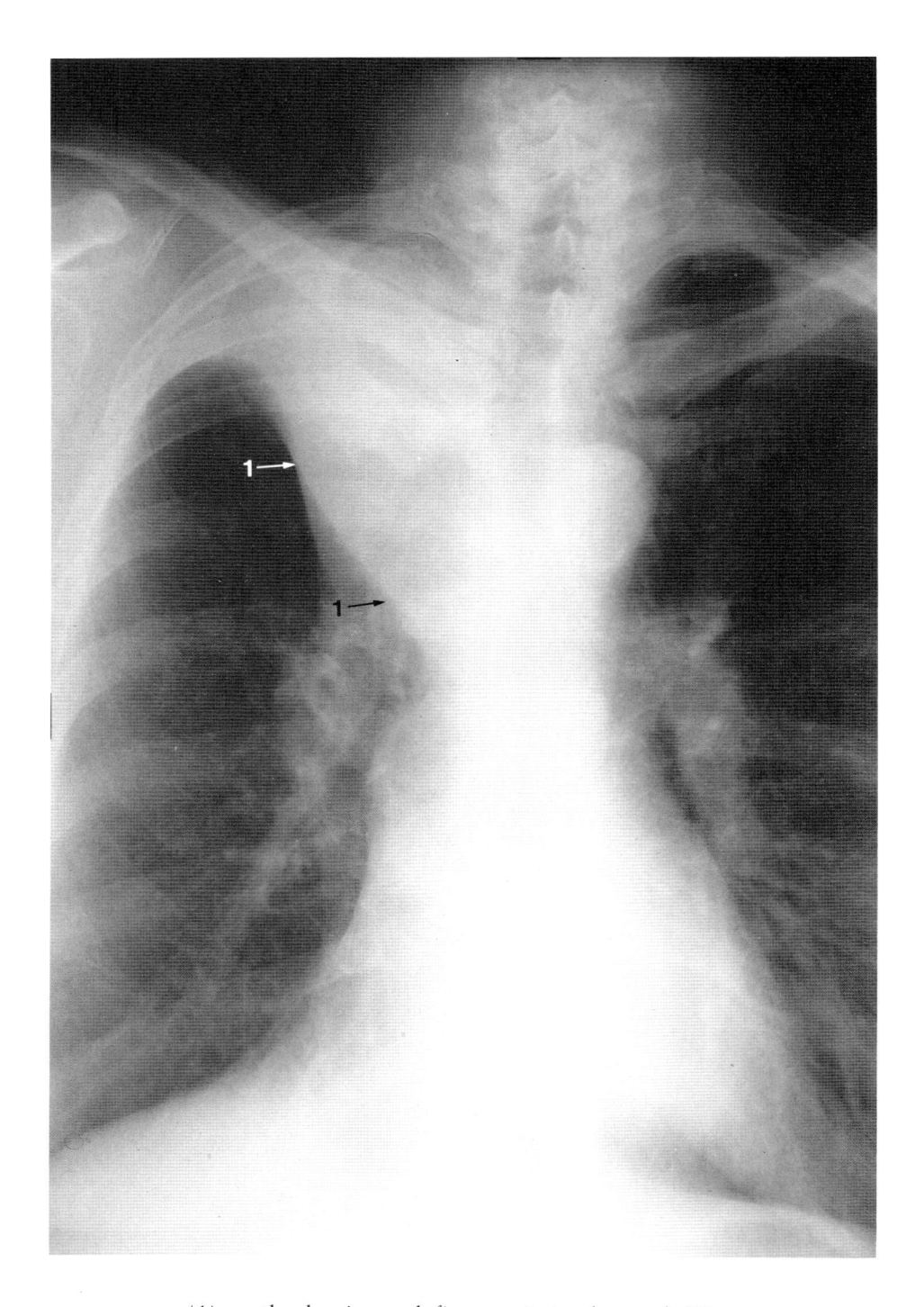

(1) = the horizontal fissure. It is elevated. The density in the right upper zone is due to collapse of the right upper lobe. (2) = a right hilar mass. The diagnosis is carcinoma of the right upper lobe bronchus.

Q24

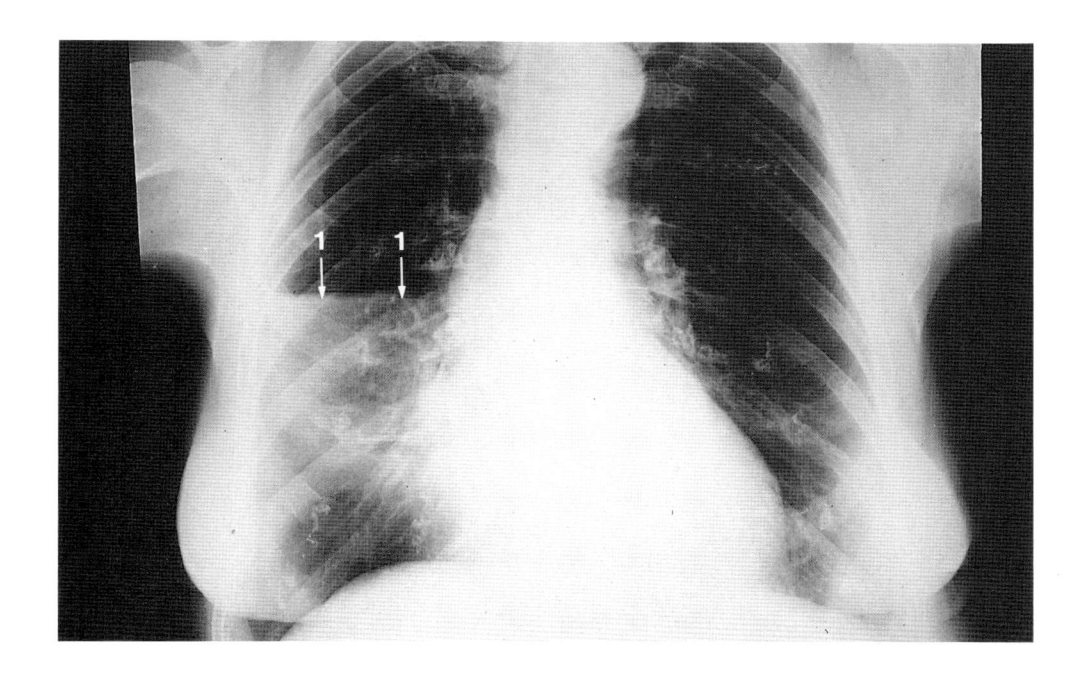

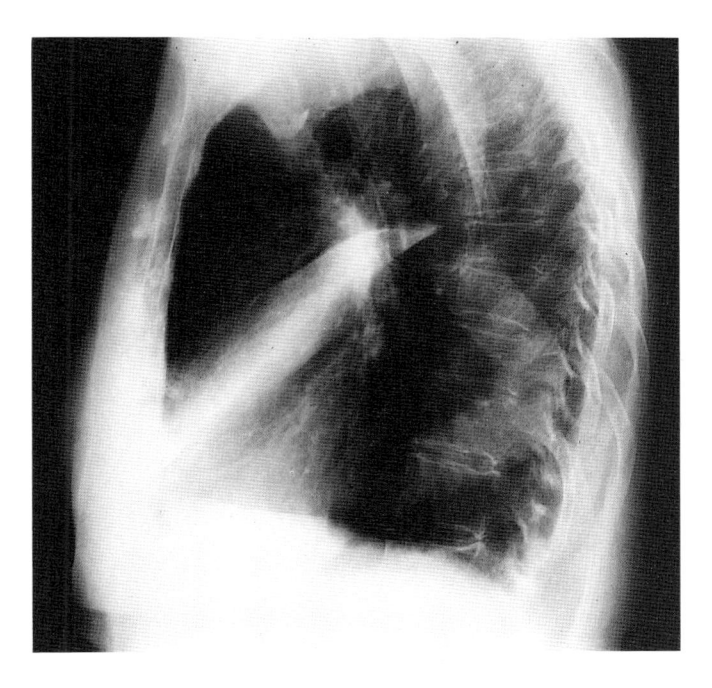

A 70-year-old woman presented with a cough.

- The right heart border is not seen clearly. What does this mean?
- What is this structure (1)?
- What does the lateral film show?

A24

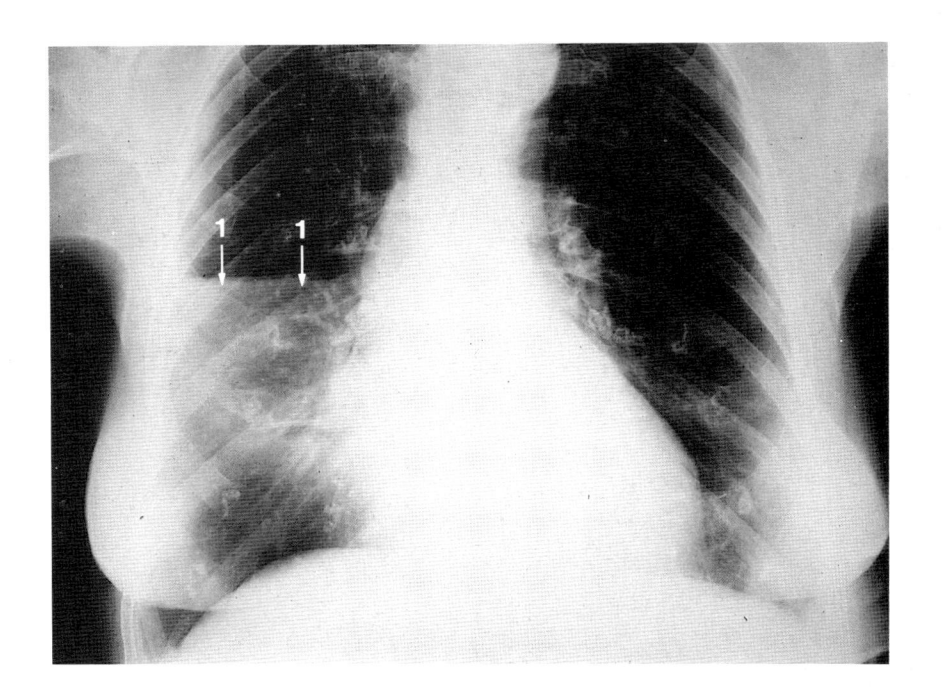

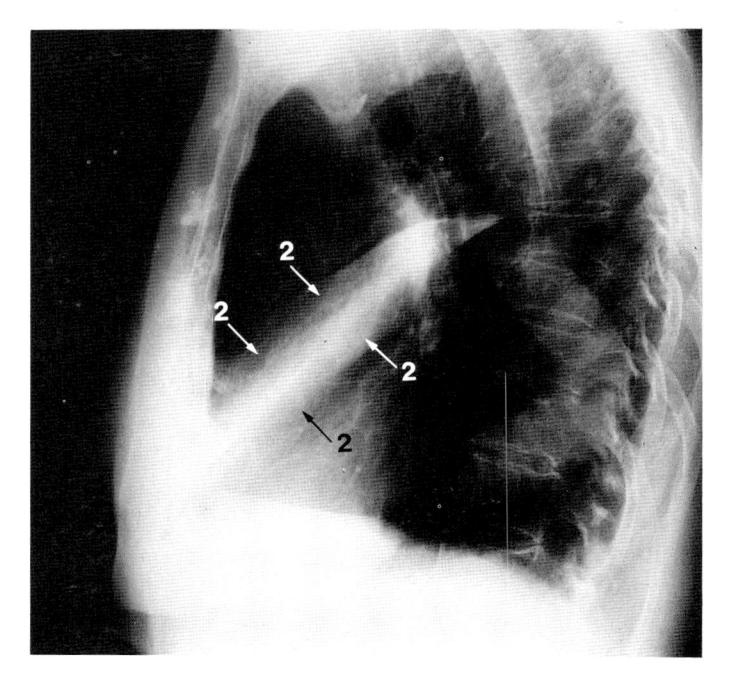

The indistinctness of the right heart border indicates that the right middle lobe (which is the part of the lung adjacent to the right heart border) is not properly aerated. (1) = the horizontal fissure. The lateral film shows collapse of the right middle lobe (2).

Q25

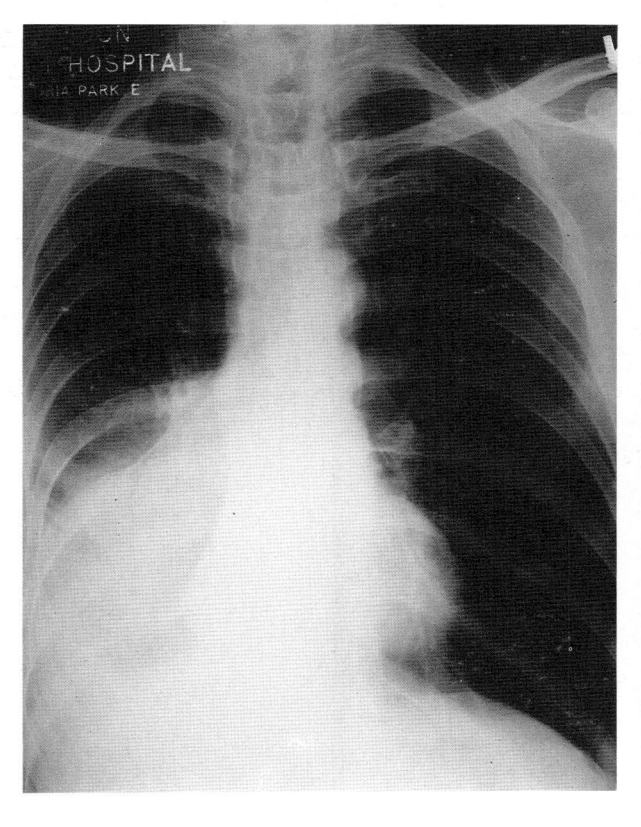

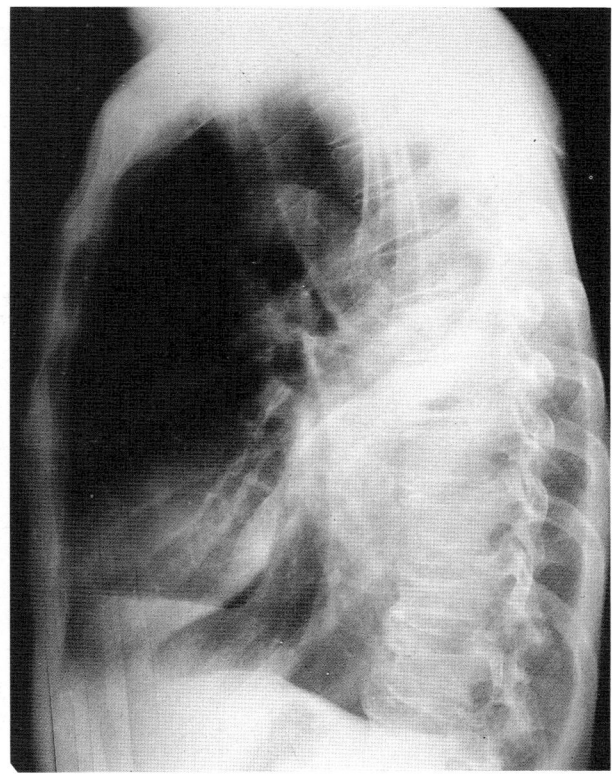

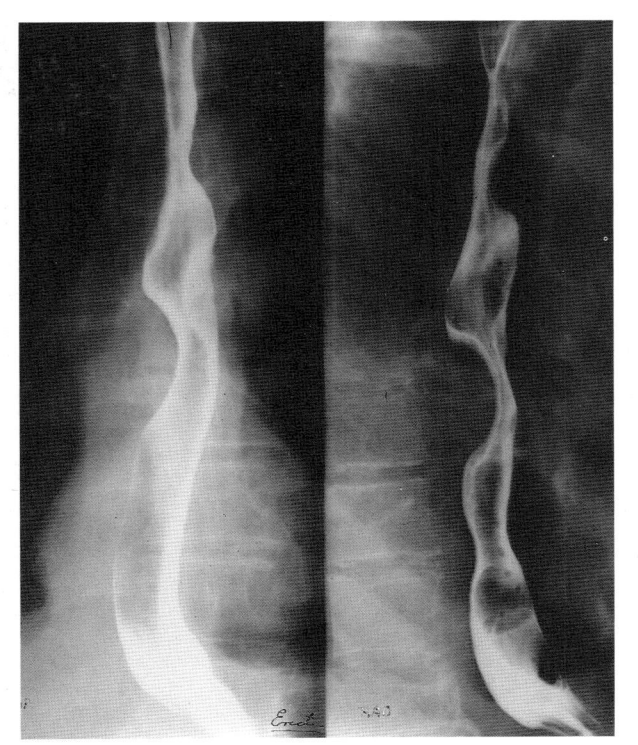

A 58-year-old man presented with a chronic cough and recent dysphagia.

- Comment on the position of the horizontal fissure.
- Is the right heart border clearly visible? What does this mean?
- Is the right hemi-diaphragm visible? What does this mean?
- What is the cause of the right lower zone opacification?

Squamous cell carcinoma occluding the right lower lobe bronchus was found at bronchoscopy.

- What does the barium swallow show?

A25

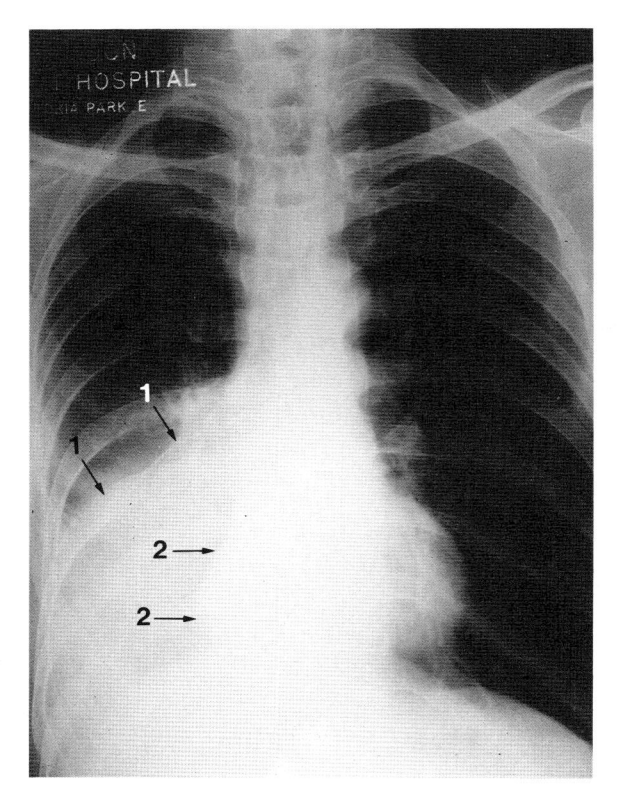

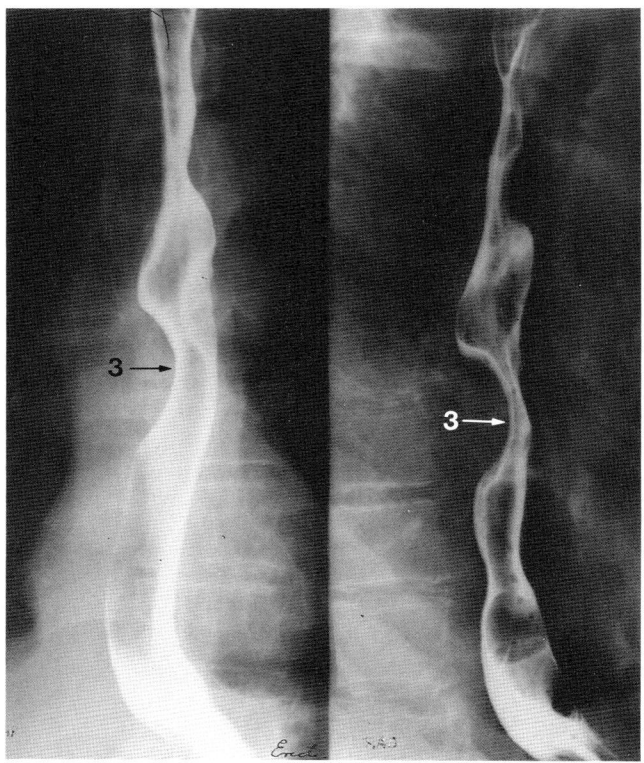

The horizontal fissure is depressed (1). The right heart border is clearly visible (2), indicating that the right middle lobe is normally aerated. The right hemi-diaphragm is not visible, indicating that aerated lung is not in contact with the diaphragm. The right lower zone opacification is due to right lower lobe collapse. The barium swallow shows extrinsic compression (3) of the mid-oesophagus due to sub carinal lymph node involvement.

Q26

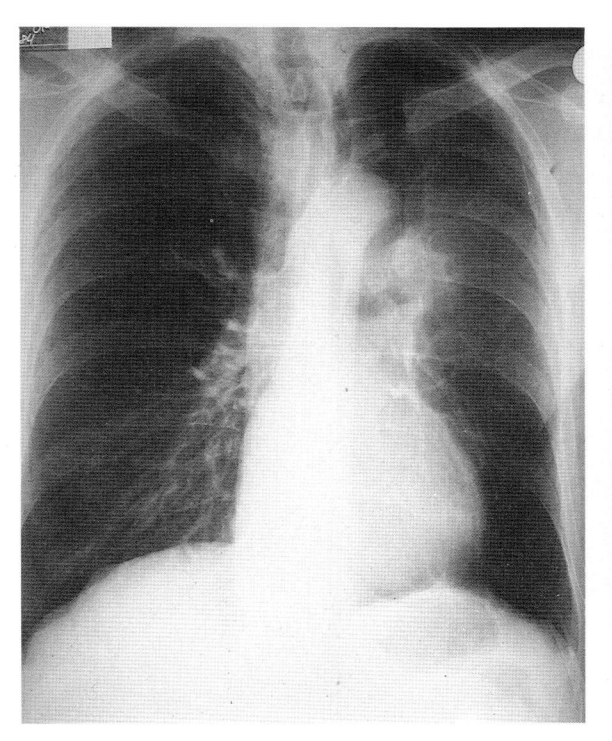

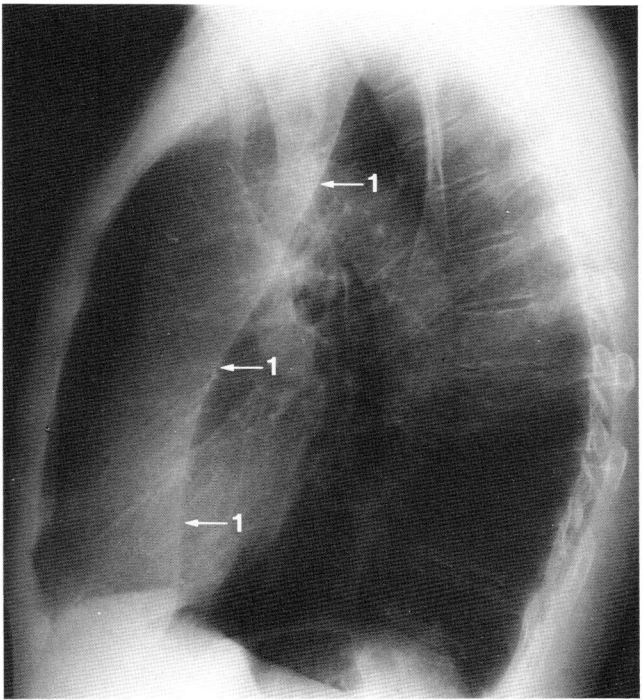

A 68-year-old chronic bronchitic presented with recent haemoptysis.

- Comment on the position of the trachea.
- Comment on the position and appearance of the left hilum.
- What is this structure (1)? Is its position normal?
- What is the cause of the increased density of the left upper zone?

A26

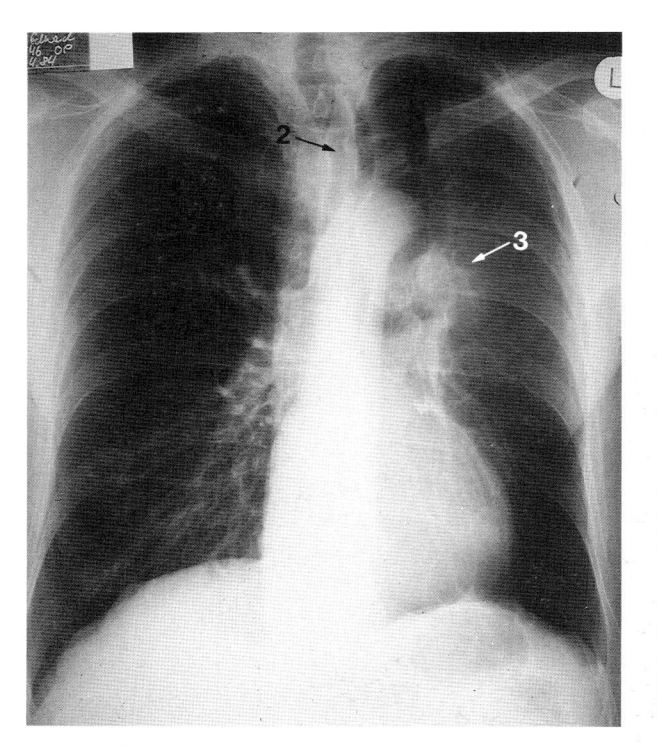

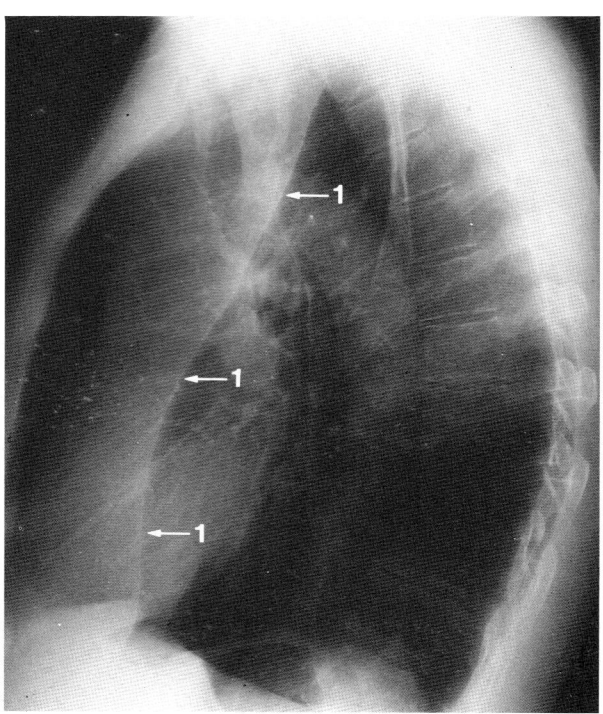

The trachea is deviated to the left (2). The left hilum (3) is elevated and enlarged. (1) = the left oblique fissure. It is displaced anteriorly. The left upper lobe anterior to it is denser than usual, and the lower lobe posteriorly is hyperinflated. The increased density of the left upper zone is caused by collapse of the left upper lobe due to a carcinoma of the bronchus.

Q27

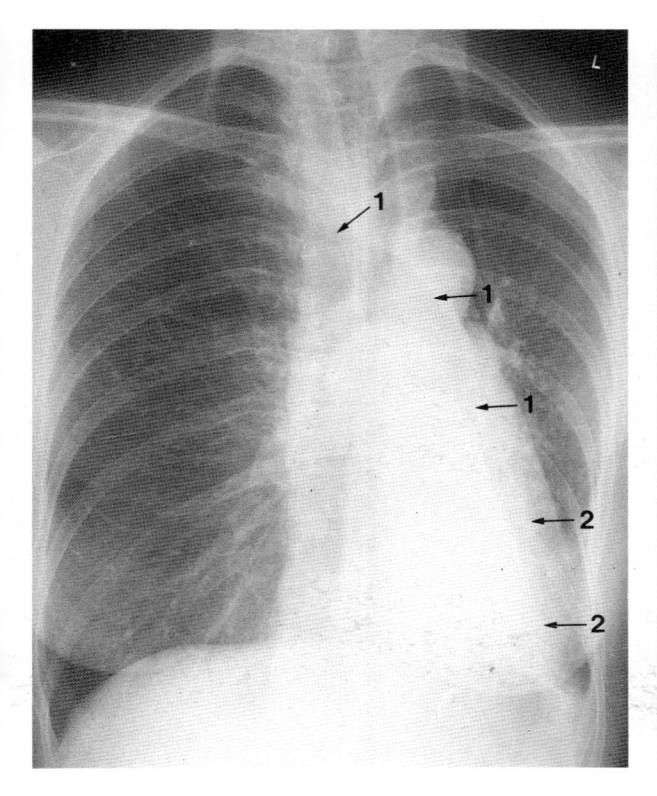

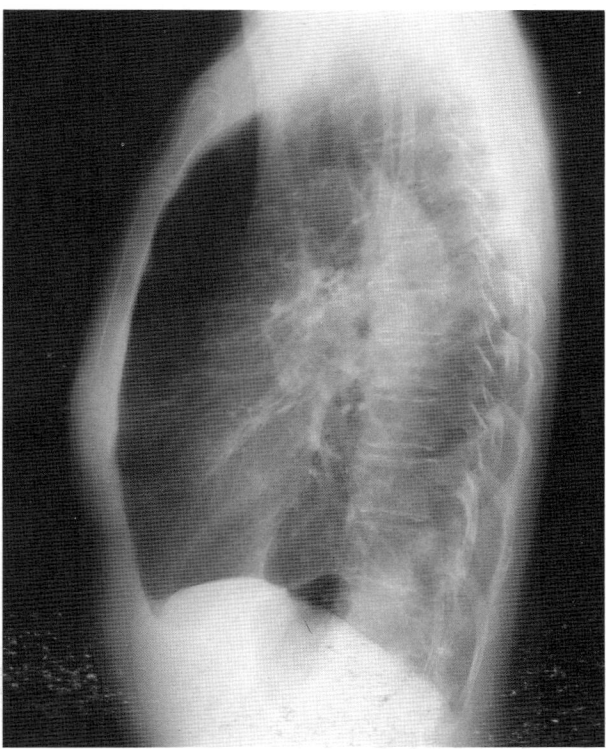

A 55-year-old man presented with a chronic cough and recent weight loss.

- Is the mediastinum in normal position?
- What is this structure (1)?
- Is the left hemi-diaphragm visible?
- What is this density (2) superimposed over the heart?

A27

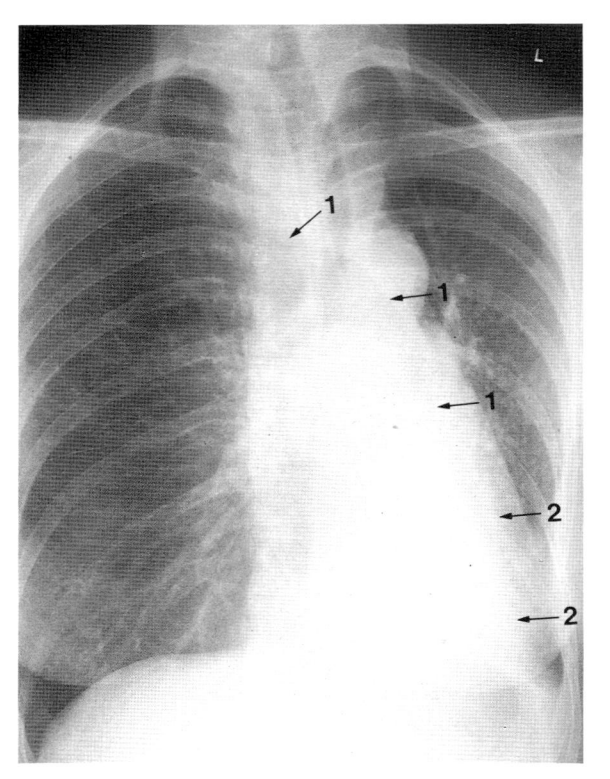

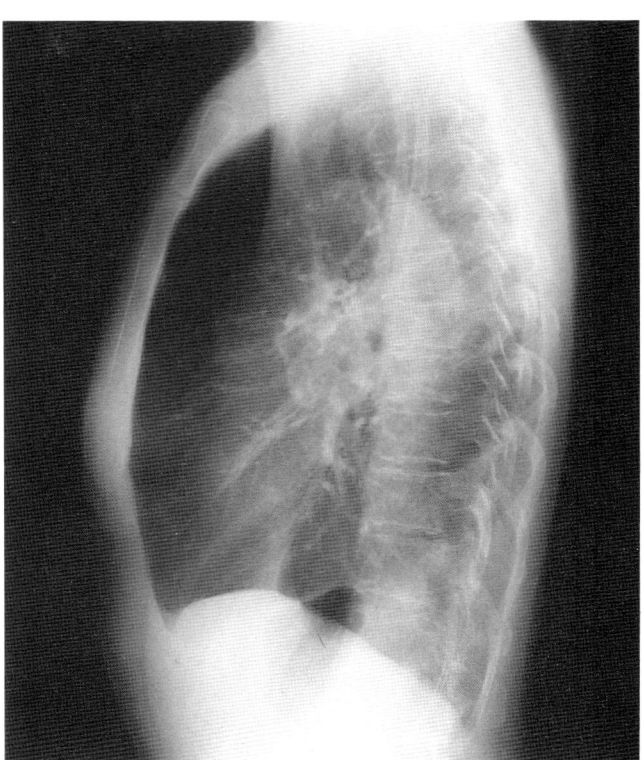

The mediastinum is not in normal position. It is displaced to the left. (1) = the edge of the right lung, which has herniated across the mid-line. The left hemi-diaphragm is not visible. (2) = the collapsed left lower lobe. At bronchoscopy a large cell carcinoma of the bronchus was occluding the left lower lobe bronchus.

Q28

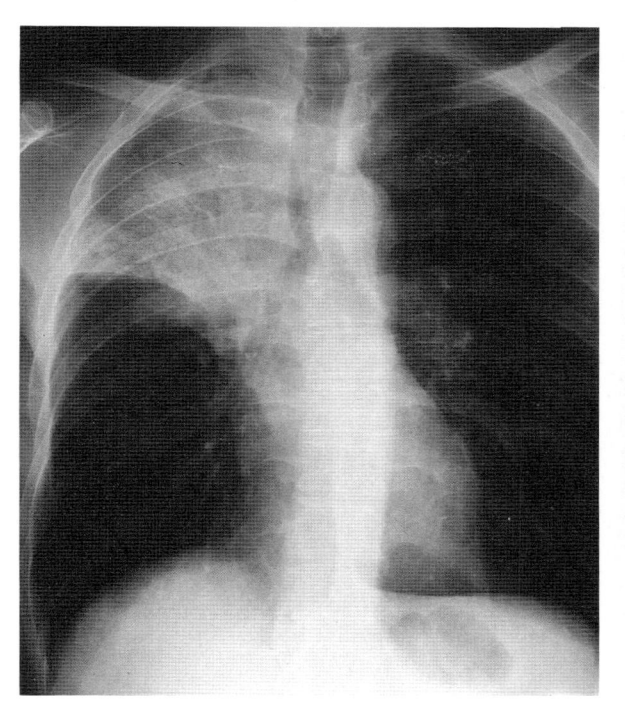

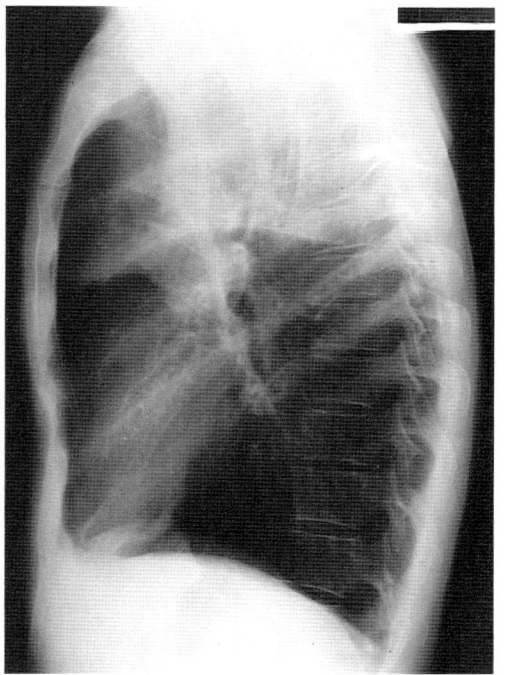

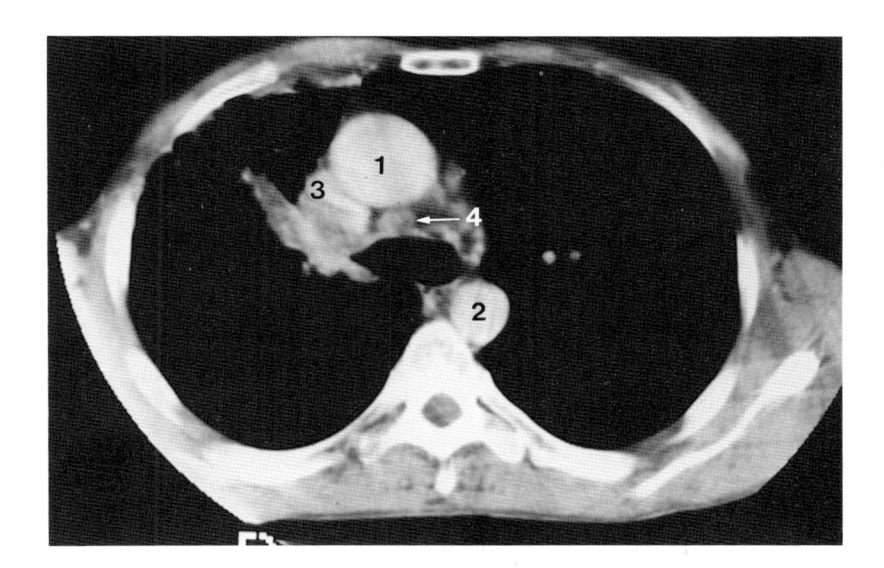

A 52-year-old man presented with a chronic cough and recent weight loss.

- What does the CXR show?

Further investigation showed a large cell carcinoma of the right upper lobe bronchus. A CT scan was performed with contrast medium enhancement.

- What are structures (1) and (2)?
- What is (3)? Is it normal?
- What is (4)?
- Is the tumour curable by operation?

A28

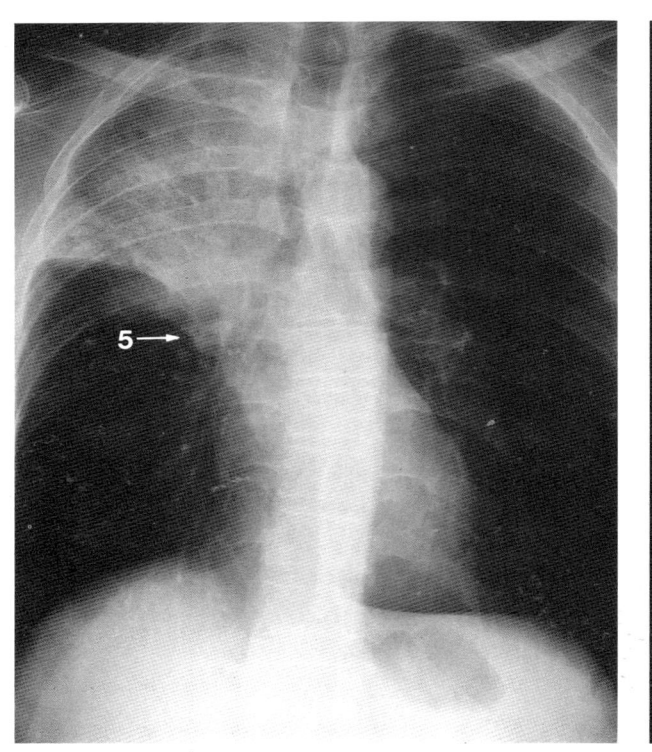

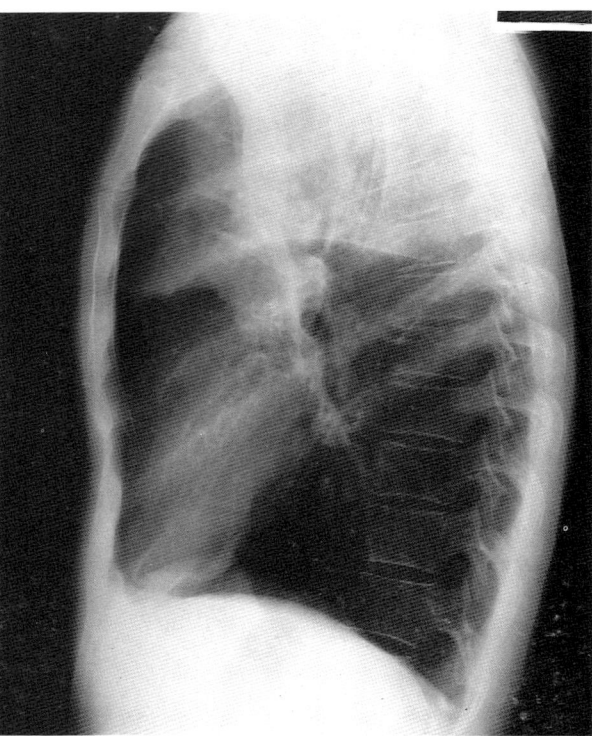

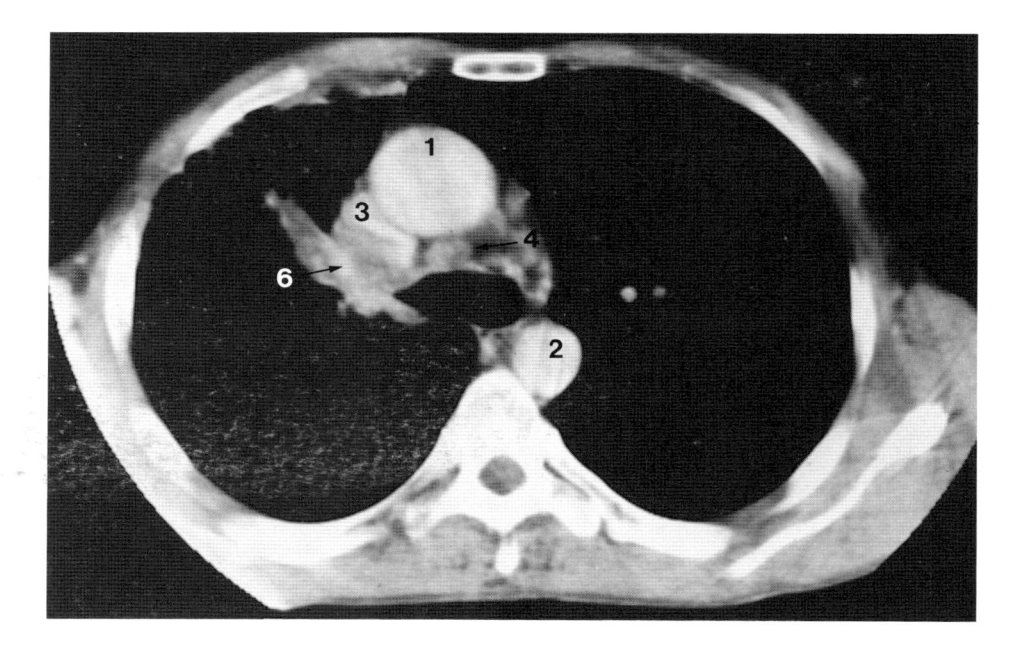

The CXR shows that the right upper lobe is consolidated and a mass is present at the right hilum (5). (1) = the ascending aorta and (2) = the descending aorta. (3) = the superior vena cava. It is compressed by the tumour (6). (4) = a pre-tracheal lymph node. It is enlarged. The mediastinal involvement demonstrated by CT makes the tumour inoperable.

Q29

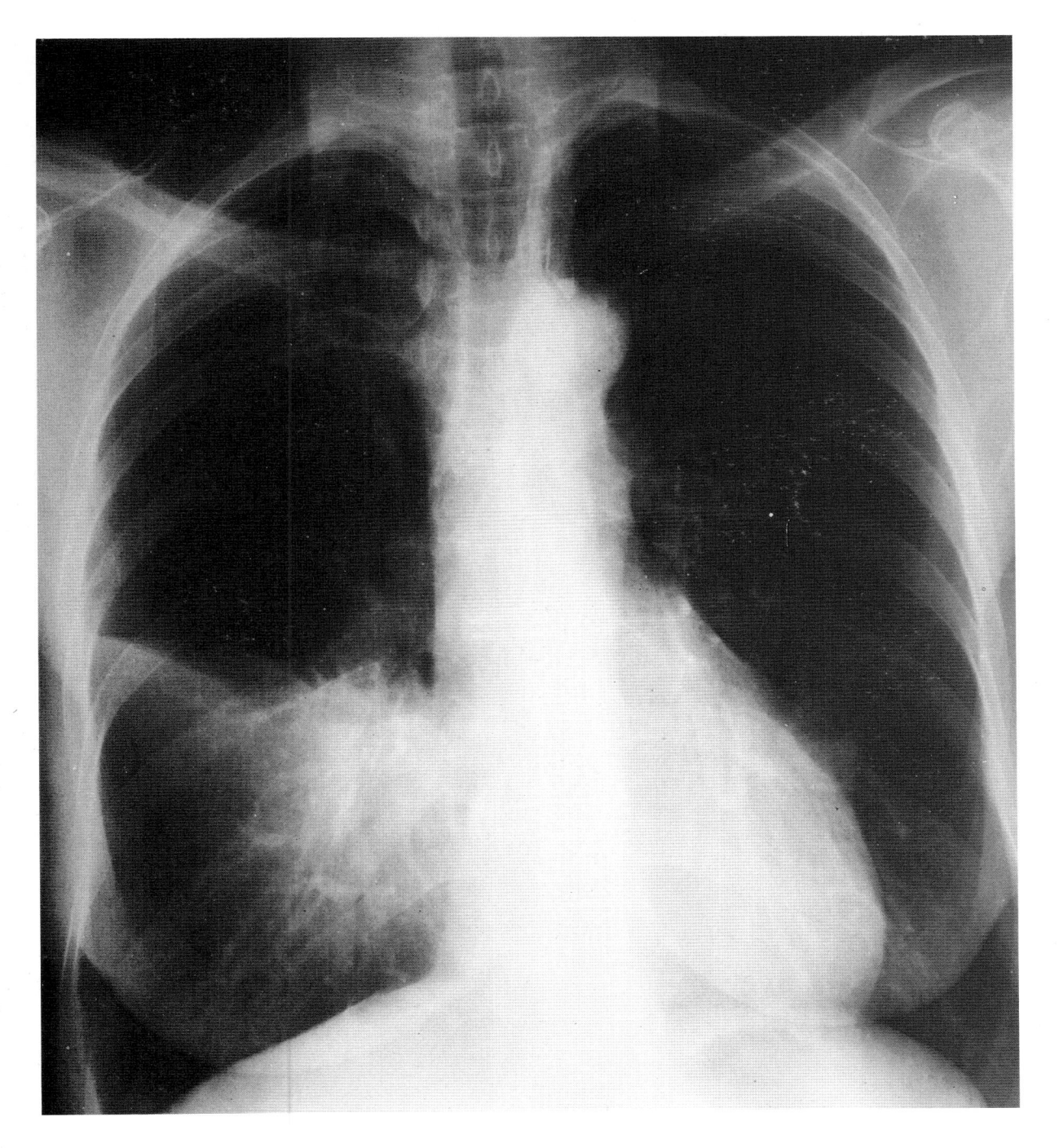

A 76-year-old woman presented with cough and fever of recent onset.

- What does the CXR show?
- Is a lateral film necessary for interpretation?

A29

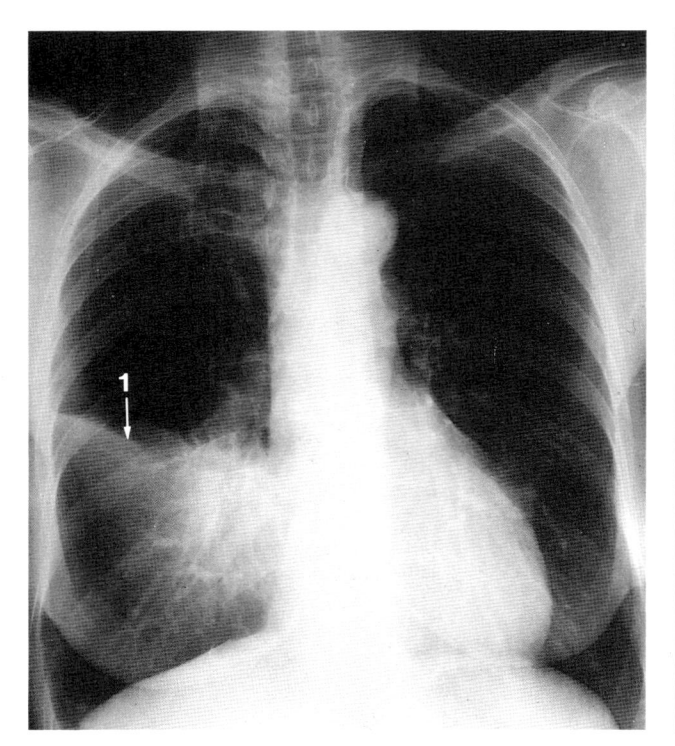

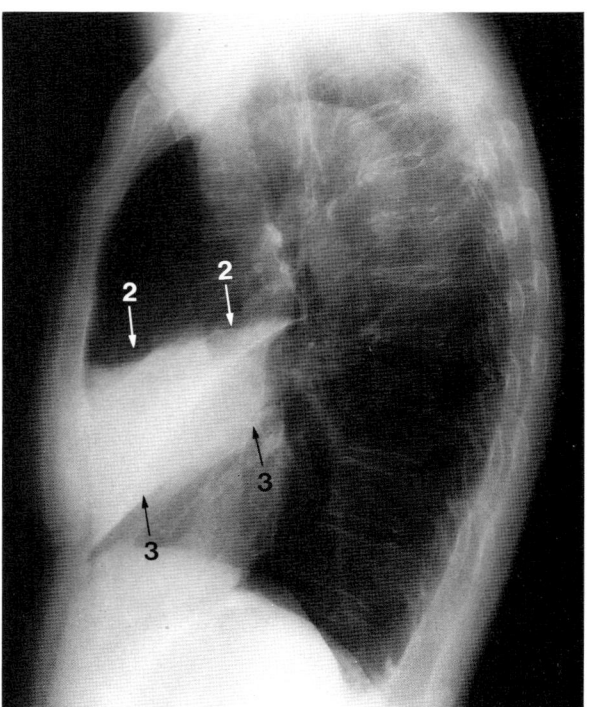

The CXR shows consolidation of the right middle lobe. The area of increased density obscures the right heart border and is limited by the horizontal fissure (1). A lateral film is not necessary for interpretation. However, the lateral film confirms consolidation of the right middle lobe, between the horizontal (2) and oblique (3) fissures, but does not further the diagnosis.

This was an acute pneumonia. The causative organism was not identified.

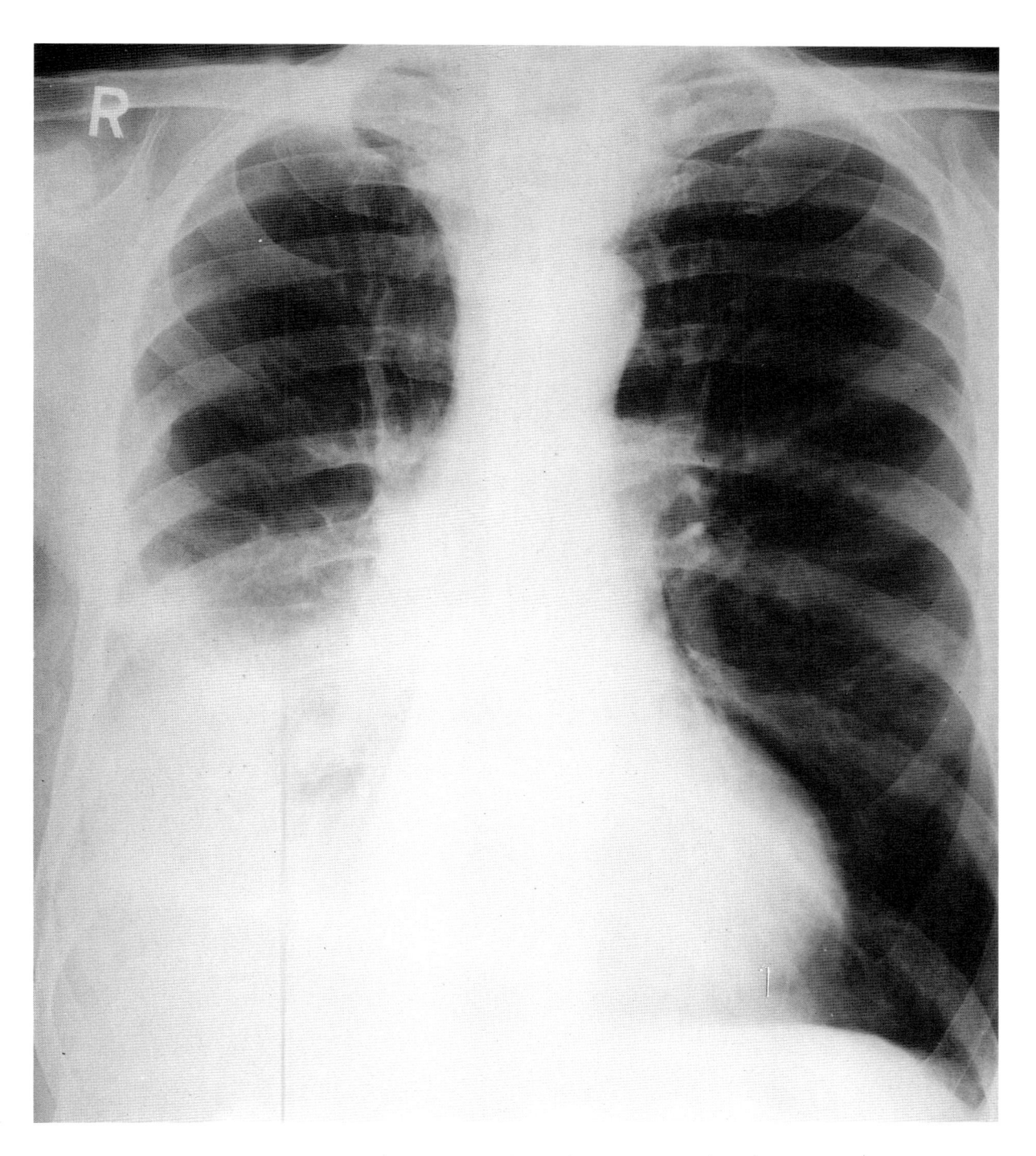

A 69-year-old chronic bronchitic presented with fever, right-sided pleuritic chest pain, and purulent sputum.

- What does the CXR show?

A30

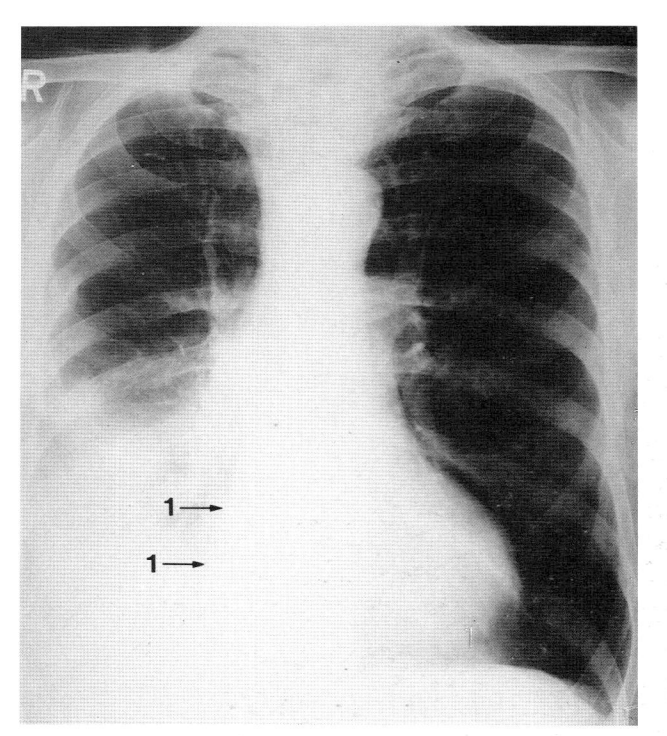

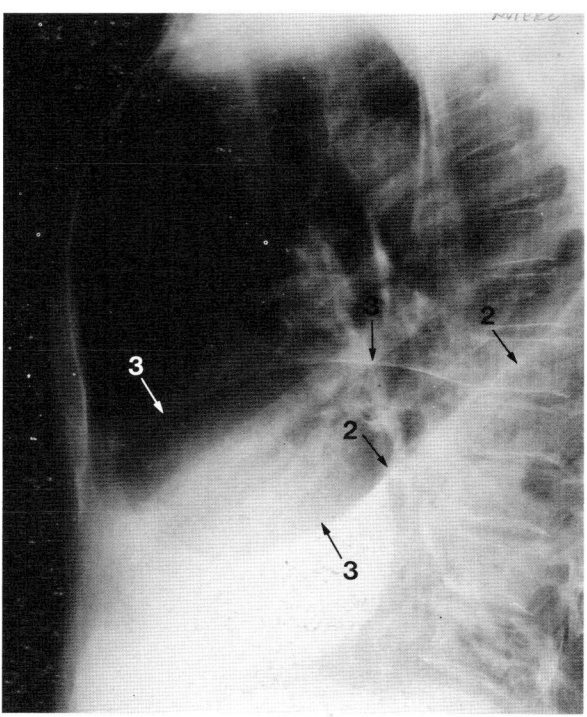

The CXR shows right lower lobe consolidation. The right basal density obscures the right hemi-diaphragm, but not the right heart border (1). The lateral film shows that the consolidation is posterior to the oblique fissure (2). The normally aerated middle lobe (3) is well demonstrated. Sputum culture revealed *Klebsiella aeruginosa*.

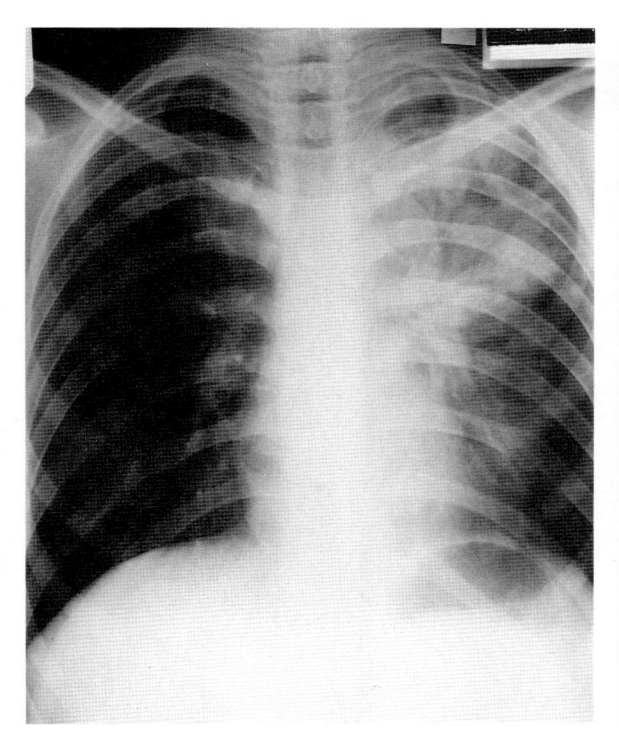

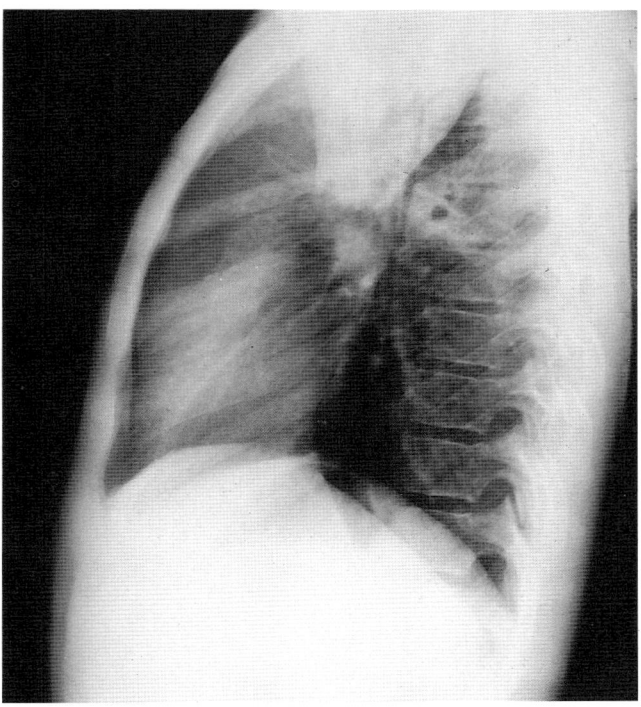

A 15-year-old male presented with a chronic cough and fever.

- Which part of the left lung is abnormal?
- Describe the left upper zone shadowing.
- Is this due to collapse or consolidation?
- What test should be done next?

A31

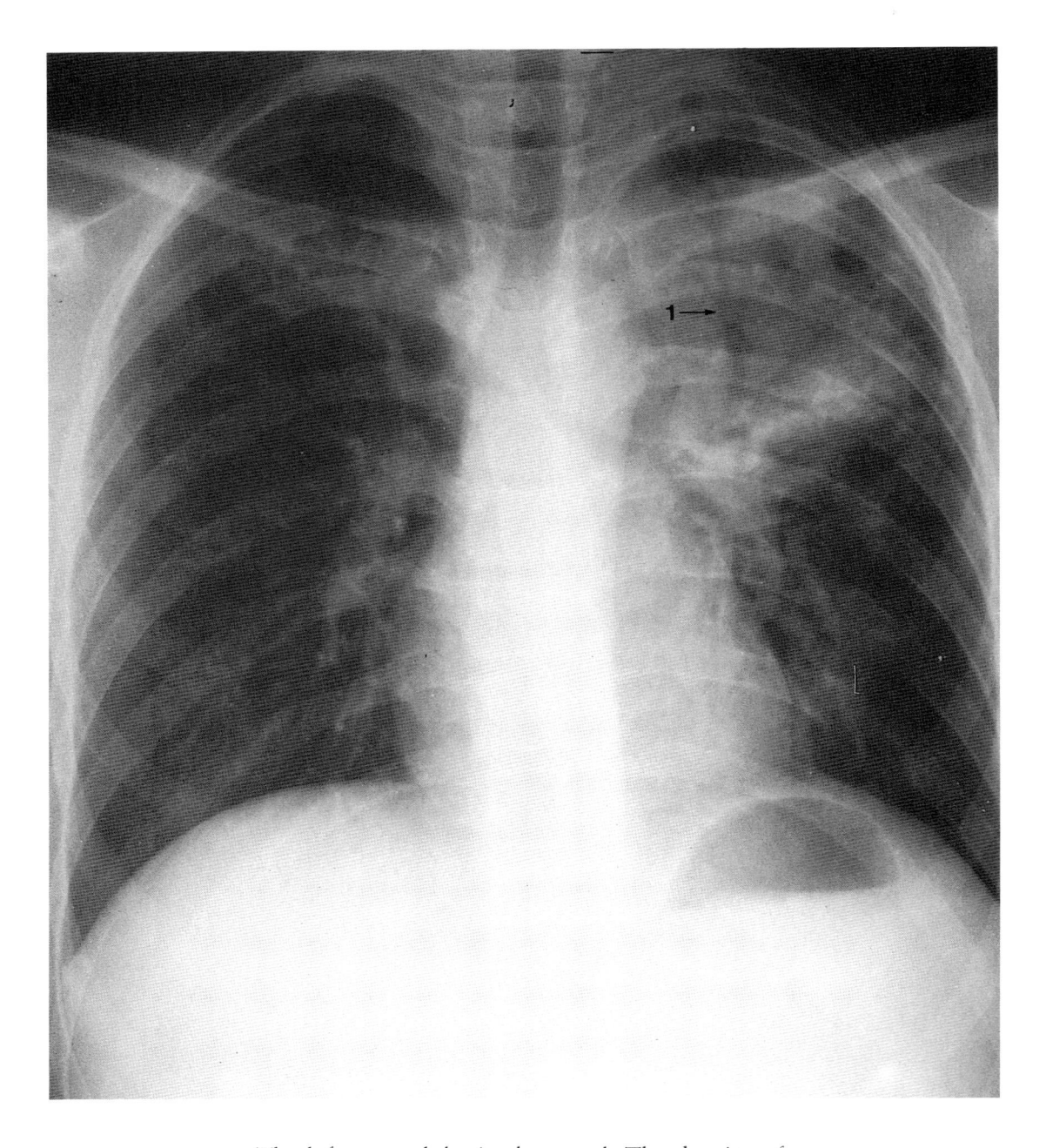

The left upper lobe is abnormal. The density of the left upper lobe is not uniform; an air bronchogram (1) is present, which is even better seen on this CXR of two days later. These branching lucencies represent patent bronchi surrounded by non-aerated alveoli. An air bronchogram almost always indicates consolidation. The sputum should be examined bacteriologically. This showed tuberculosis.

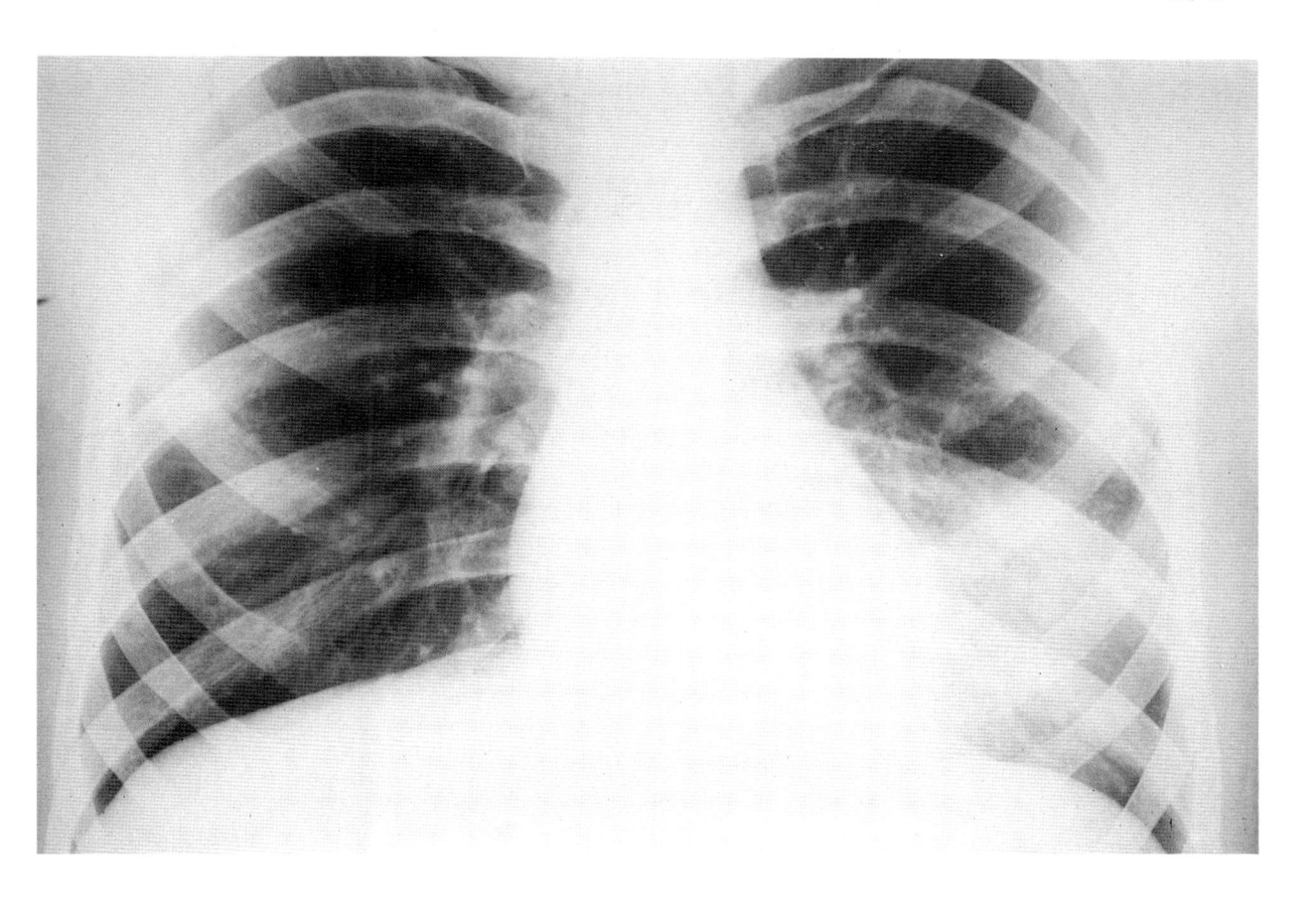

A 22-year-old male presented with acute onset of cough, fever and left pleuritic pain.

- What is the abnormality?

A32

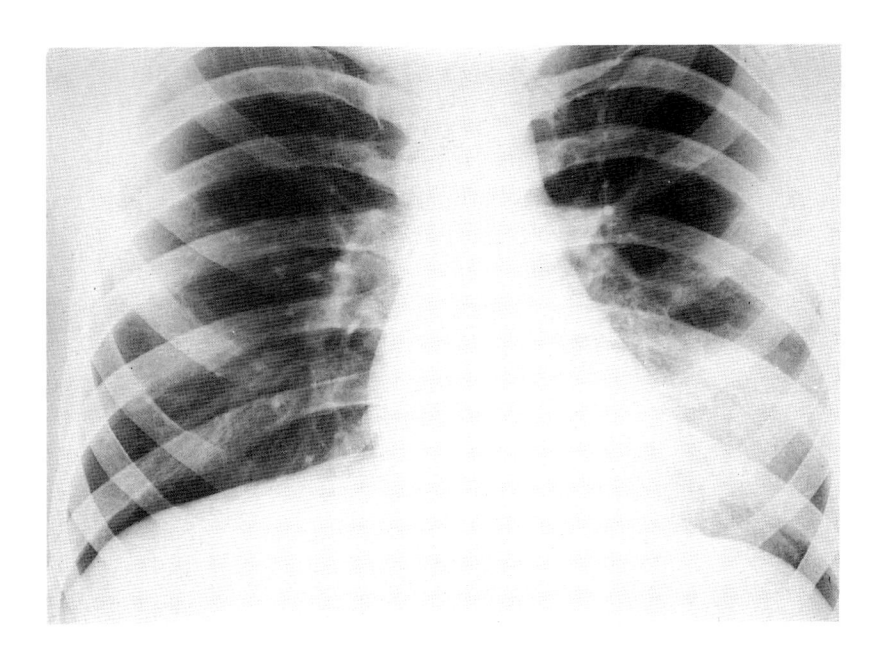

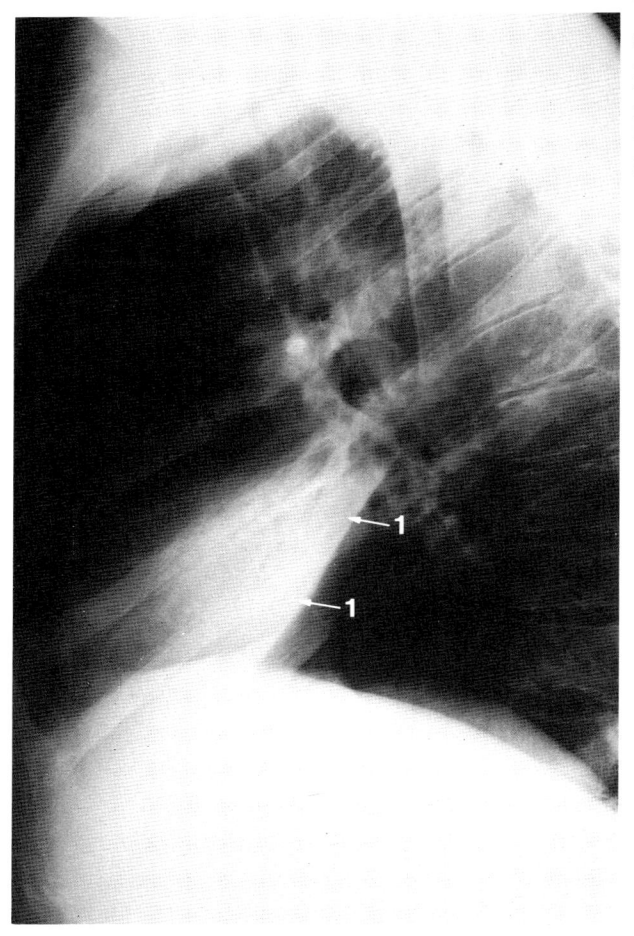

There is lingular consolidation. Left lower zone shadowing obscures the left heart border, but not the diaphragm. This is confirmed on the lateral film. The consolidation is anterior to the lower half of the oblique fissue (1). *Streptococcus pneumoniae* was isolated from the sputum.

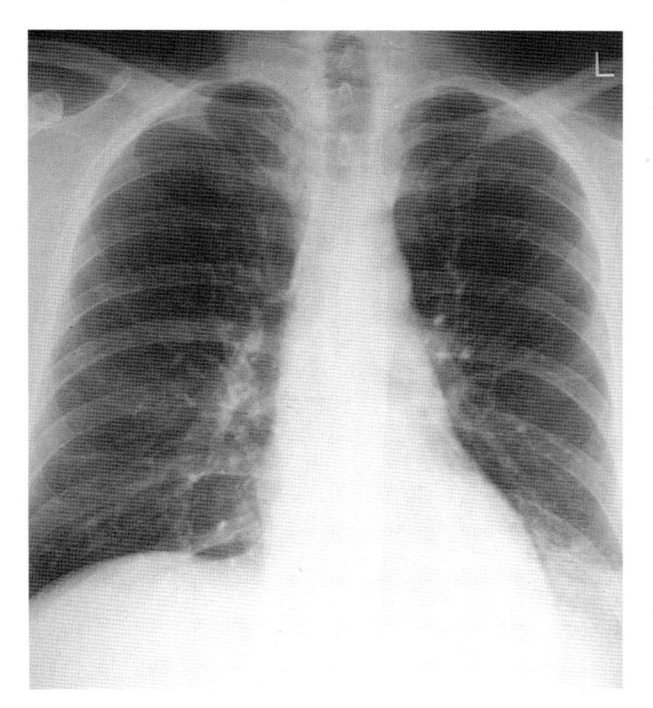

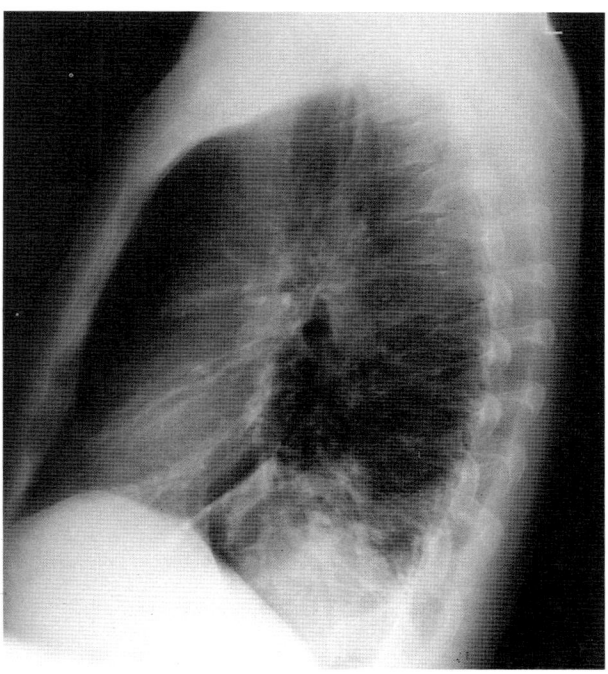

A 40-year-old male presented with a productive cough and left-sided chest pain.

- What is the abnormality?

A33

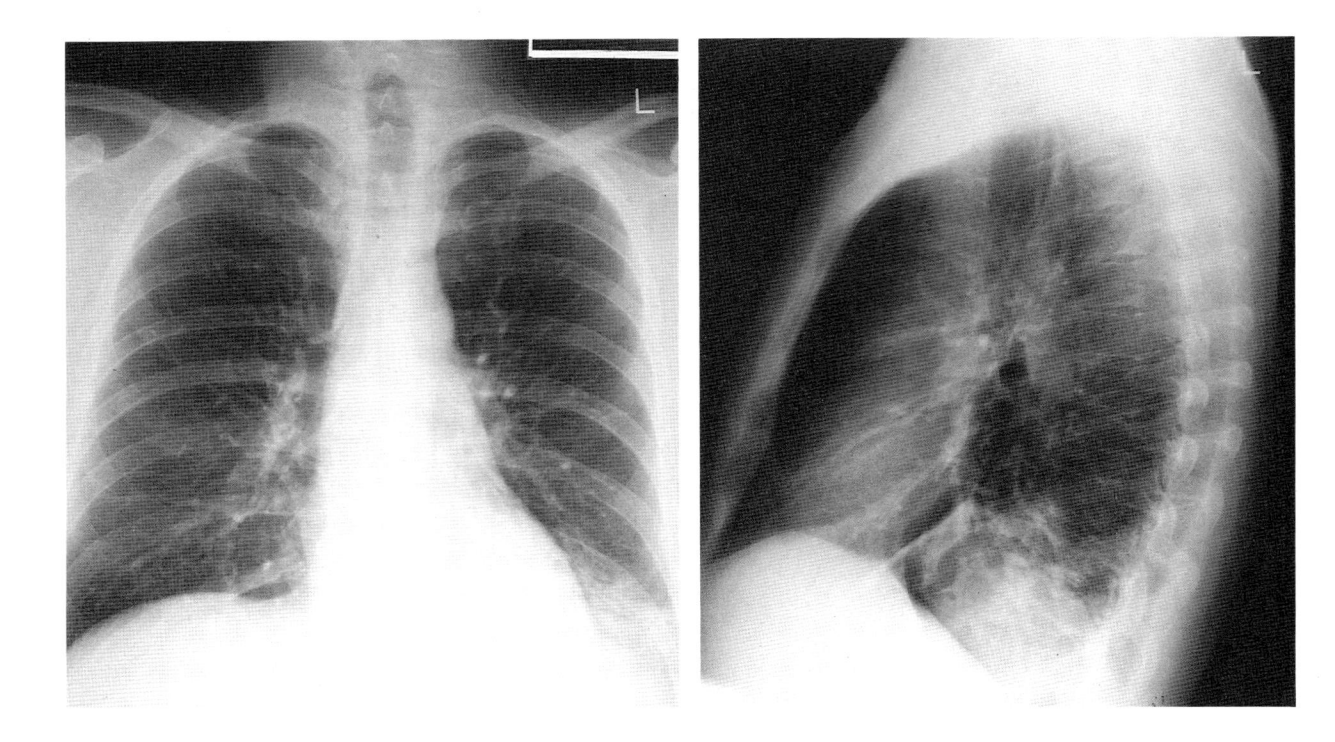

There is consolidation of the posterior basal segment of the left lower lobe. The left hemidiaphragm is obscured, but the left heart border is clearly visible.

Q34

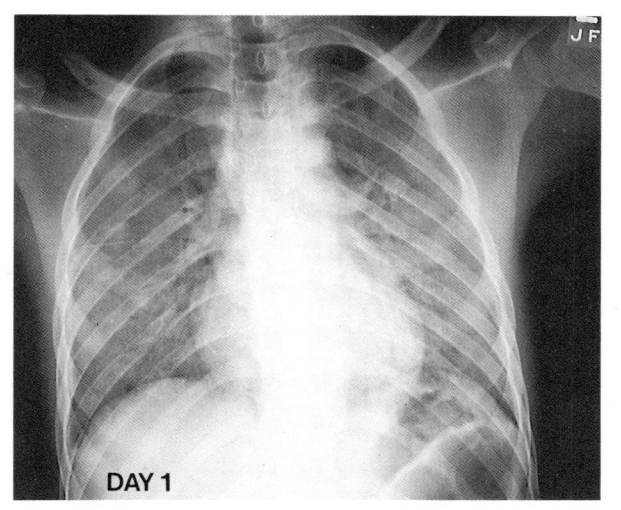

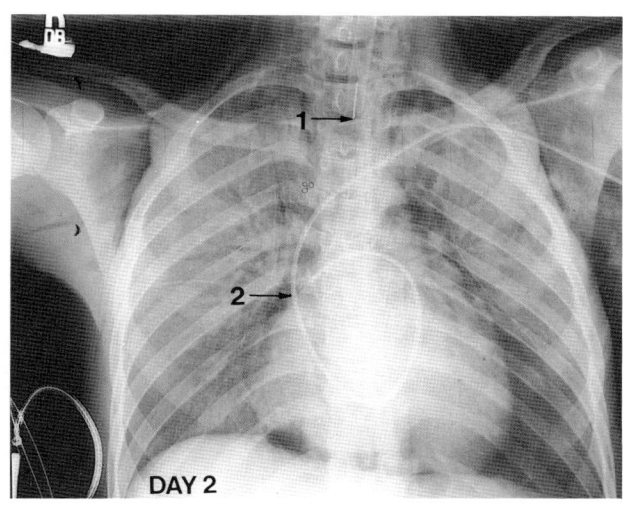

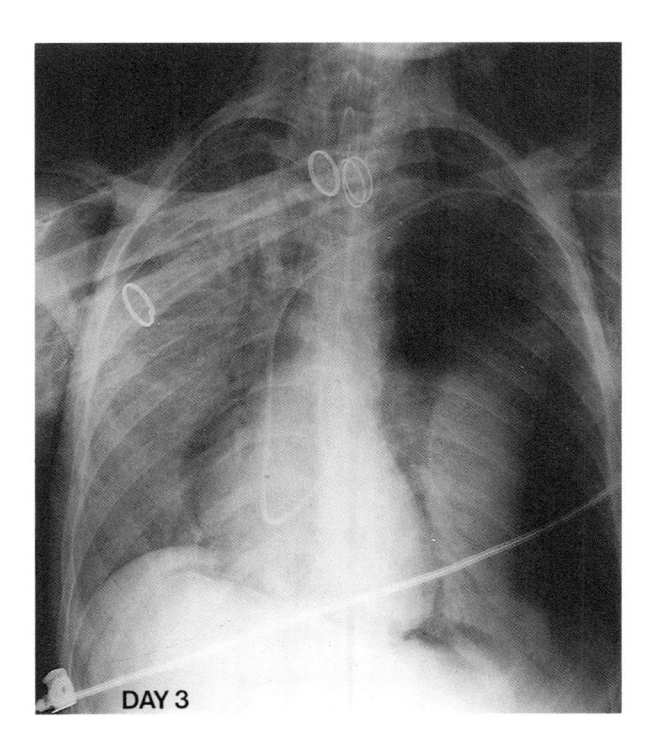

DAY 1

DAY 2

DAY 3

A 15-year-old male presented with a severe viral pneumonia. The CXRs were taken on successive days.

The first CXR shows diffusely increased density of both lungs.

- Is this due to pleural fluid, atelectasis or consolidation? It became necessary to ventilate the patient.
- What is (1)?
- What complication has occurred?
- What is (2)?
- What further complication is seen on the last film?

A34

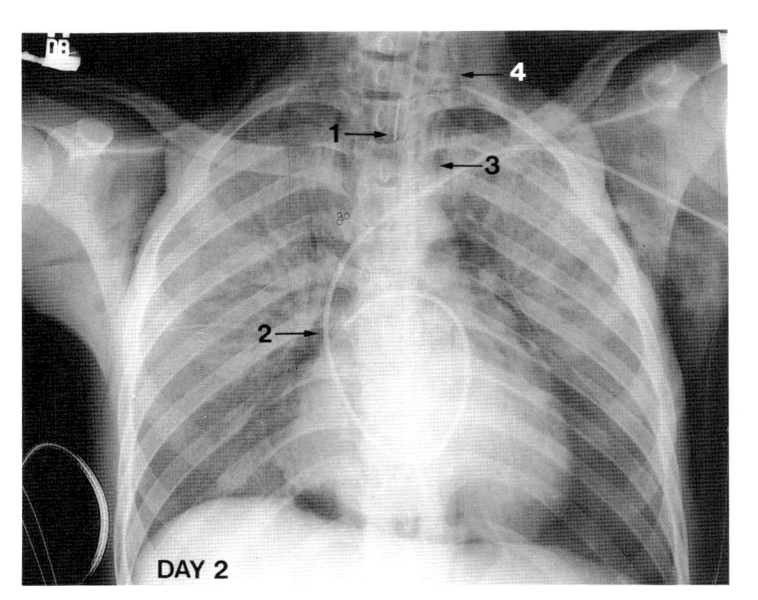

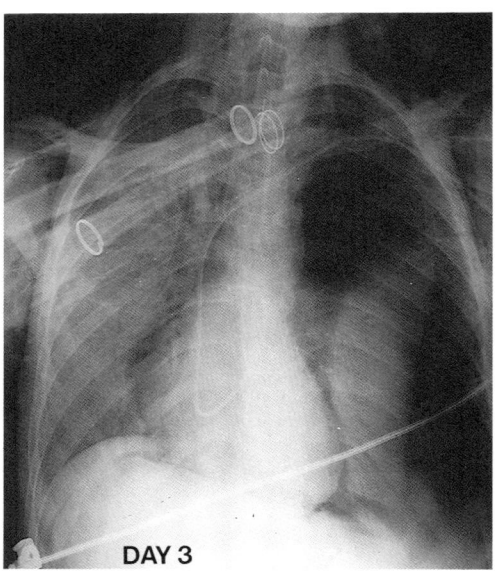

DAY 2

DAY 3

The diffusely increased density is due to consolidation. The volume of both lungs is normal, and air bronchograms are widely visible. (1) = the tip of the endotracheal tube. Pneumomediastinum has occurred. Air is present in the soft tissue planes of the mediastinum (3) and around the heart. Air has also tracked up into the neck (4) and over the chest wall, causing surgical emphysema. (2) = a Swan-Ganz catheter. A left tension pneumothorax is seen on the last film. The left lung has collapsed, and the mediastinum is pushed to the right.

Q35

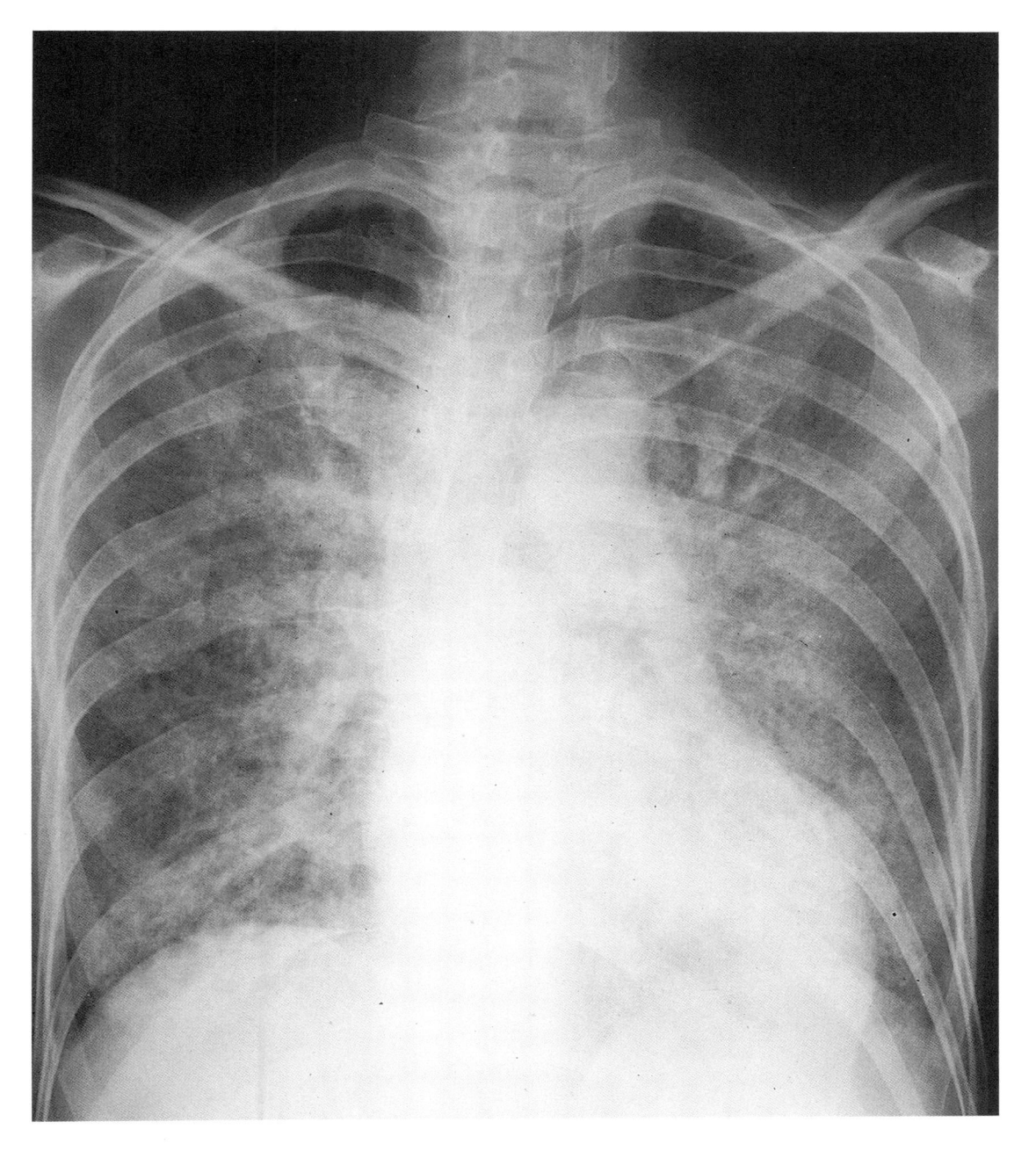

A 25-year-old male with acquired immune deficiency syndrome (AIDS) presented with shortness of breath.

- What does the CXR show?
- What is the differential diagnosis?
- How would you make the diagnosis?

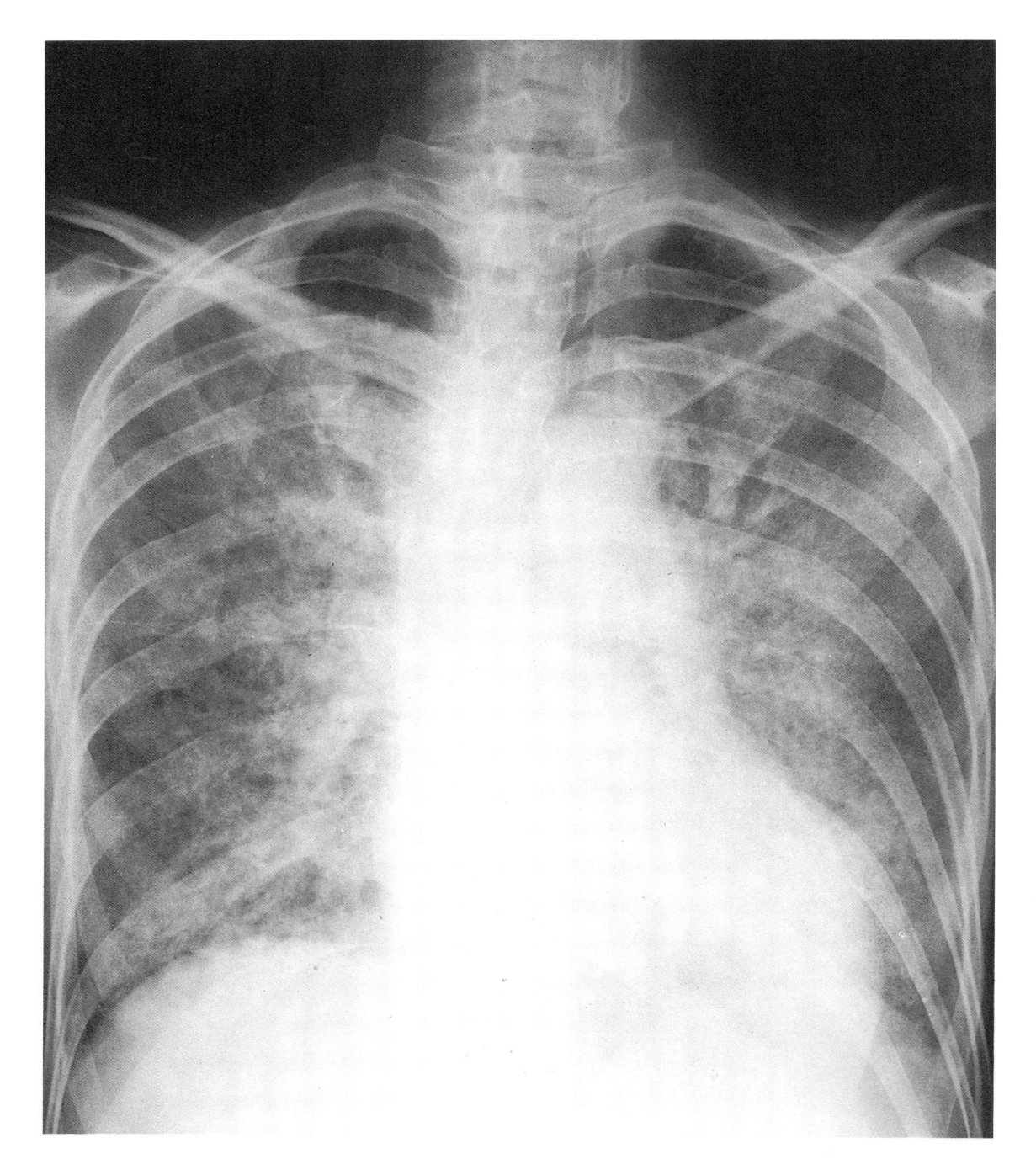

The CXR shows diffuse shadowing throughout both lungs, consistent with widespread consolidation. The differential diagnosis is an opportunistic infection, including pneumocystis, cytomegalovirus, and fungal infection. Bronchoalveolar lavage revealed *pneumocystis carinii*.

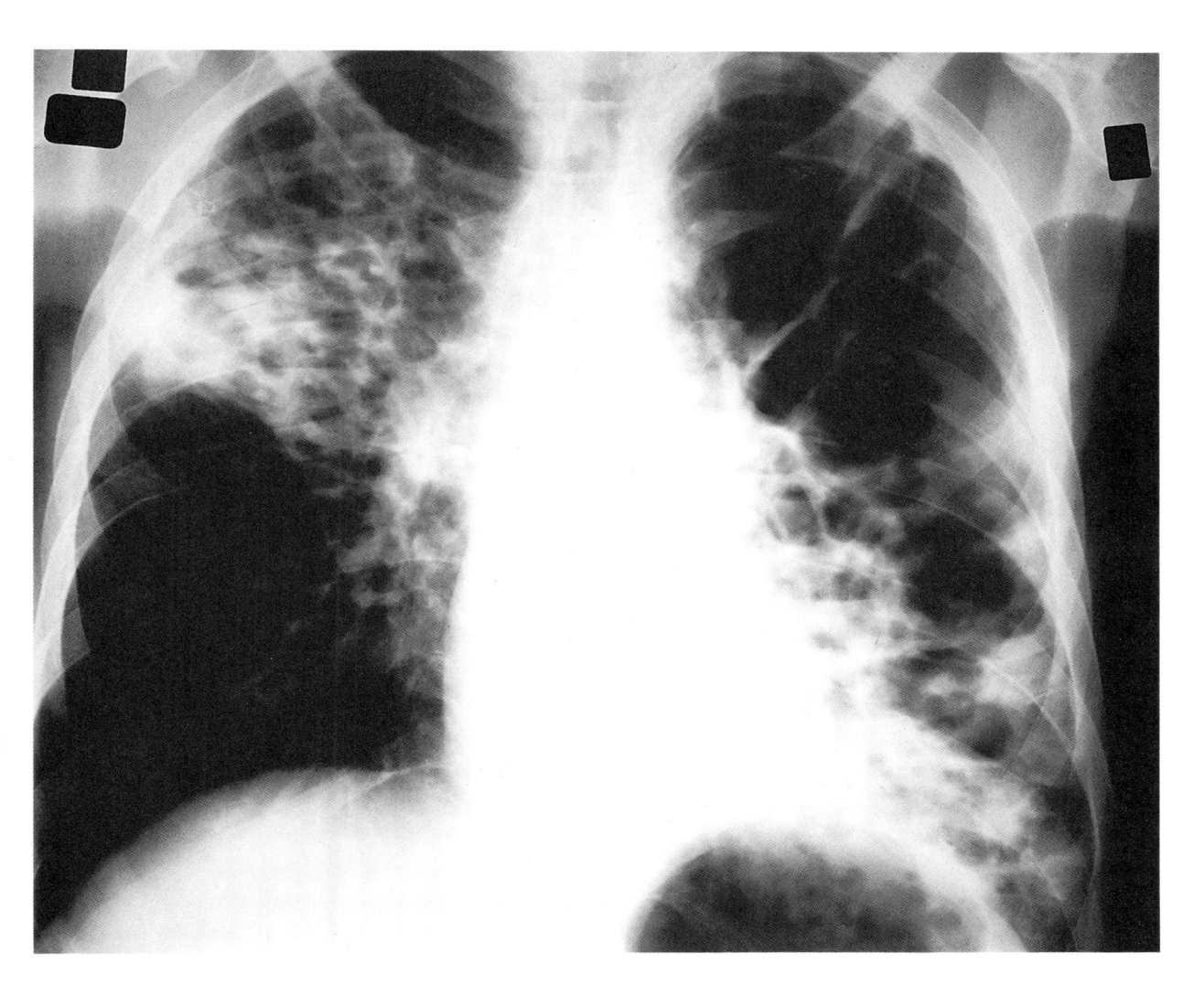

A 28-year-old intravenous heroin abuser presented with a cough, fever, and general debility.

- What does the CXR show?
- What is the probable diagnosis?
- How would you confirm the diagnosis?

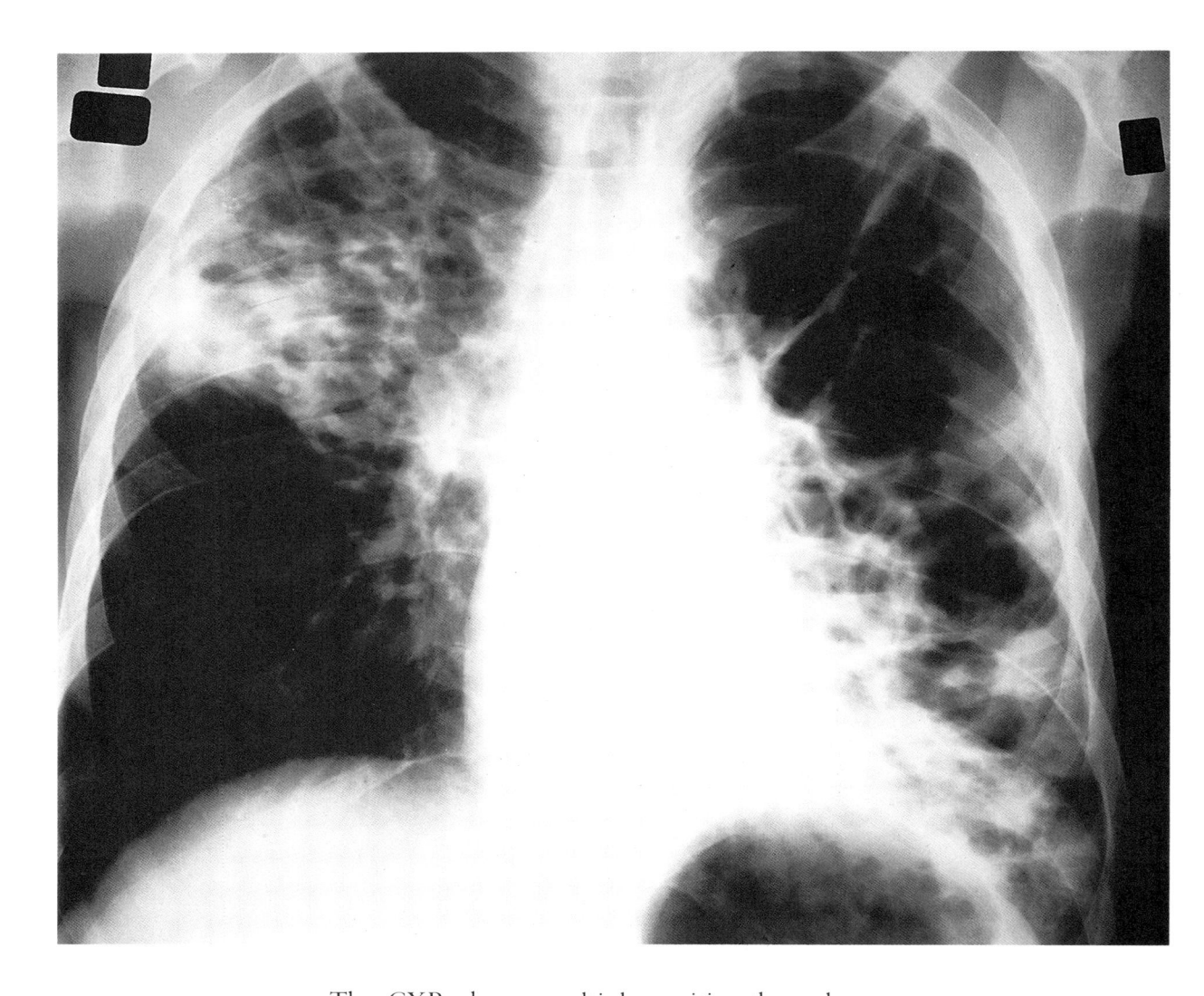

The CXR shows multiple cavities throughout both lungs. Pulmonary tuberculosis (or possibly a staphylococcal pneumonia) is the probable diagnosis. Examination of the sputum showed acid fast bacilli.

Q37

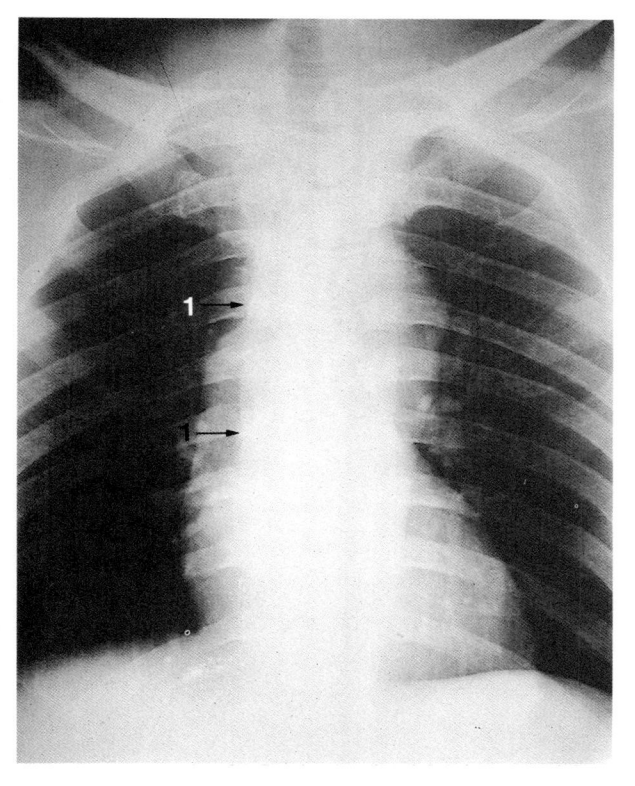

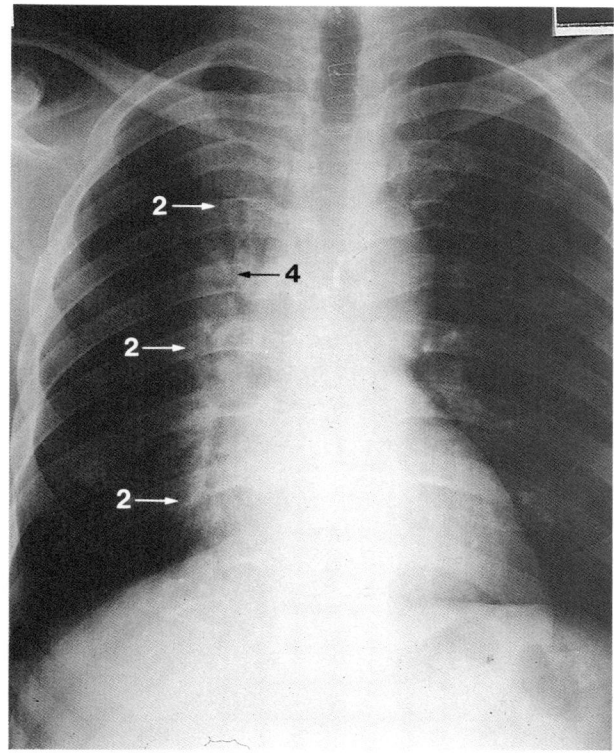

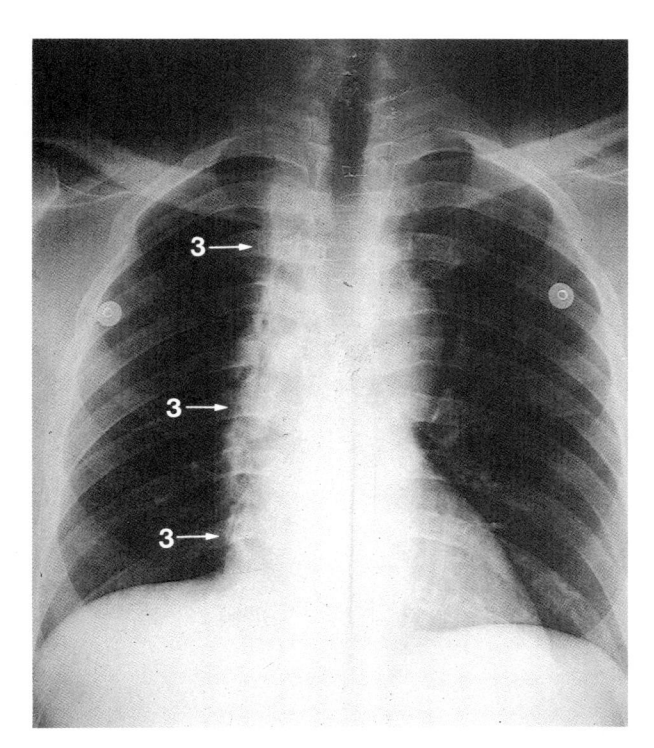

A 45-year-old male presented with diffuse histiocytic lymphoma. At the time of the first CXR there were clinical signs of thoracic spinal cord compression. Displacement of the right paraspinal line (1) is present. Following surgical decompression the entire spine was irradiated.

- Explain the appearance (2) on the CXR 10 weeks later.
- Explain the appearance (3) on the CXR a further four weeks later.

A37

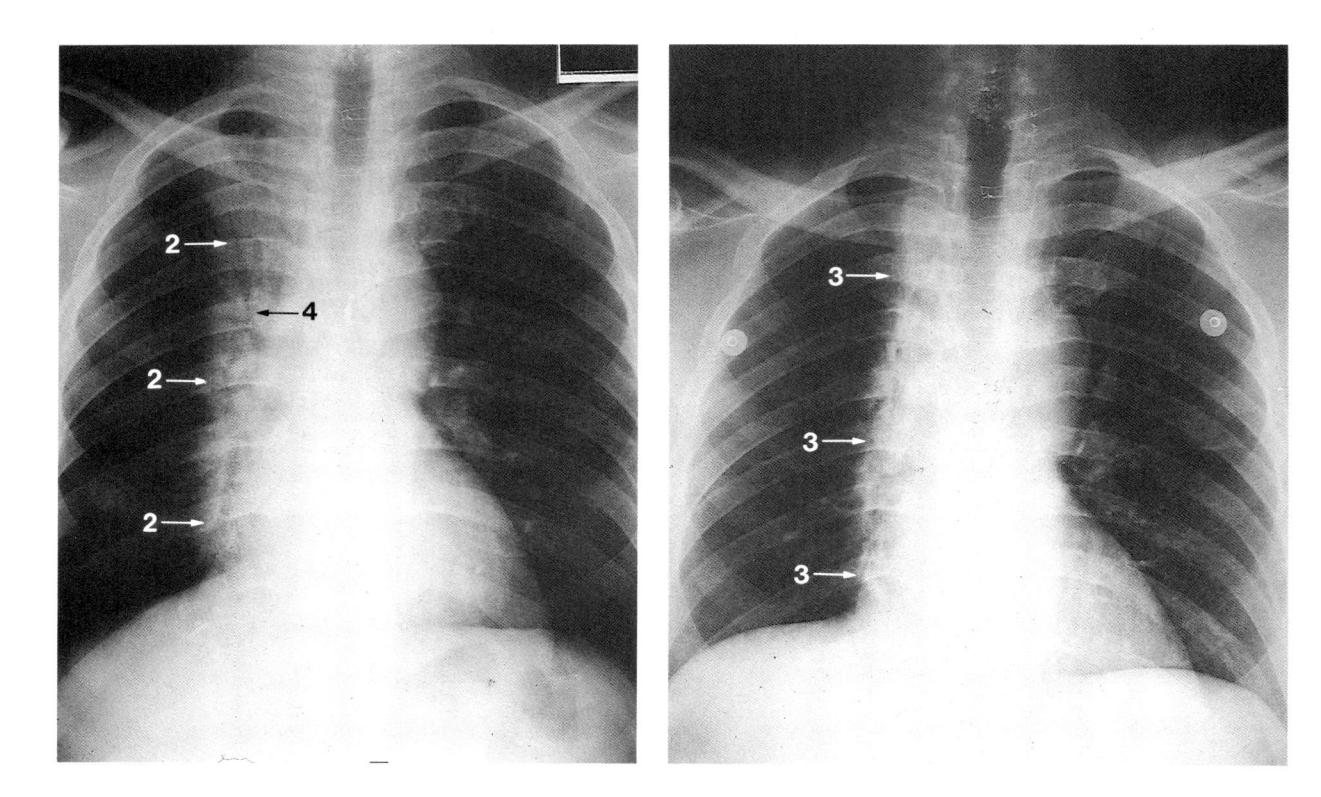

The CXR 10 weeks after irradiation shows extensive right paramediastinal shadowing. An air bronchogram (4) is visible, indicating that this is consolidation. The consolidation is non-segmental and corresponds to the shape of the radiotherapy portal. It represents the exudative phase of radiation pneumonitis. Four weeks later the consolidated lung has contracted due to radiation fibrosis.

Q38

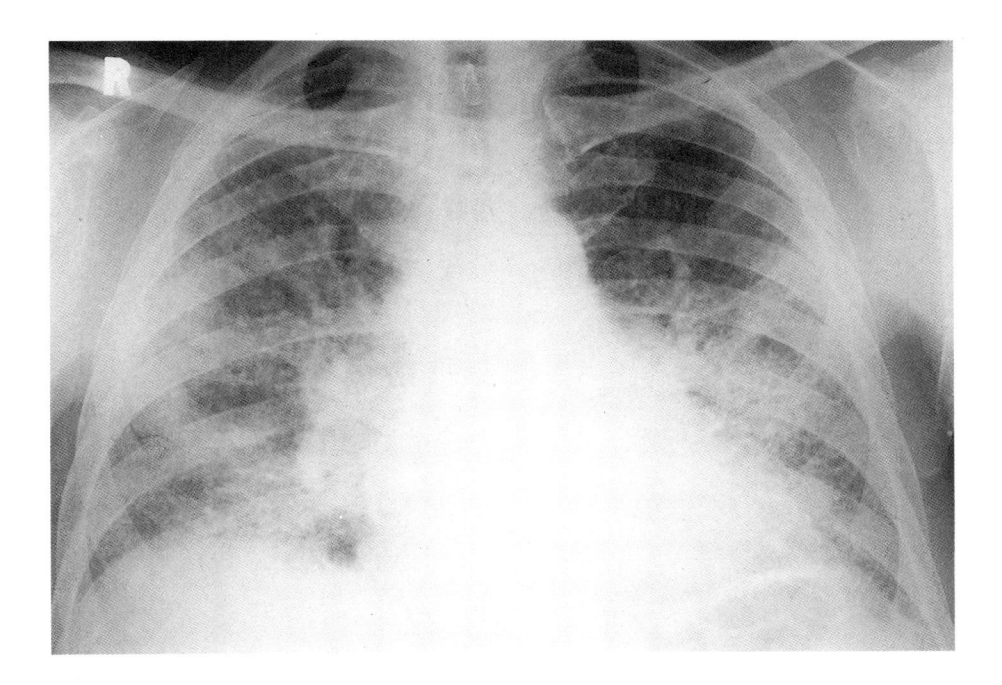

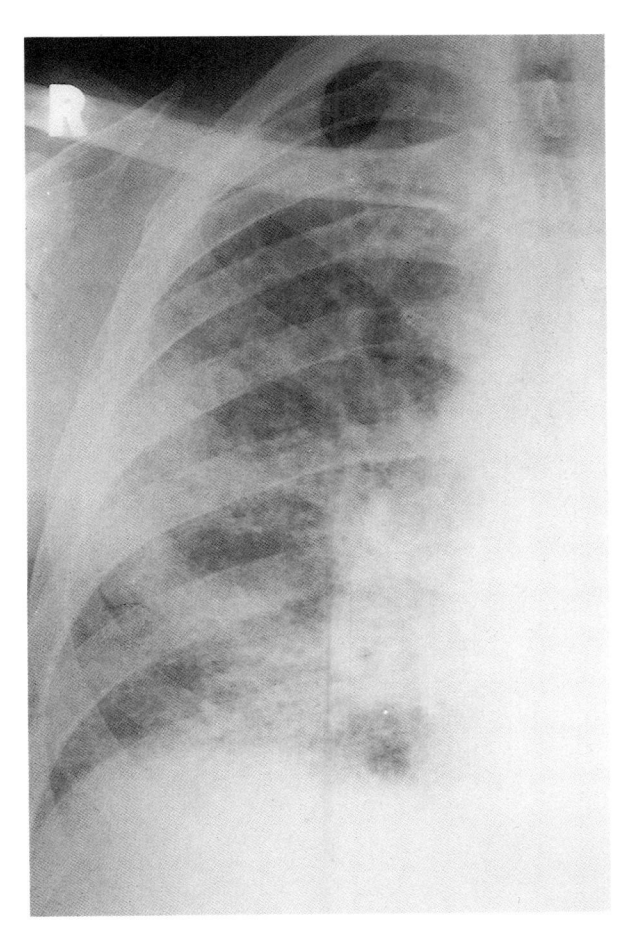

A 69-year-old male presented with progressive shortness of breath and a non-productive cough. Physical examination revealed central cyanosis, finger clubbing, and widespread crackles in the chest.

- Comment on the lung volumes.
- Describe the shadowing in the lungs.
- What is the probable diagnosis?
- How could it be confirmed?

A38

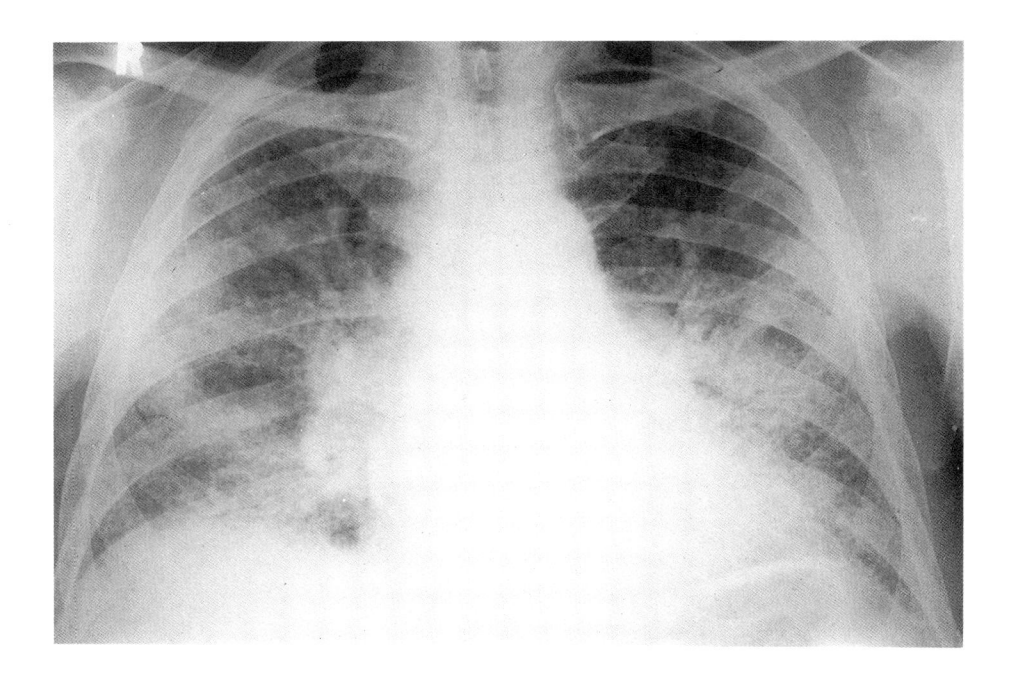

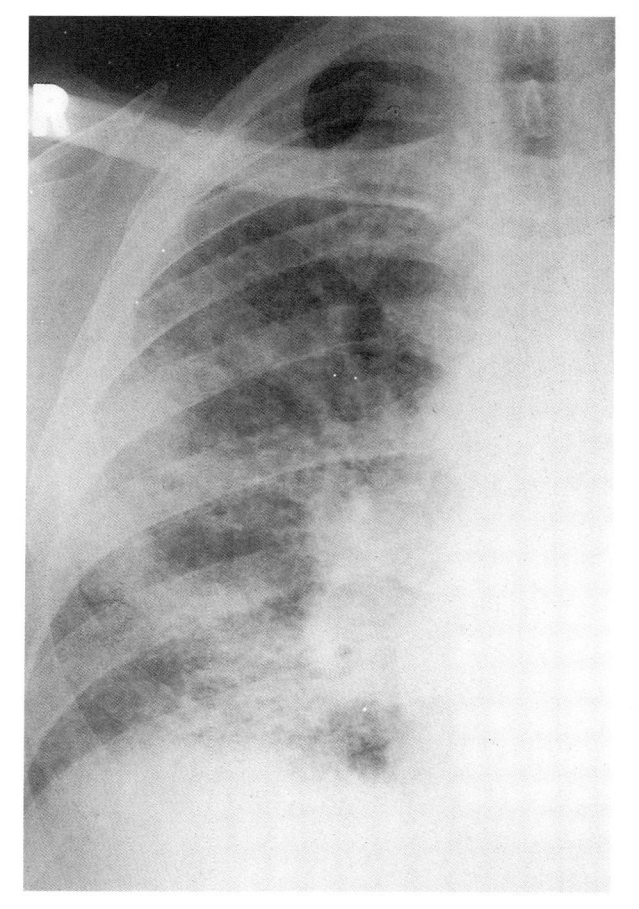

The lung volumes are decreased. The shadowing is diffuse but densest in the mid and lower zones, and comprises a ground glass appearance, with superimposed fine nodular and honeycomb opacities. The probable diagnosis is cryptogenic fibrosing alveolitis. It could be confirmed by drill or open biopsy of the lung.

Q39

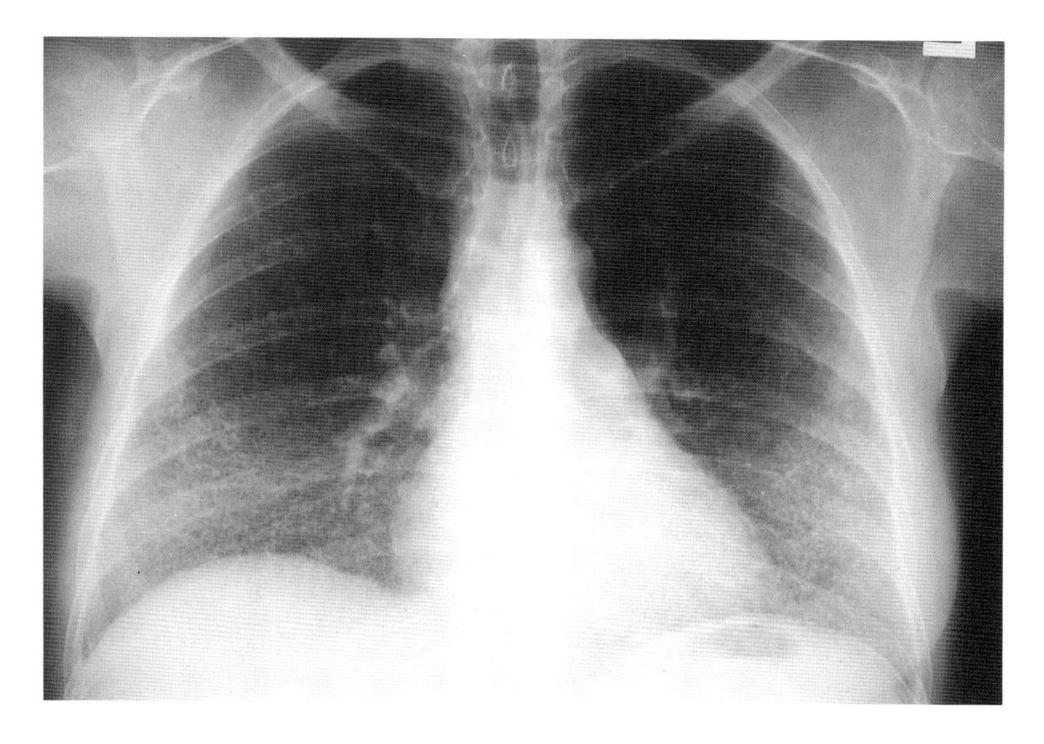

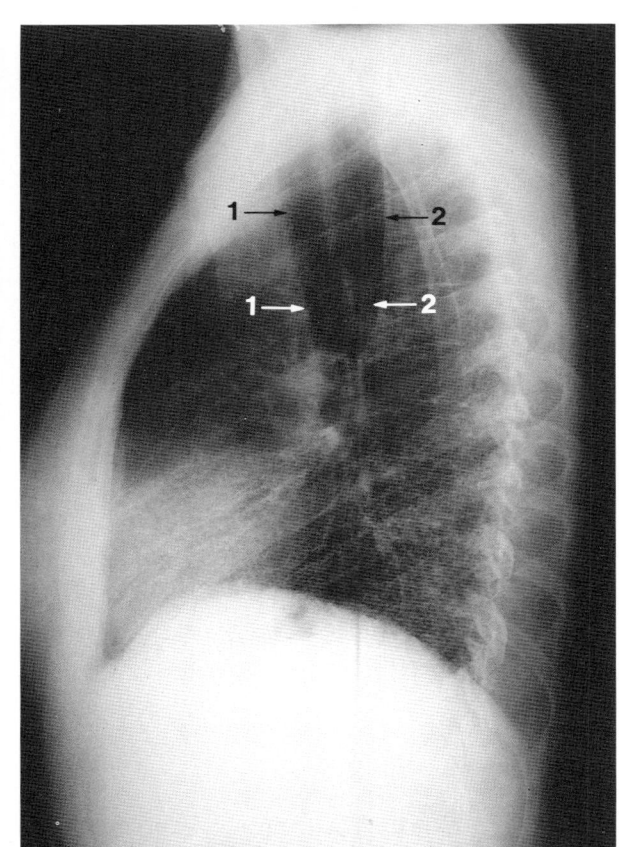

A 37-year-old female presented with arthritis, dysphagia, and a dry cough.

- Describe the changes in the lungs.
- What is structure (1)?
- What is structure (2)? Is it normally visible in a CXR?
- What is the diagnosis and what other part of the patient would you x-ray?

A39

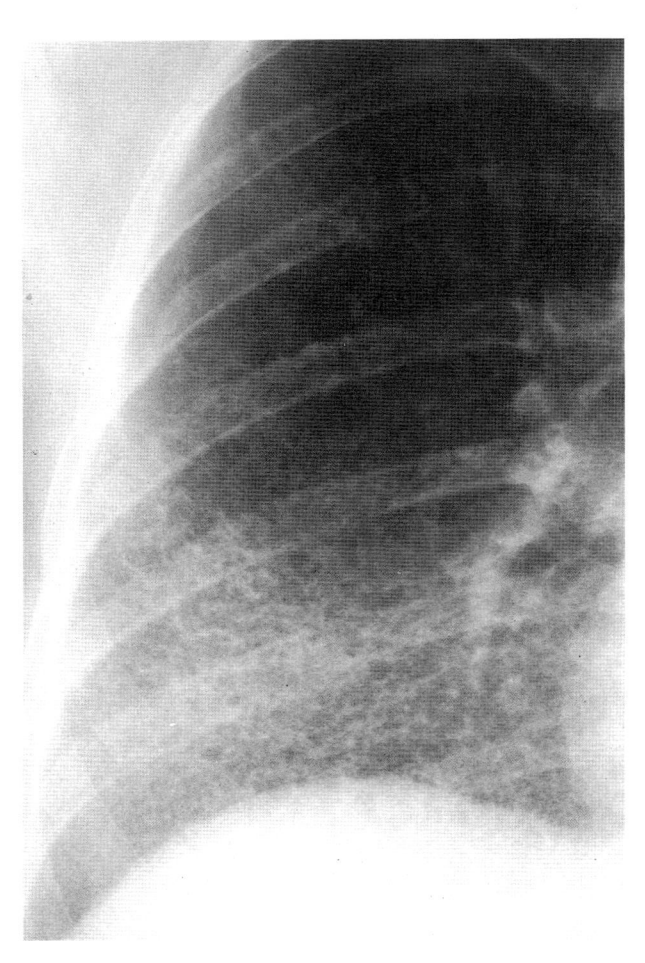

Fine reticulo-nodular shadowing is present in both lower zones, consistent with pulmonary fibrosis. (1) = the trachea. (2) = the oesophagus. It is not normally visible, but in this case it is dilated and air-filled. The diagnosis is scleroderma. X-ray of the hands may show changes typical of scleroderma. Note the deforming arthropathy, acro-osteolysis (3) and soft tissue calcification (4).

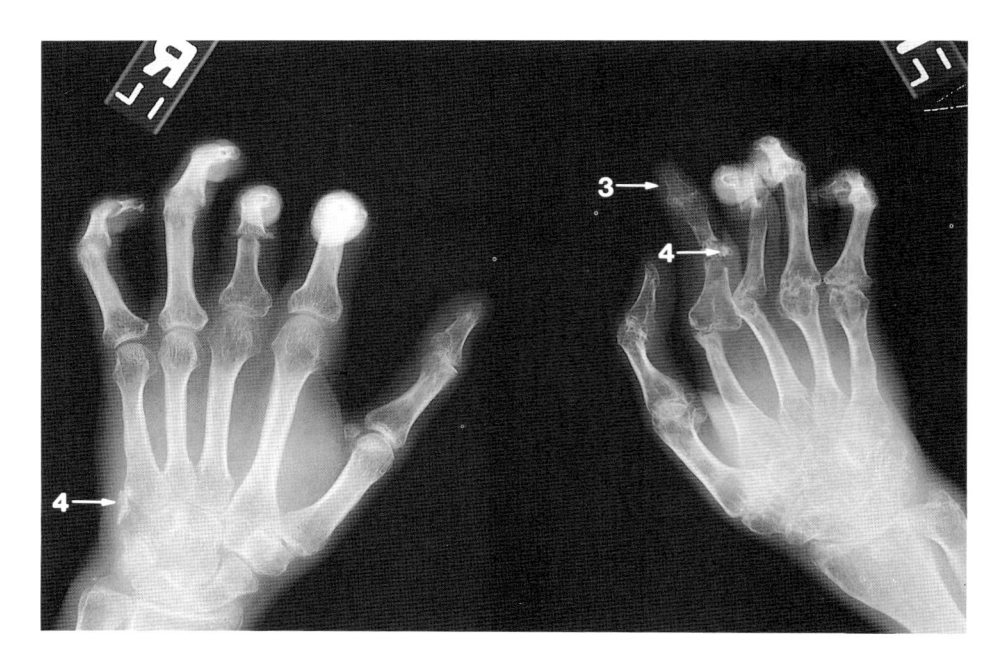

Q40

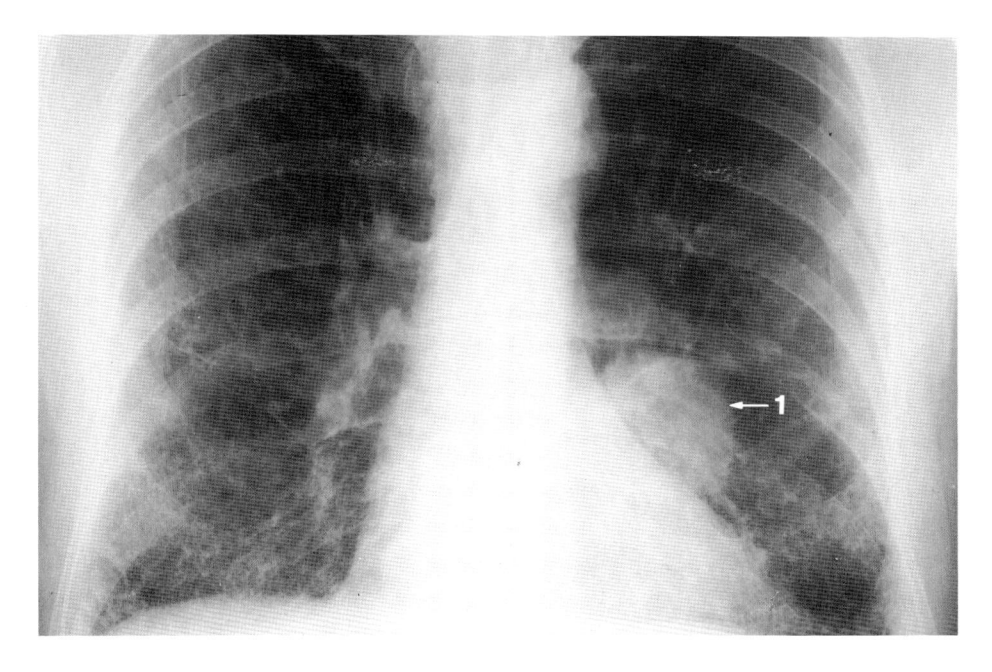

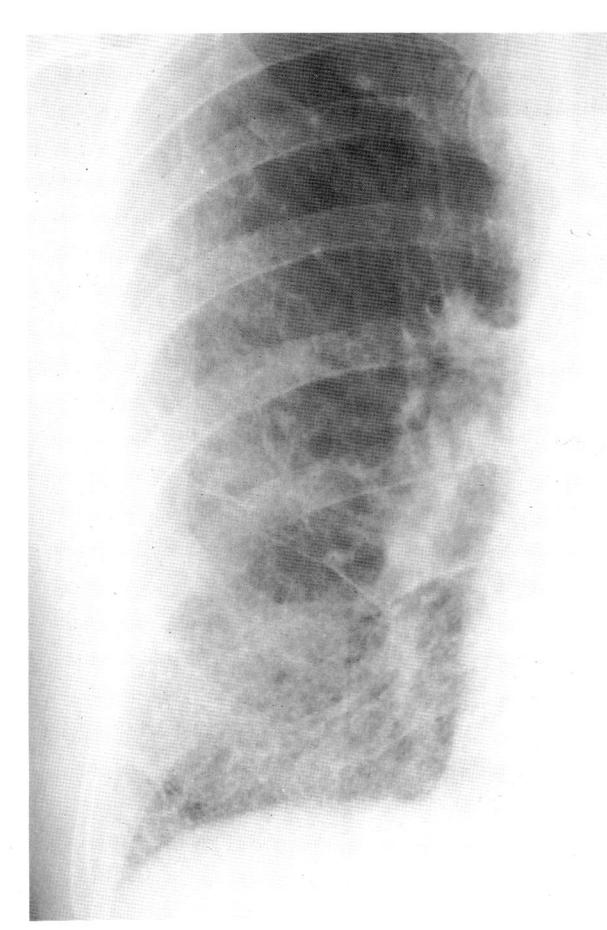

A 69-year-old retired dockyard worker presented with a chronic cough and recent haemoptysis. His work involved contact with asbestos.

- What widespread changes are seen in the lungs?
- Where is the opacity (1) located?
- What is this opacity?
- How would you confirm the diagnosis?

A40

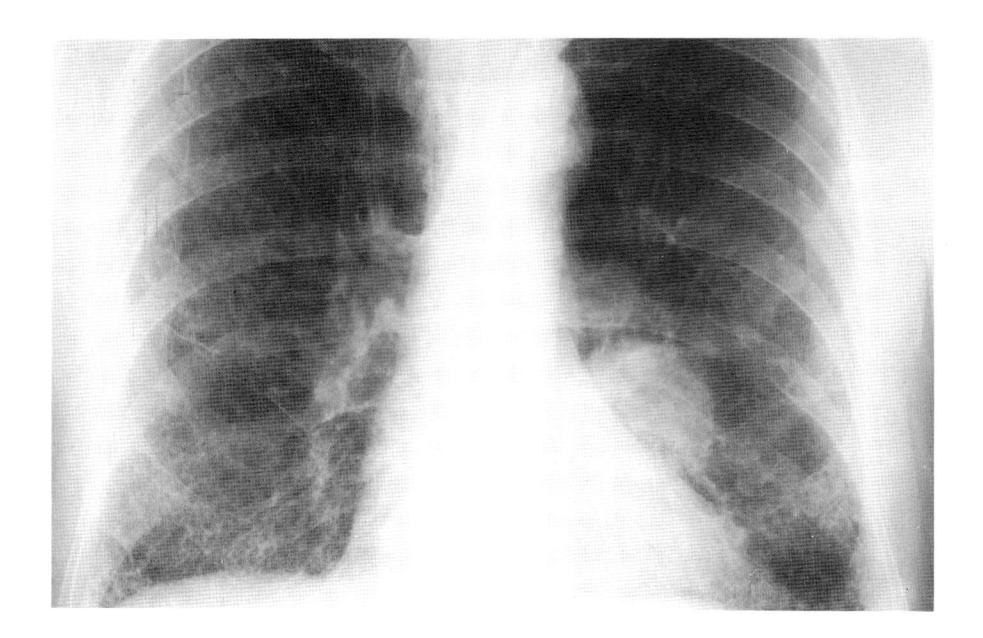

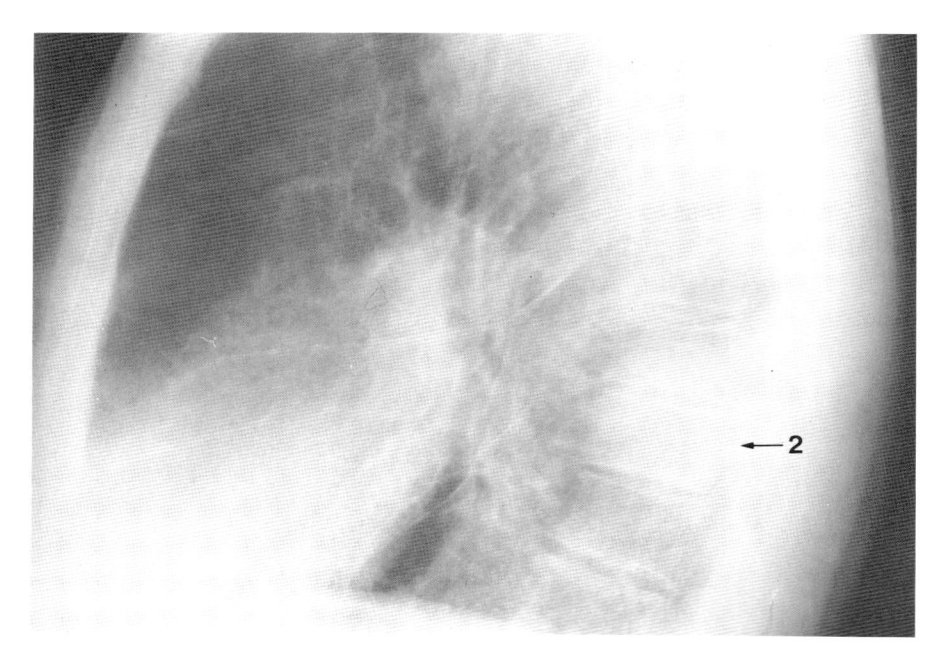

Reticulo-nodular shadowing is present throughout both lungs, with a basal predominance. It is due to asbestosis.

Since (1) does not obscure the left heart border, it must be in the lower lobe. This is confirmed (2) on the lateral film. (1) = a bronchogenic carcinoma. Percutaneous needle biopsy showed a squamous cell carcinoma.

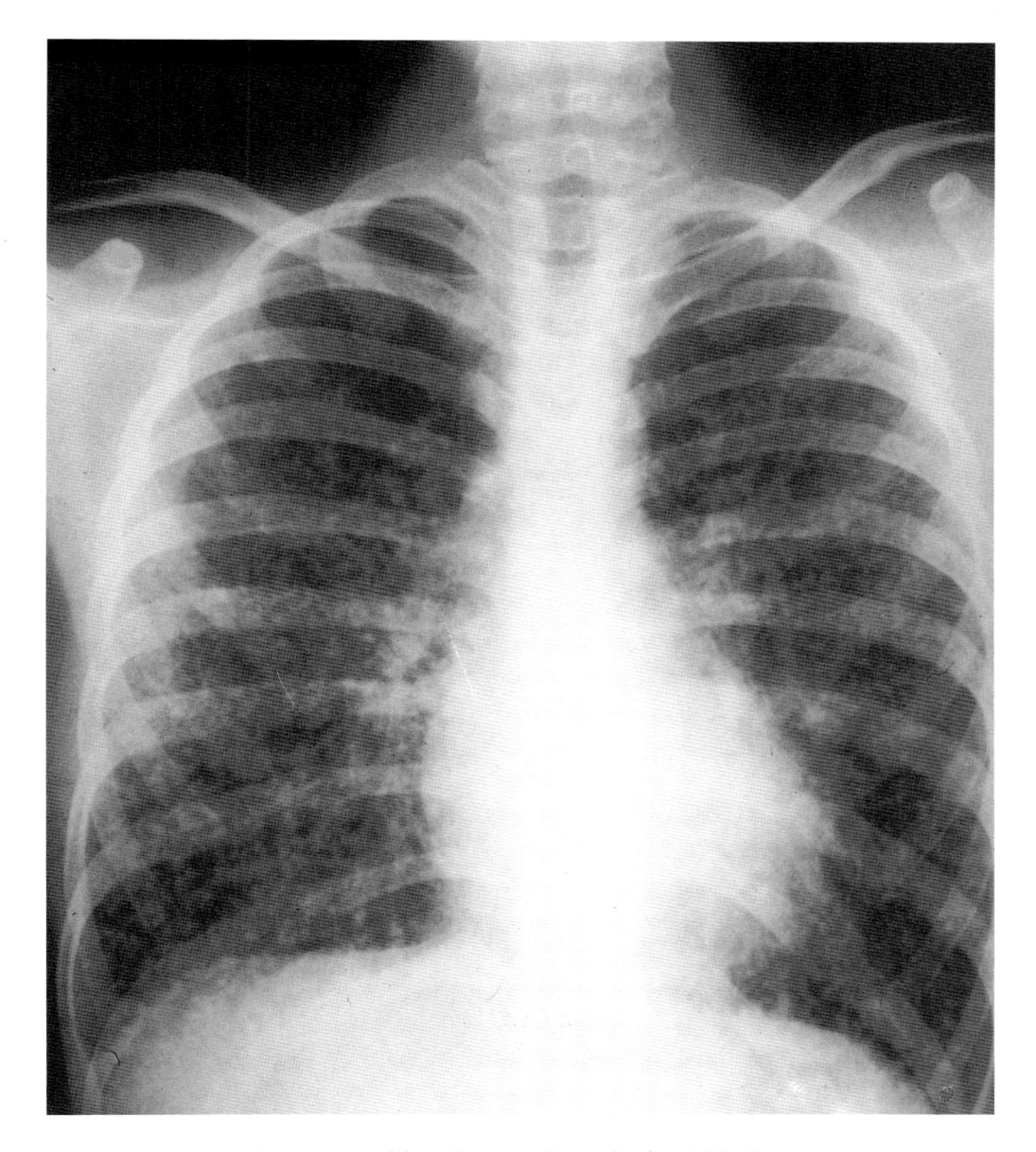

A 42-year-old male complained of mild lethargy, but had no specific symptoms.

- Describe the CXR.
- What is the differential diagnosis?

On physical examination a nodule was found in the neck.

- What is the probable diagnosis, and how would you confirm it?

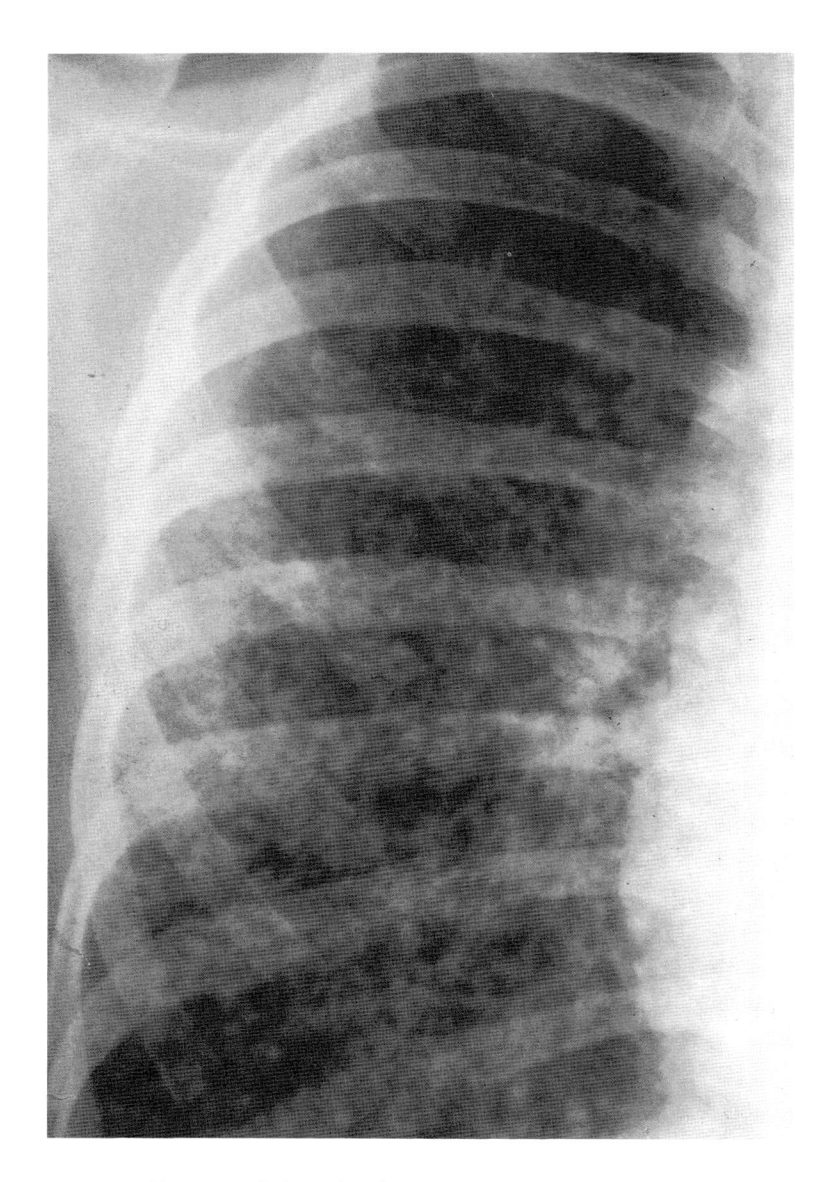

Diffuse nodular shadowing is present throughout both lungs. There is relative sparing of the apices. The nodules are small (less than 5 mm in diameter) and of soft tissue density. The differential diagnosis is tuberculosis, histoplasmosis, pulmonary metastases, sarcoidosis, and pneumoconiosis.

The probable diagnosis in this case is metastatic thyroid carcinoma. The neck nodule was excised, and shown to be a medullary thyroid carcinoma. If this had not given the diagnosis, transbronchial lung biopsy or percutaneous drill biopsy of the lung would have been performed.

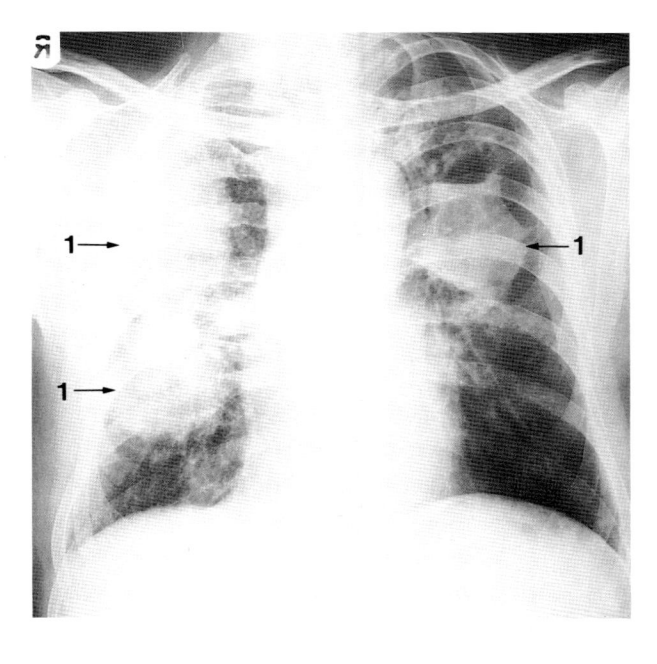

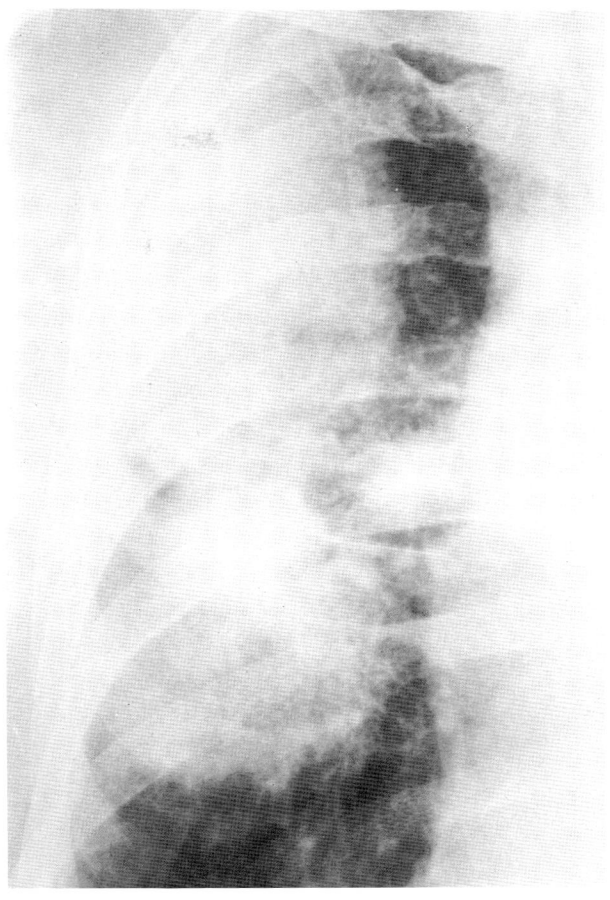

A 65-year-old coal miner presented with a chronic cough. The close-up of the CXR shows the diffuse nodular pattern of coal miner's pneumoconiosis.

- What are the larger densities (1)?
- What is their significance?
- What complication is seen in the left upper zone mass?

A42

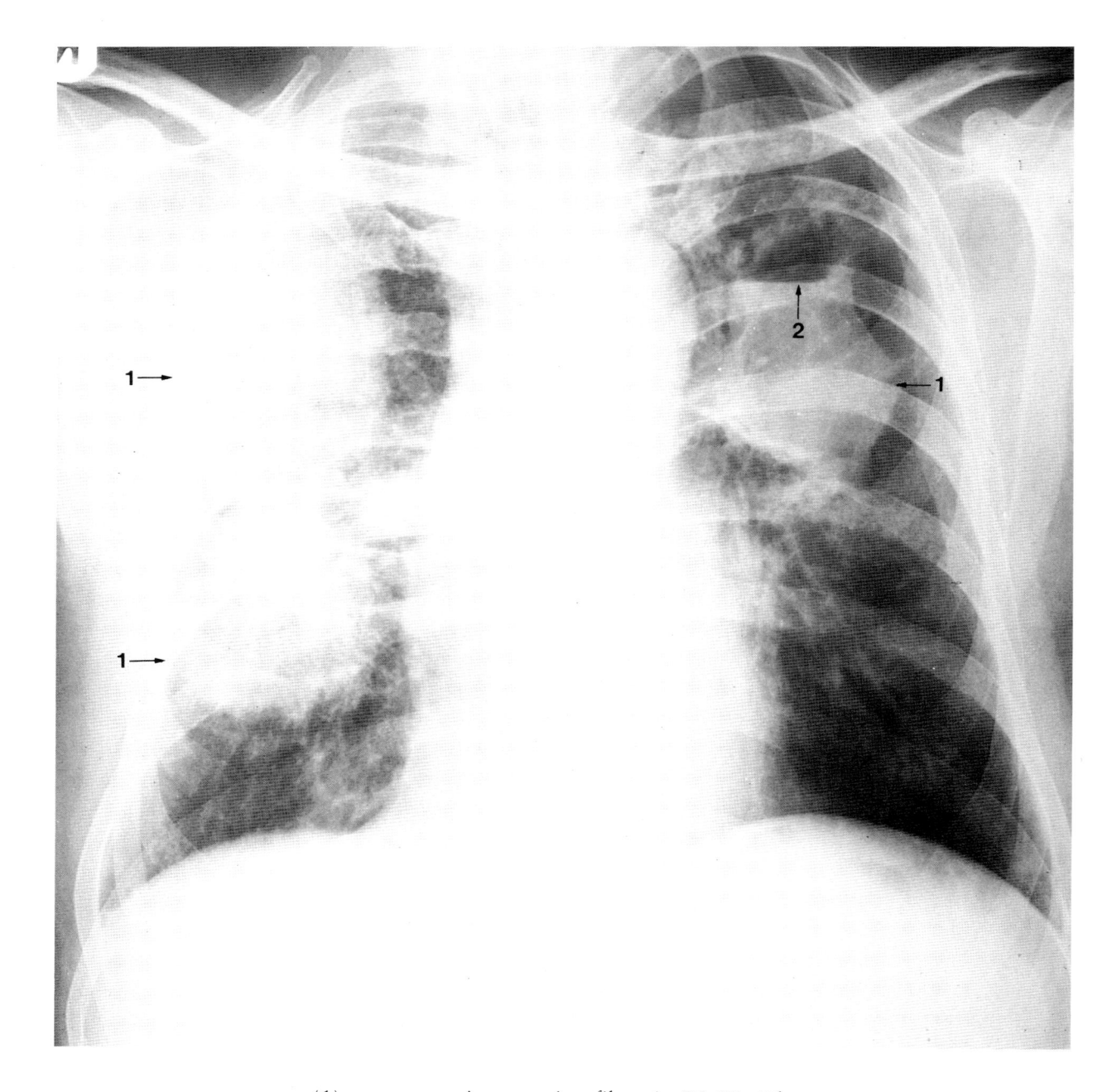

(1) = progressive massive fibrosis (PMF). They indicate that the inhaled coal dust contained fibrogenic material, probably silica. A fluid level (2) is present in the left upper zone mass, indicating cavitation. This is usually due to ischaemic necrosis or tuberculosis, but may be due to a neoplasm. In this case sputum examination for TB and malignant cells was negative.

Q43

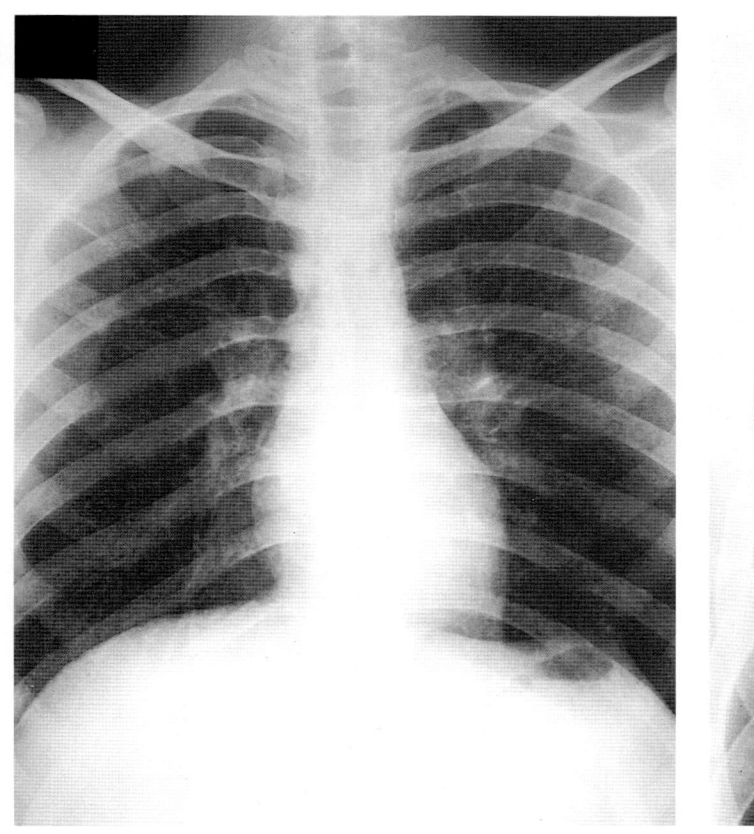

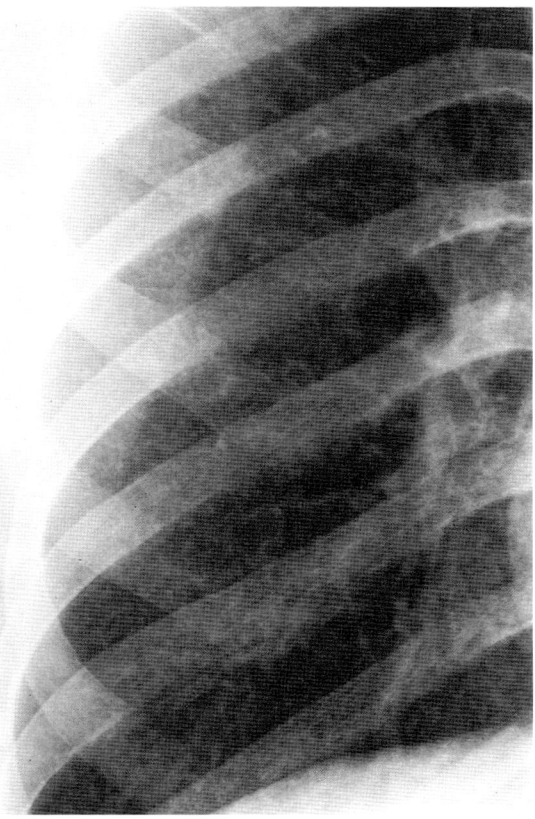

A 19-year-old presented with weight loss and fever.

- What is the diagnosis?
- Is there a differential diagnosis?

A43

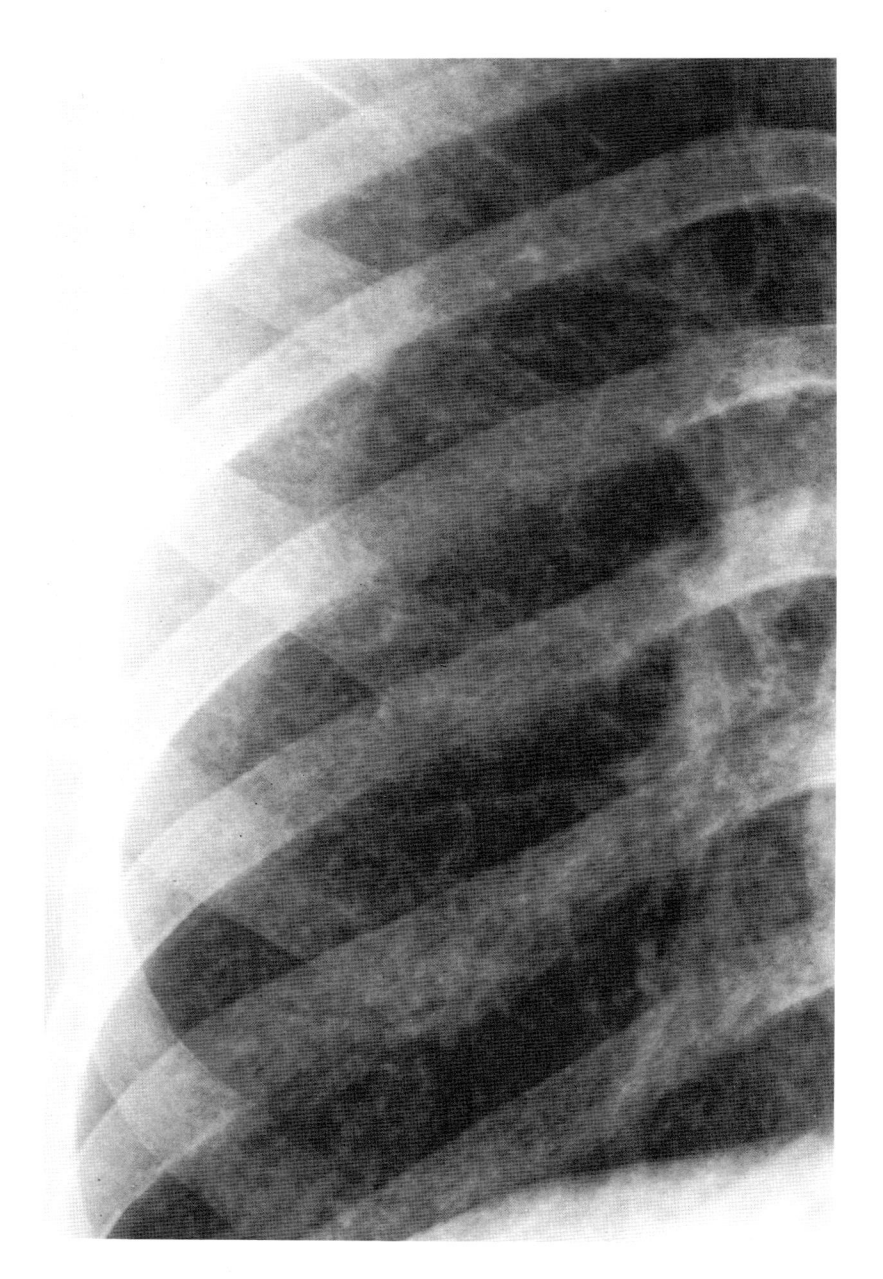

The diagnosis is miliary tuberculosis. There is not really a differential diagnosis. This detail of the CXR shows truly miliary shadowing. The nodules are very small and diffusely throughout both lungs. In sarcoidosis there is usually evidence of lymphadenopathy on the CXR, and the nodules tend to spare the apices and lower zones. In a patient from North America, a fungal infection such as histoplasmosis should be considered.

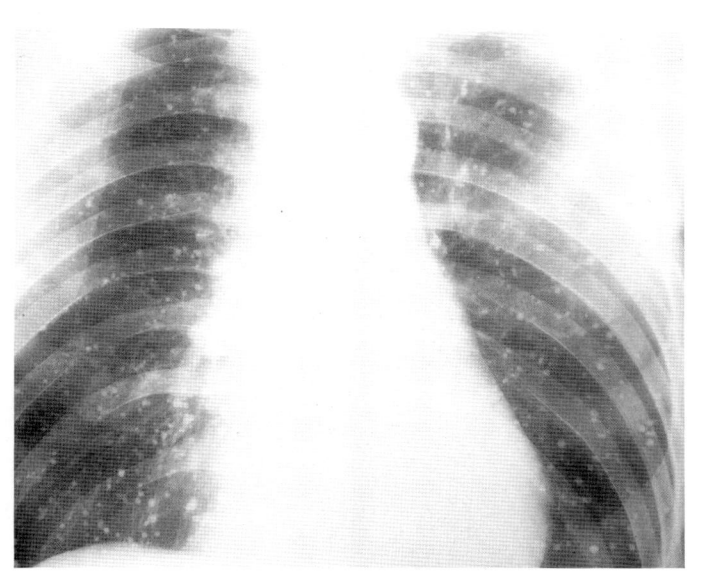

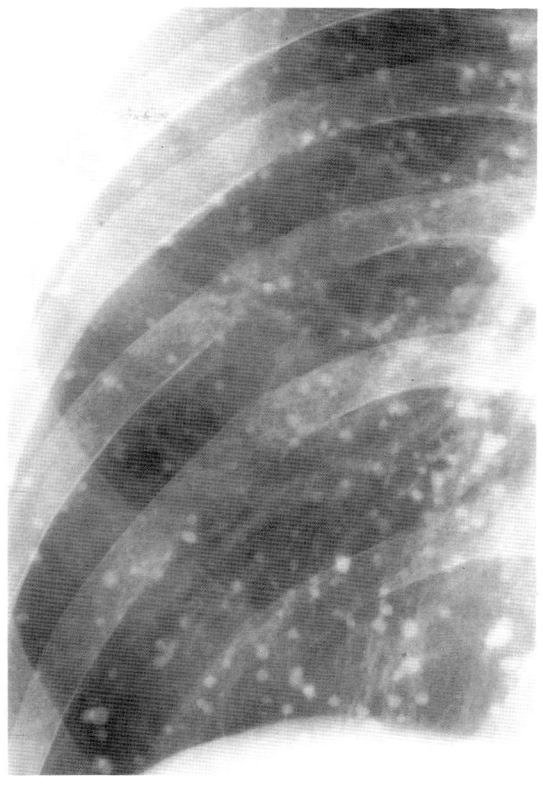

A 50-year-old male was asymptomatic. The CXR was taken for an insurance medical examination. The close-up shows the right mid and lower zones.

- Describe the CXR.
- What is the differential diagnosis?

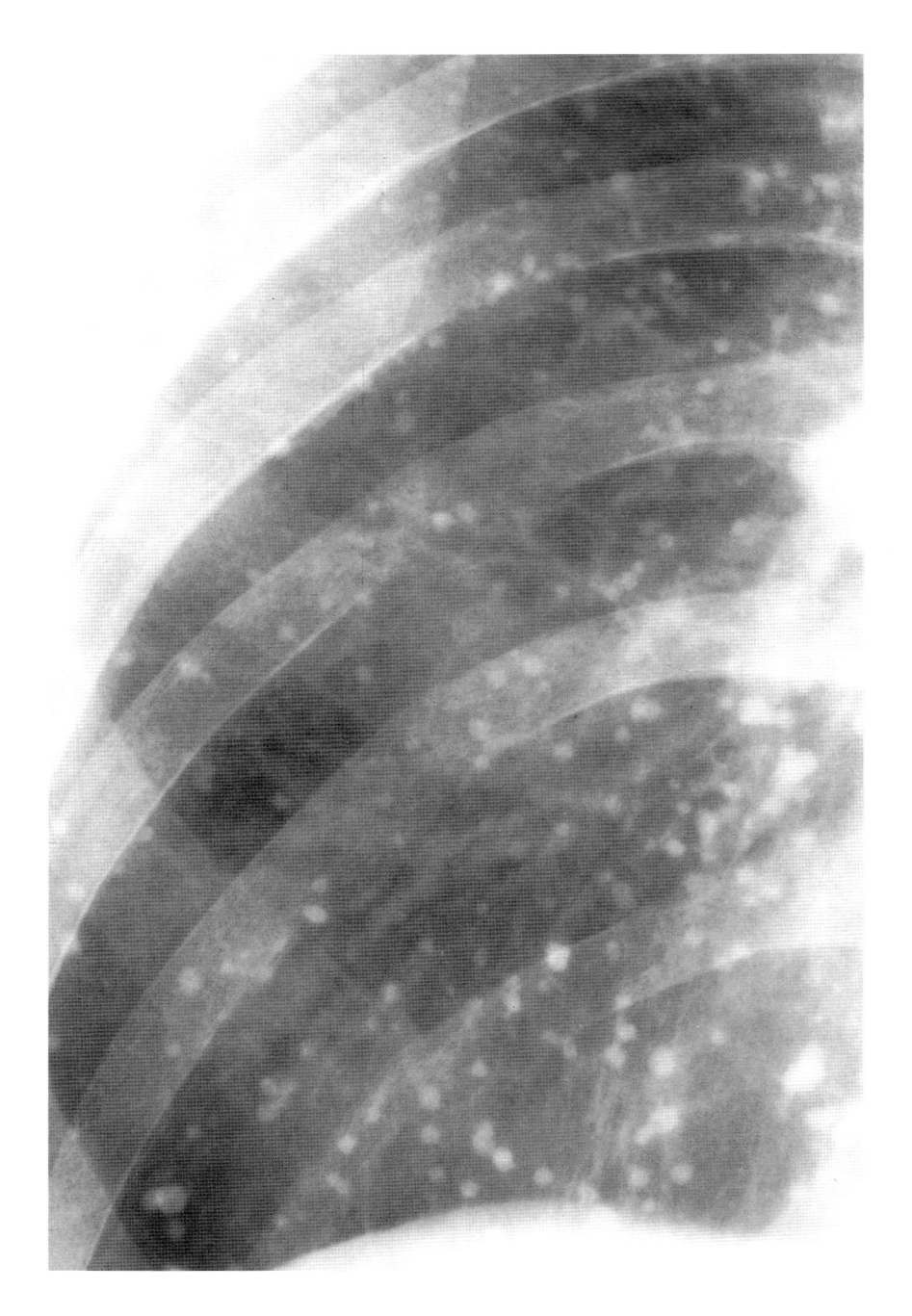

Multiple small calcified nodules are present in both lungs. In a fit asymptomatic individual the likely causes are previous varicella pneumonia, tuberculosis or histoplasmosis. In pulmonary alveolar microlithiasis the nodules are smaller. This patient gave a history of chicken pox some 20 years earlier.

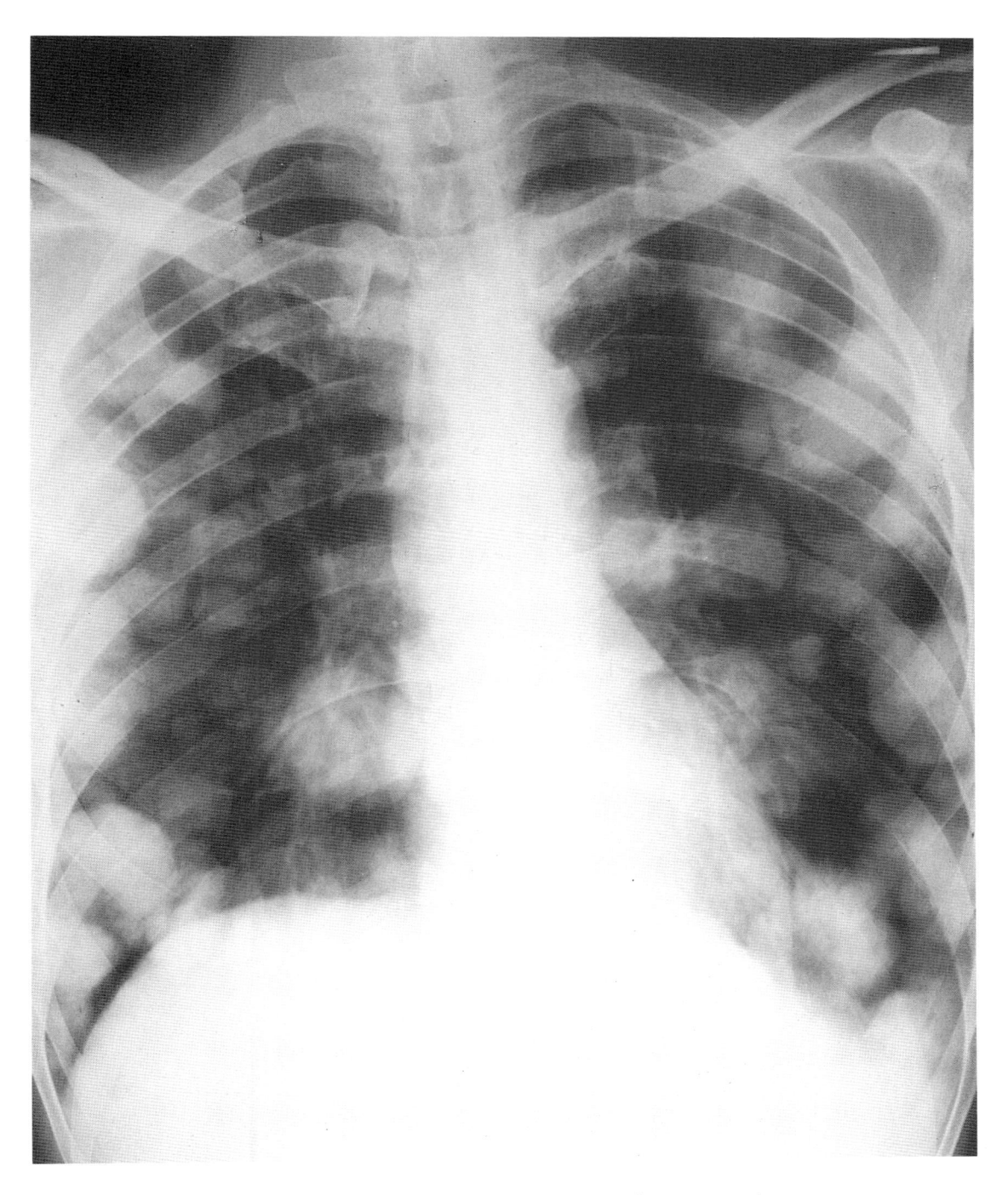

A 43-year-old male presented with a scrotal mass.

- What does the CXR show?
- What is the scrotal mass?

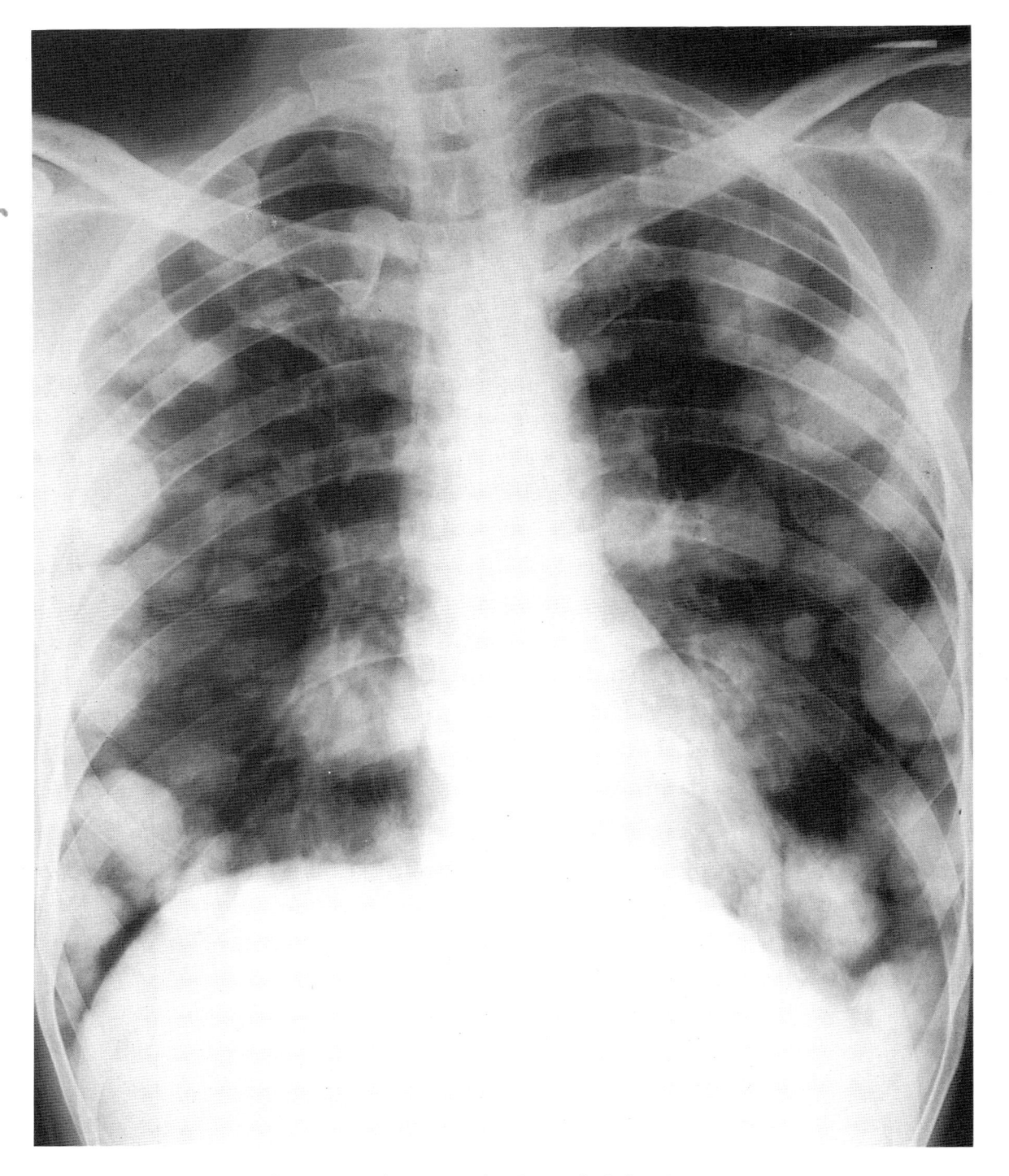

The CXR shows multiple well-defined round opacities throughout both lungs. The appearance is typical of multiple pulmonary metastases. The scrotal mass was a testicular teratoma.

Q46

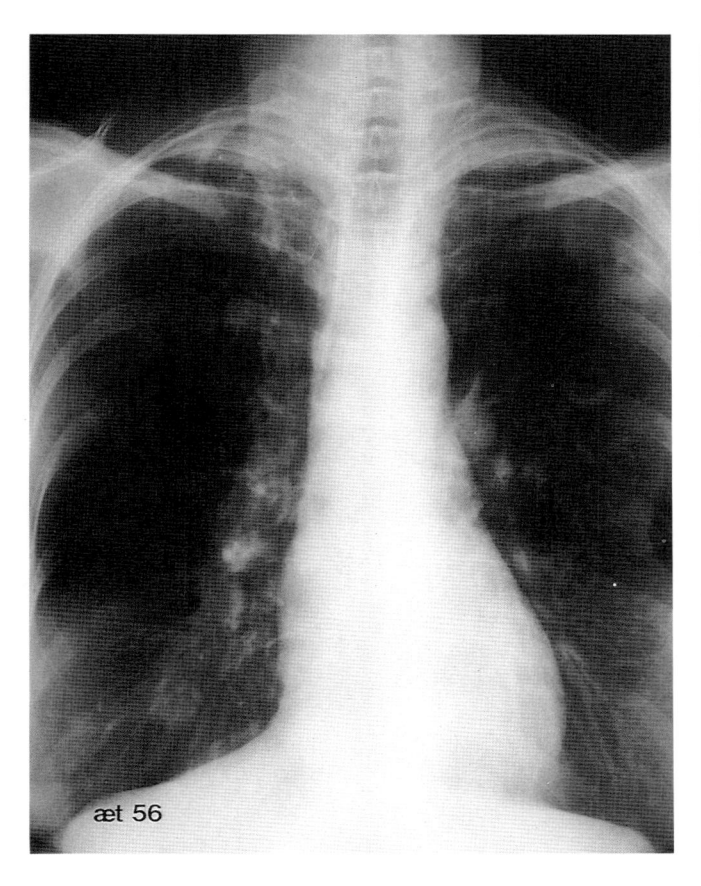

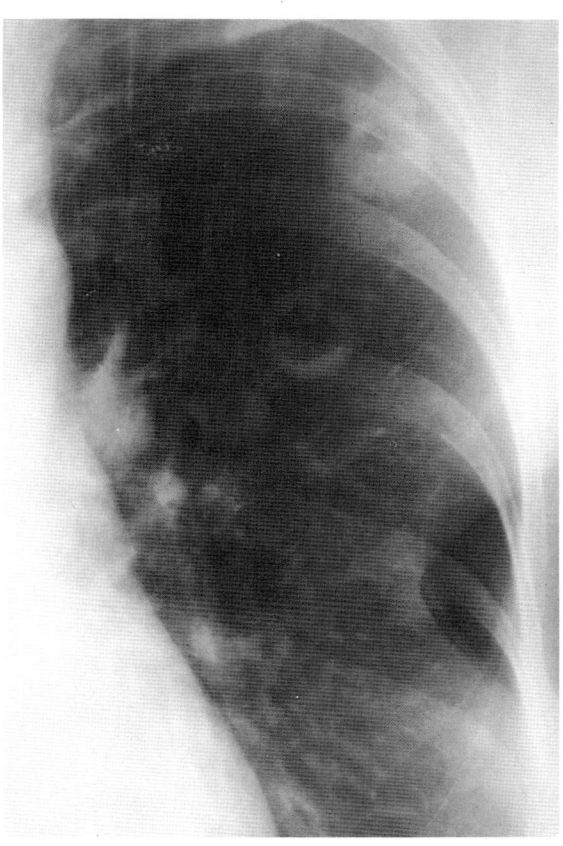

aet 56

A 56-year-old woman presented with hoarseness and weight loss.

- What does the CXR show?
- What is the differential diagnosis?
- What is the probable diagnosis in this case?

A46

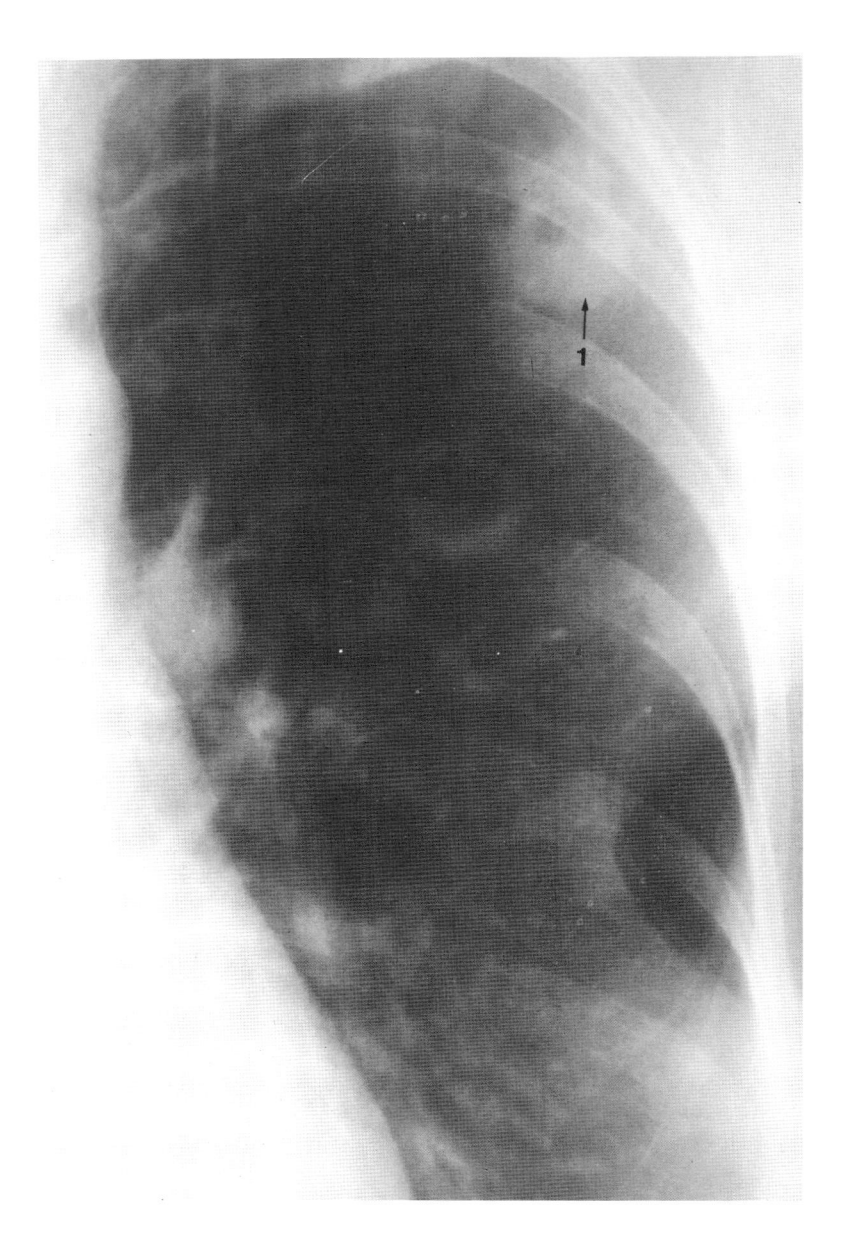

The CXR shows multiple cavitating masses in both lungs. Most are thick walled, and at least one contains a fluid level (1). Multiple pulmonary cavities may be due to abscesses, metastases, lymphoma, rheumatoid nodules, Wegener's granuloma and fungi. In this case the probable diagnosis is carcinoma of the larynx. Cavitation of pulmonary metastases may occur with any primary tumour, but it is most often seen with squamous cell tumours. Sarcomas also have a tendency to cavitate.

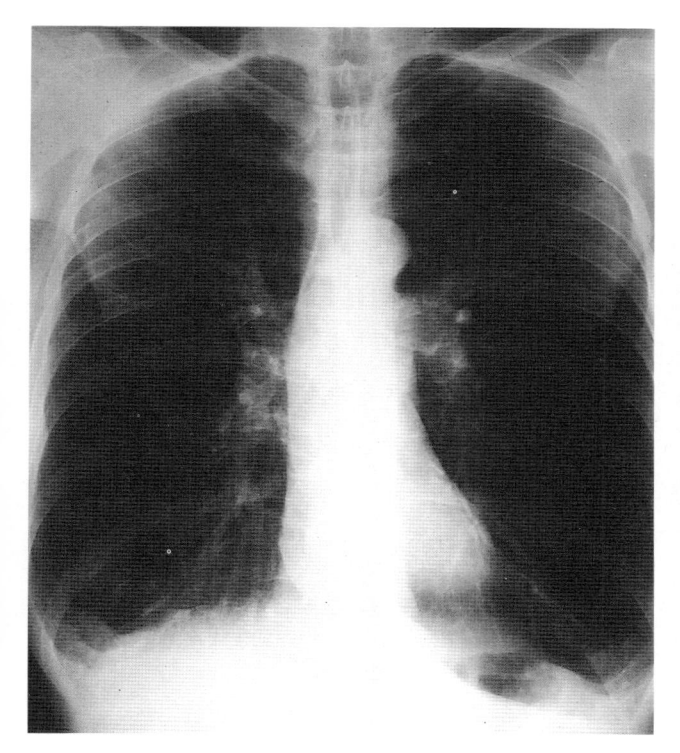

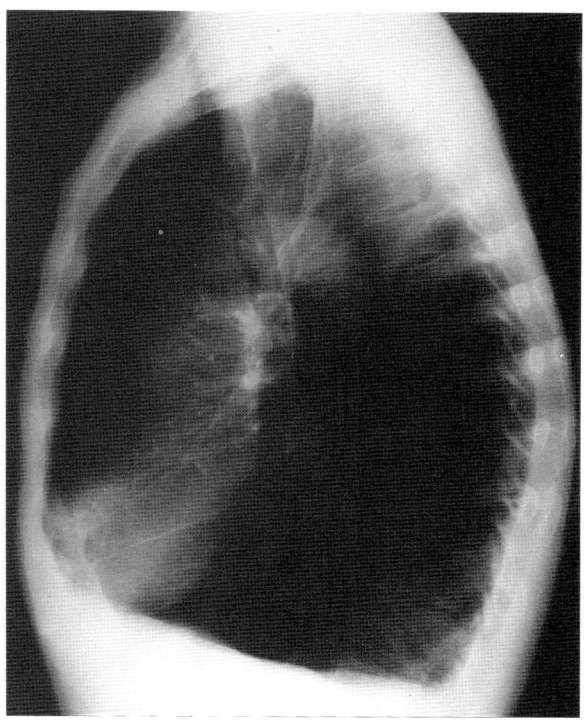

A 54-year-old man presented with shortness of breath.

- Comment on the size of the lungs.
- What is the diagnosis?
- Are the hila normal?

A47

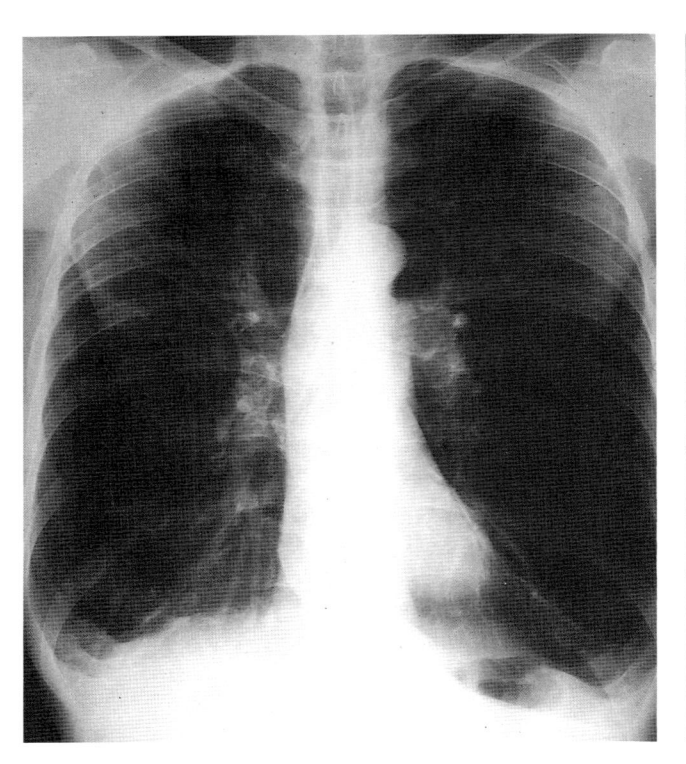

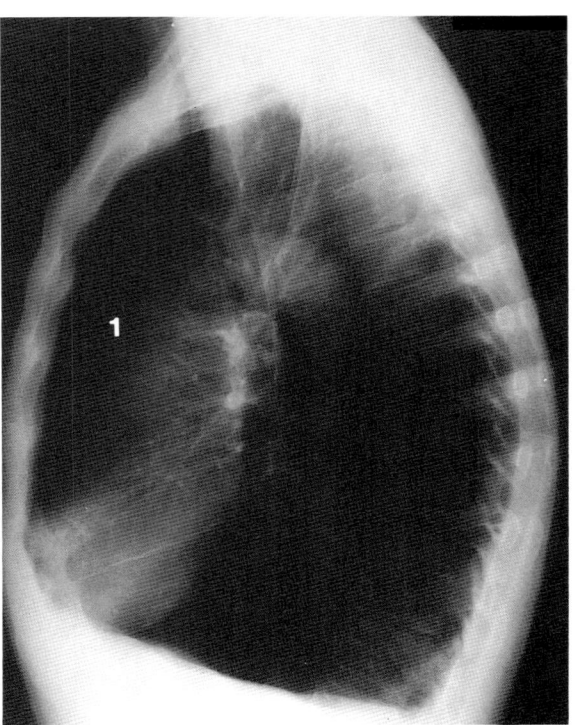

The lungs are hyperinflated. The diaphragm is low and flat; the chest is barrel-shaped; the retrosternal air-space (1) is enlarged. The diagnosis is chronic obstructive airways disease. The pulmonary vascular pattern in the right and left lower zones is attenuated by extensive emphysema. The hila are enlarged due to dilatation of the central pulmonary arteries, indicating pulmonary arterial hypertension.

Q48

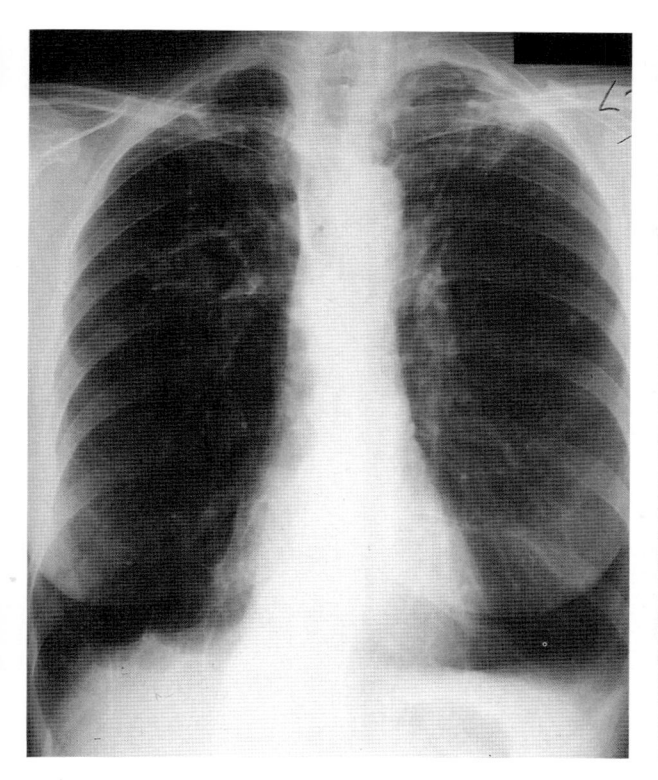

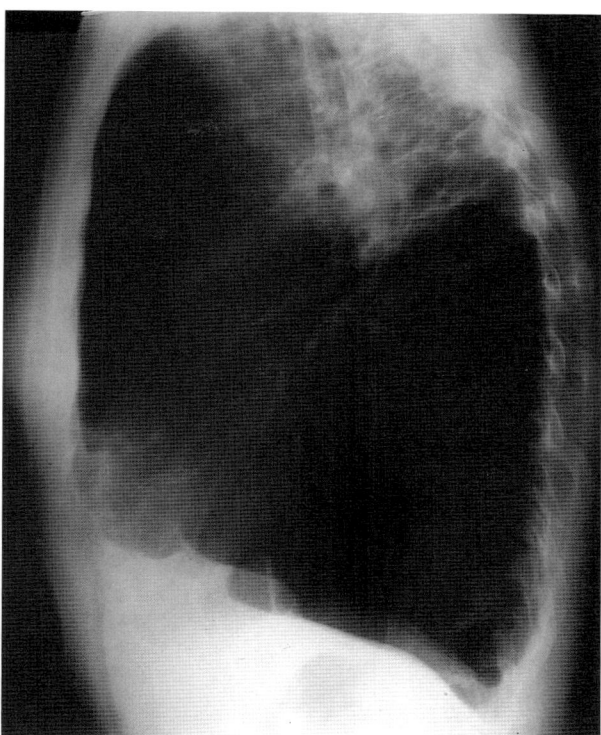

A 56-year-old woman presented with chronic obstructive airways disease. The lungs are hyperinflated and the diaphragm is low and flat.

- Are the hila in normal position?
- What other chest disease has this patient had?

A48

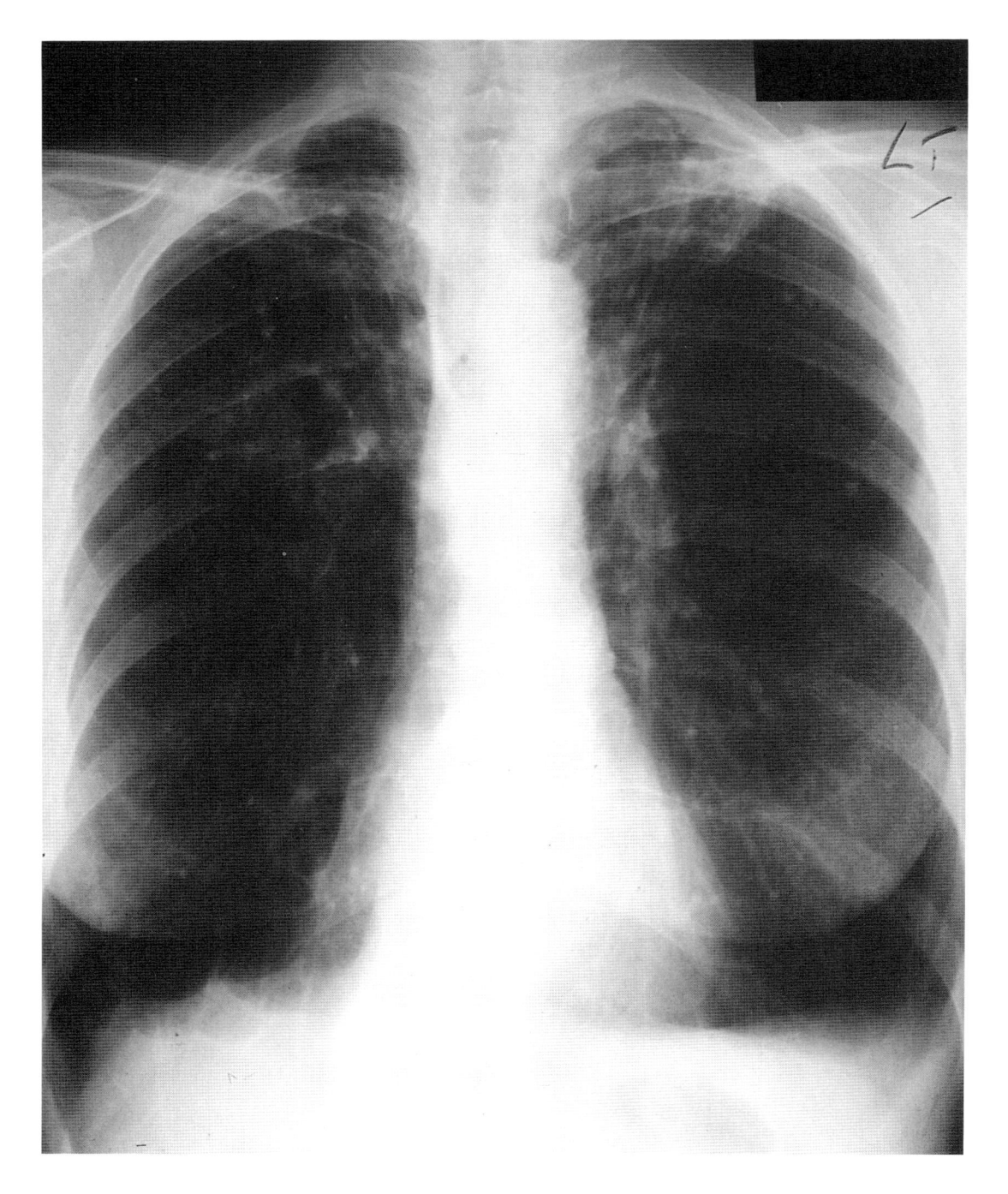

The hila are elevated. The patient has had pulmonary tuberculosis. Streaky linear shadows extending from the hila to the apices and the hila elevation are due to bilateral upper lobe fibrosis. Calcified upper zone nodules are granulomas.

Q49

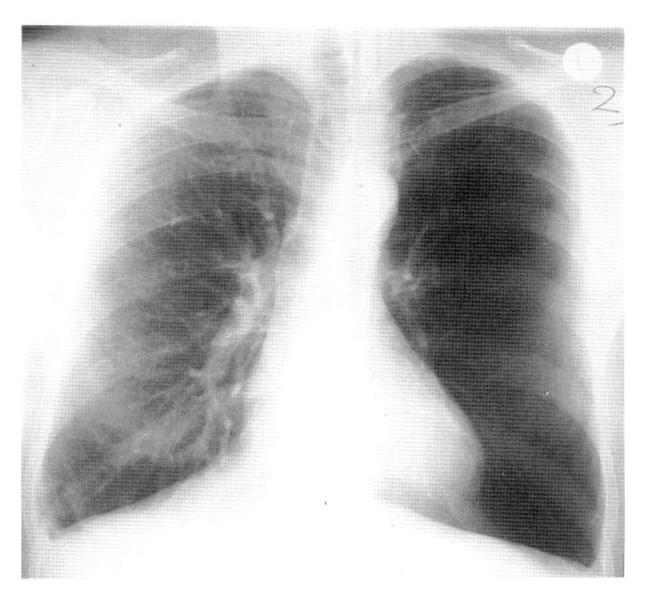

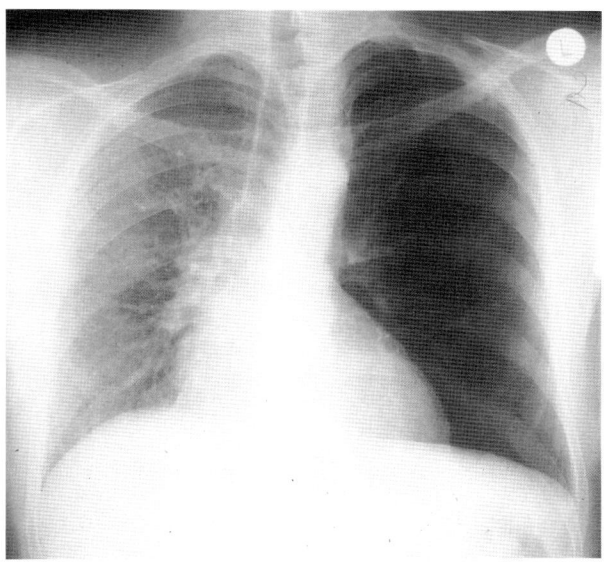

A 38-year-old asymptomatic man presented with a history of childhood infections.

- Comment on the density of the lungs and the appearance of the left hilum of the first CXR.

The second CXR was taken at end-expiration.

- How has the appearance changed?
- What is the diagnosis?

A49

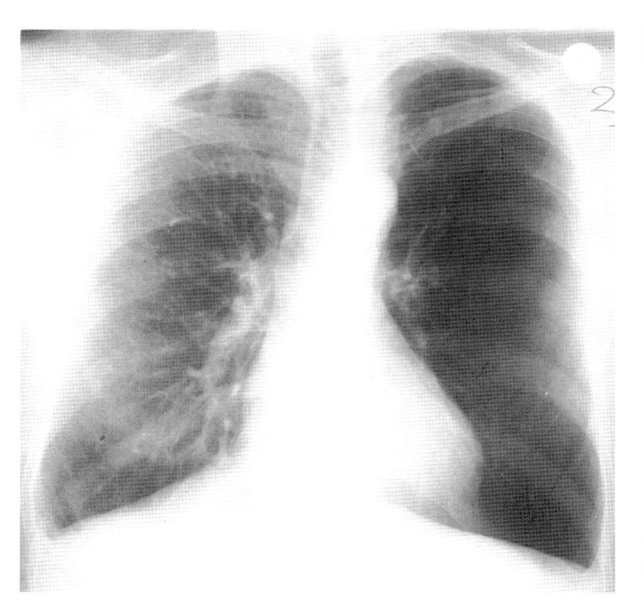

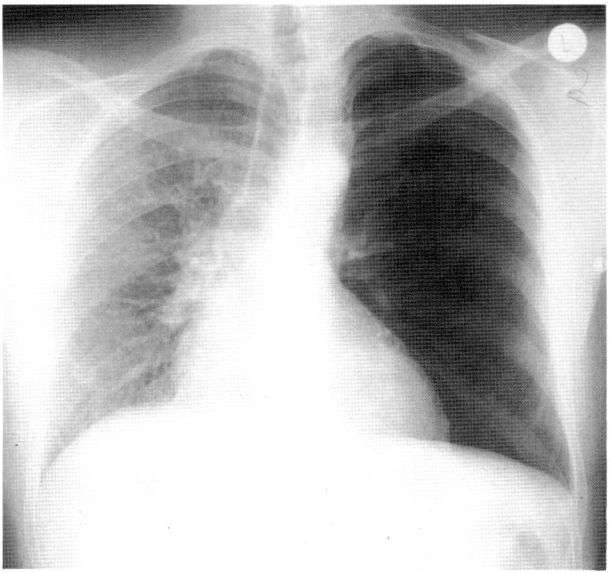

The left lung is hypertransradiant, and the left hilum is small. On the second CXR the mediastinum has moved to the right; the right hemidiaphragm has risen, but not the left. These appearances indicate air-trapping in the left lung. The diagnosis is unilateral emphysema, also known as Macleod's or Swyer-James' Syndrome.

Q50

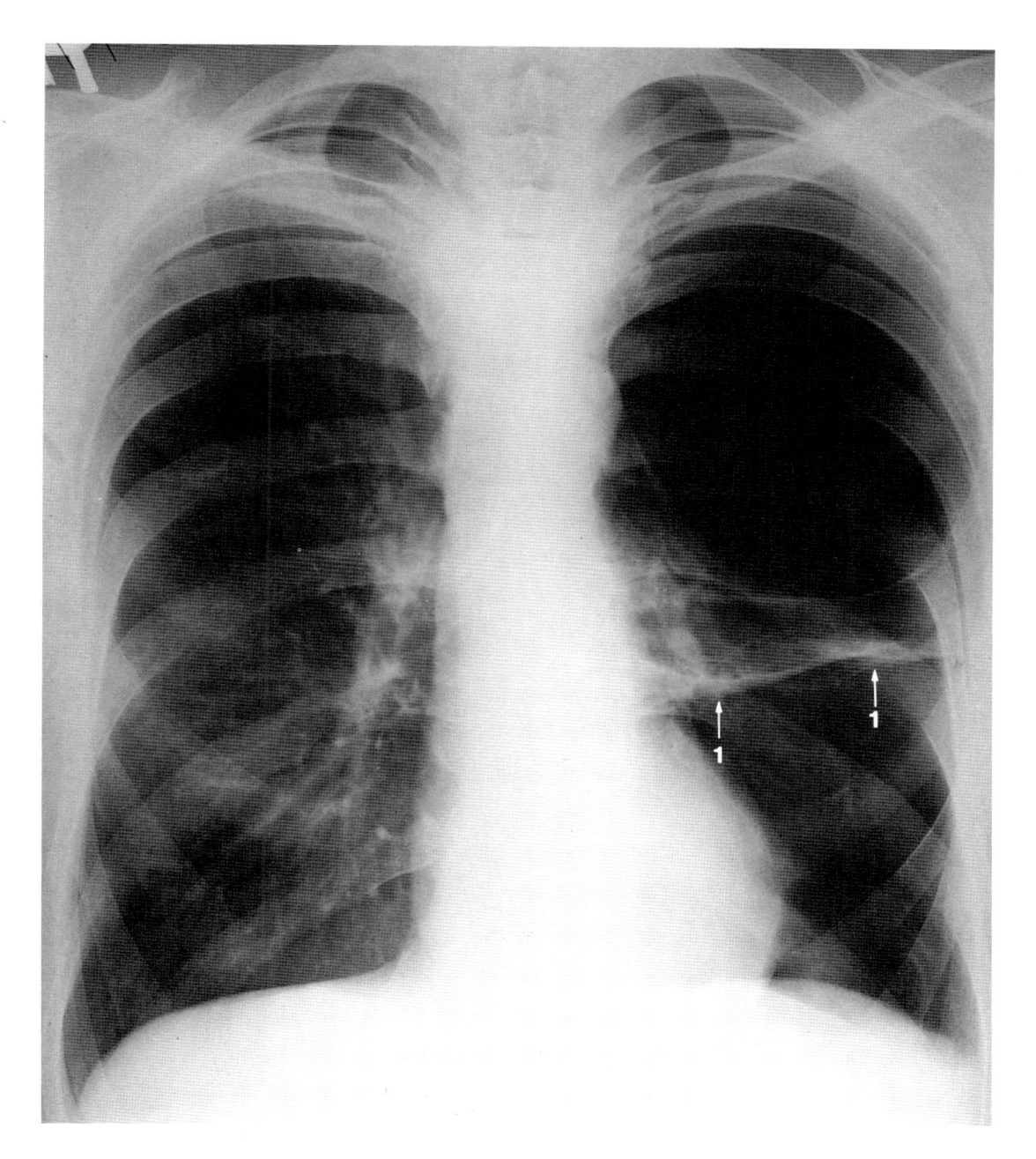

A 37-year-old man presented with increasing shortness of breath.

- Describe the appearance of the left upper zone.
- What are the horizontal band shadows (1) in the left mid zone?
- What is the diagnosis?

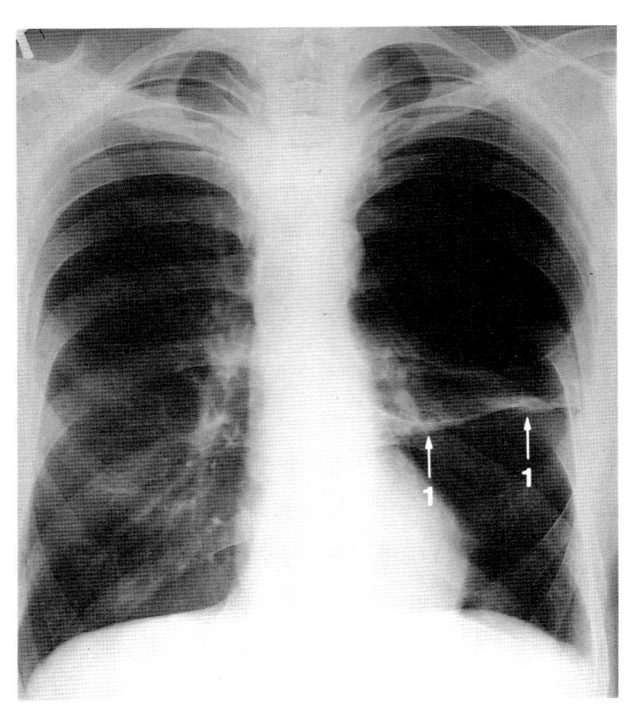

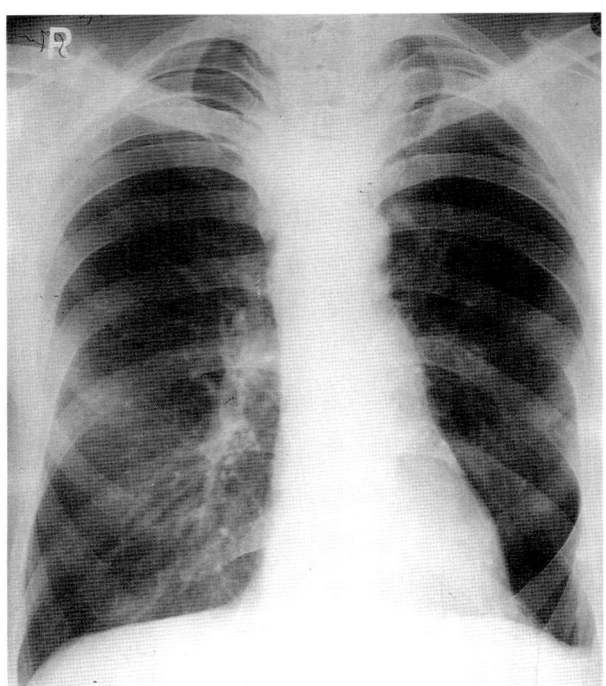

A large round cyst occupies the left upper zone, with complete absence of pulmonary vessels. (1) = compressed lung. The diagnosis is a large emphysematous cyst of the left upper lobe. The second CXR was taken after removal of the cyst. The compressed lung has re-expanded.

Q51

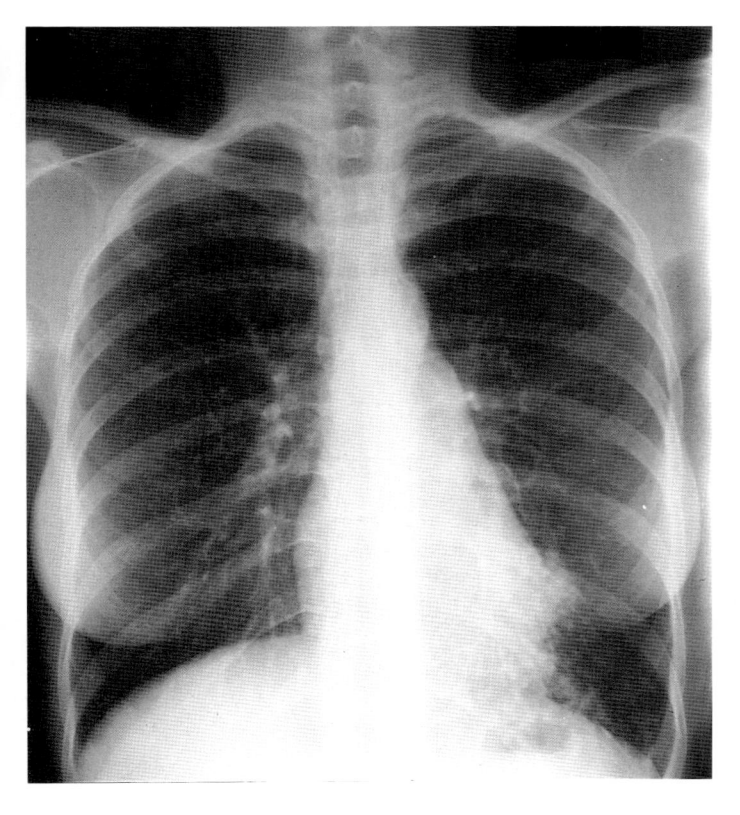

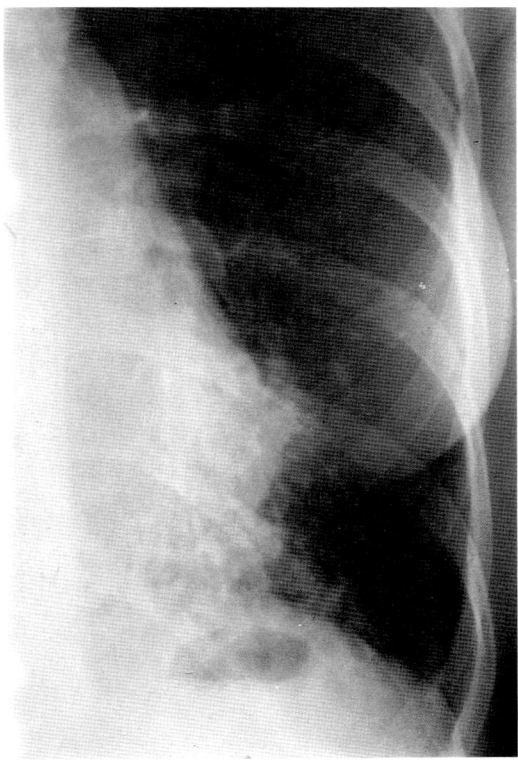

A 26-year-old female presented with a chronic cough producing half a cupful of purulent sputum daily.

- What is the clinical diagnosis?
- What does the CXR show?
- What is the radiological diagnosis?
- Is further investigation indicated?

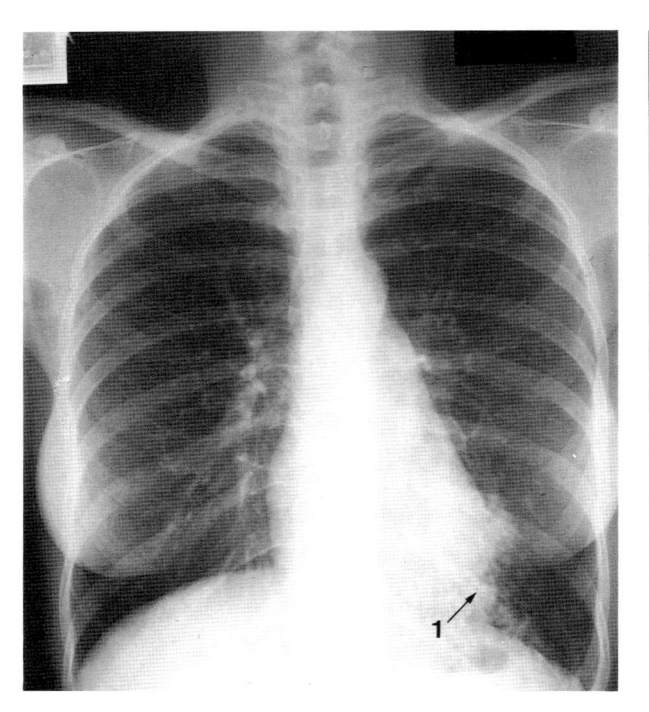

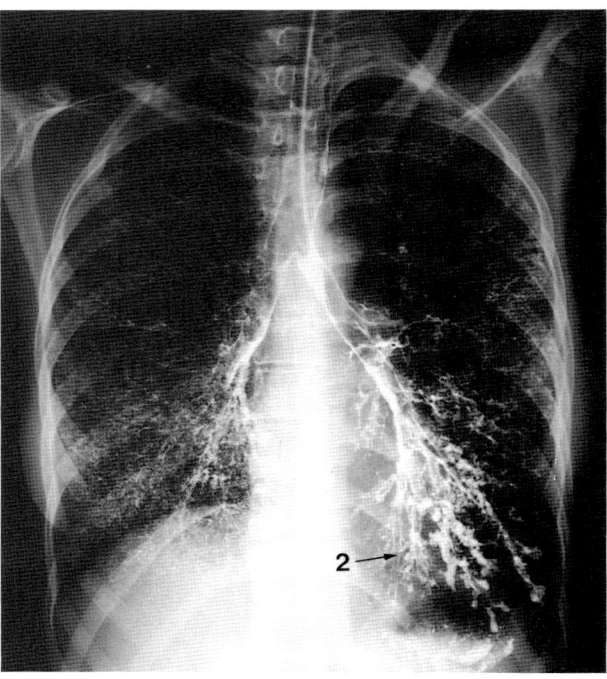

The clinical diagnosis is bronchiectasis. The CXR shows branching tubular shadows (1) in the left lower zone. They represent dilated, fluid-filled bronchi. The radiological diagnosis is also bronchiectasis.

If surgery is planned, it is essential to know the extent of the bronchiectasis. Bronchography was performed in this case, and demonstrated dilated left lower lobe bronchi, some of which contain retained secretions (2). Narrow section CT will also demonstrate bronchiectasis, and is probably the method of choice.

Q52

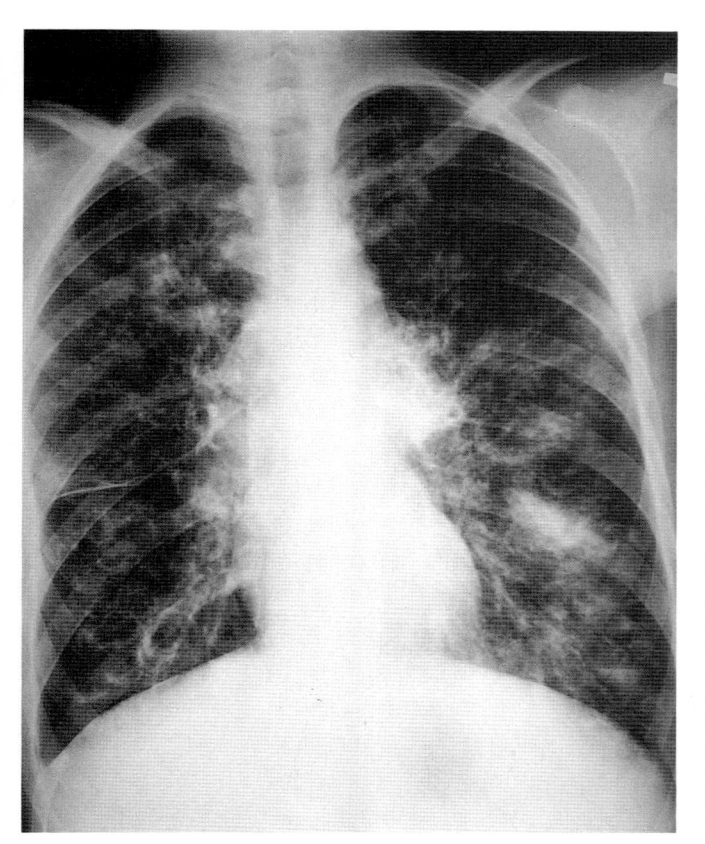

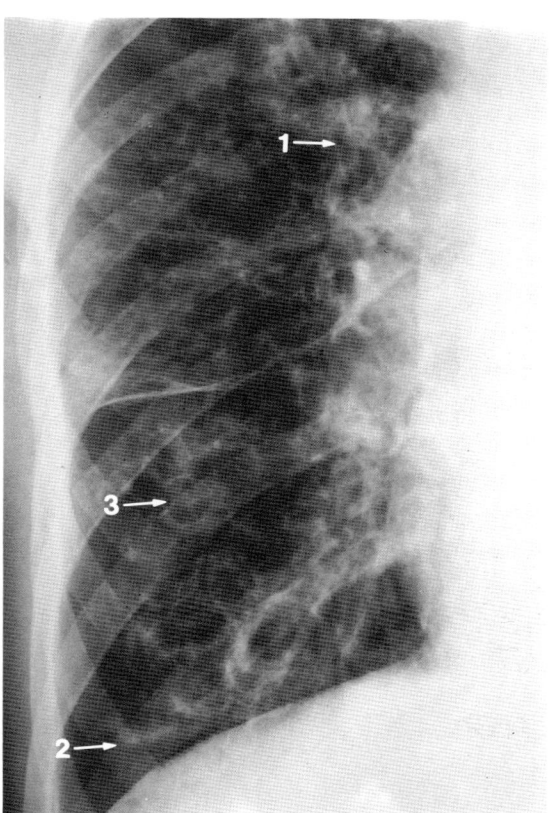

A 16-year-old male presented with a chronic cough and progressive shortness of breath.

- Does the diaphragm look normal?
- Comment on the hila.
- Describe the abnormal lung shadows (1-3).
- What is the diagnosis?

A52

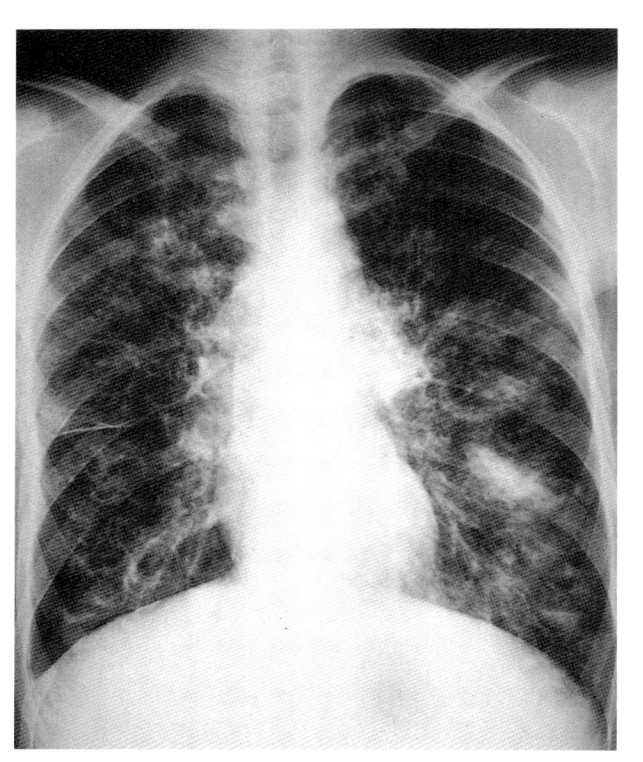

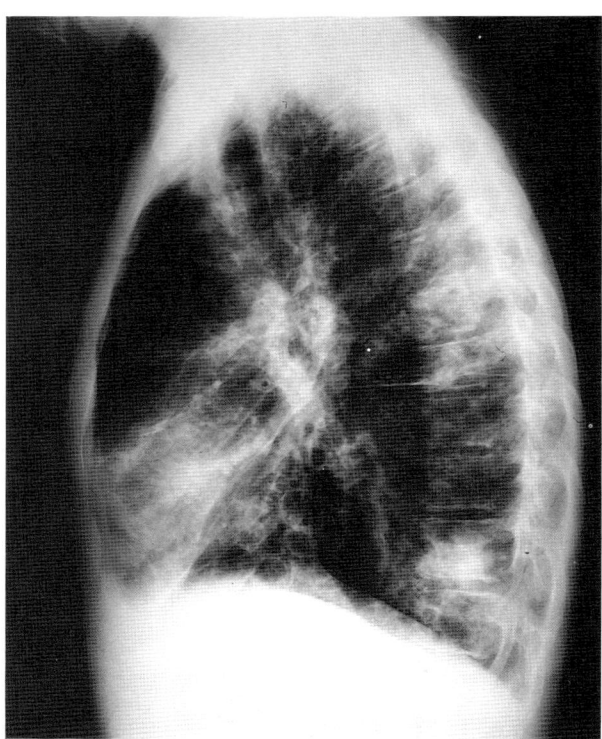

The diaphragm is flattened, indicating that the lungs are hyperinflated. The hila are enlarged. This is probably due to both lymph node and pulmonary artery enlargement. (1) = tram lines, indicating bronchial wall thickening; (2) = band shadows, representing peripheral atelectasis; (3) = ring shadows, indicating cystic bronchiectasis. The diagnosis is cystic fibrosis.

Q53

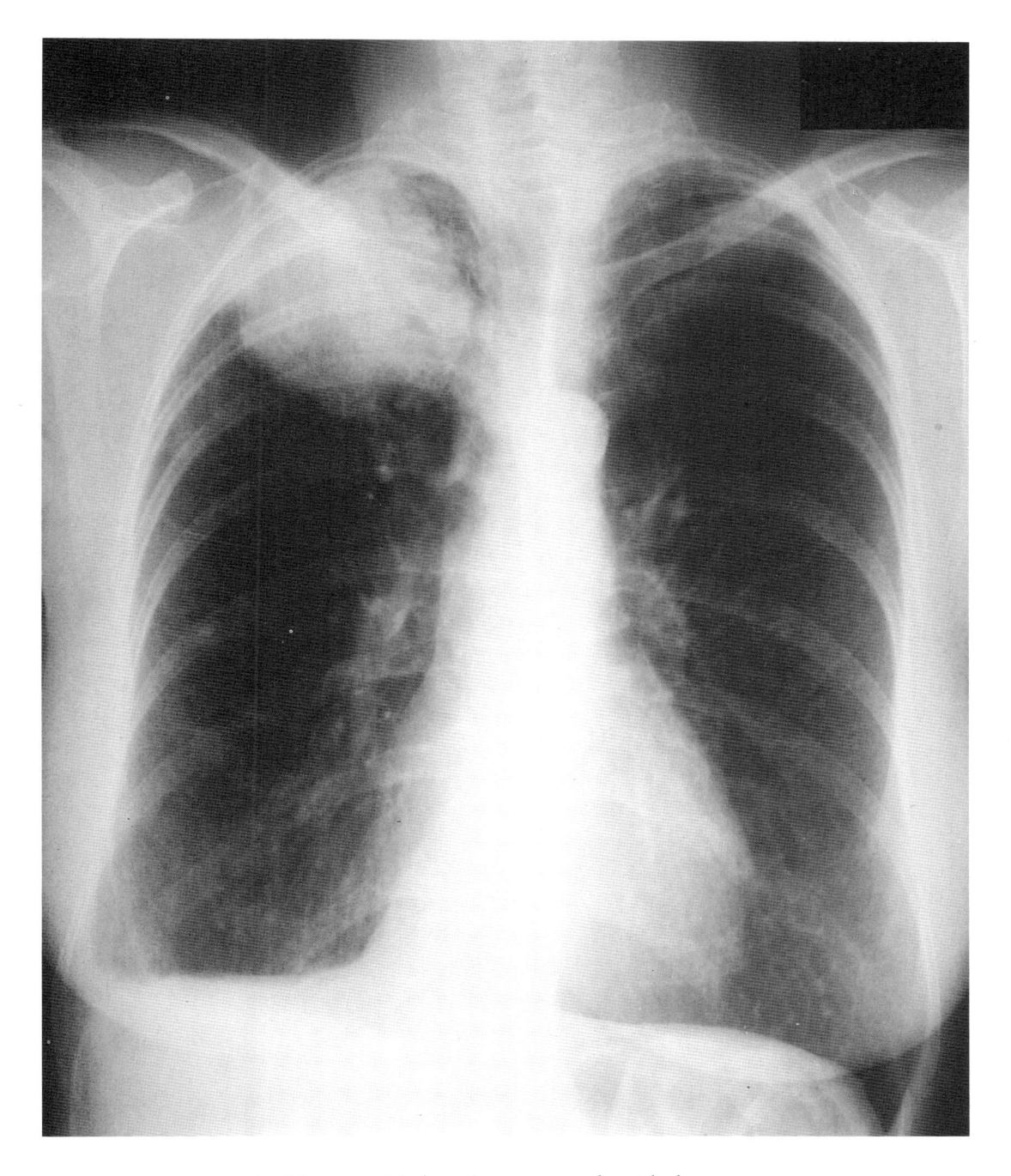

A 55-year-old female presented with haemoptysis.

- Describe the CXR.
- What is the probable diagnosis?
- What further investigations are indicated?

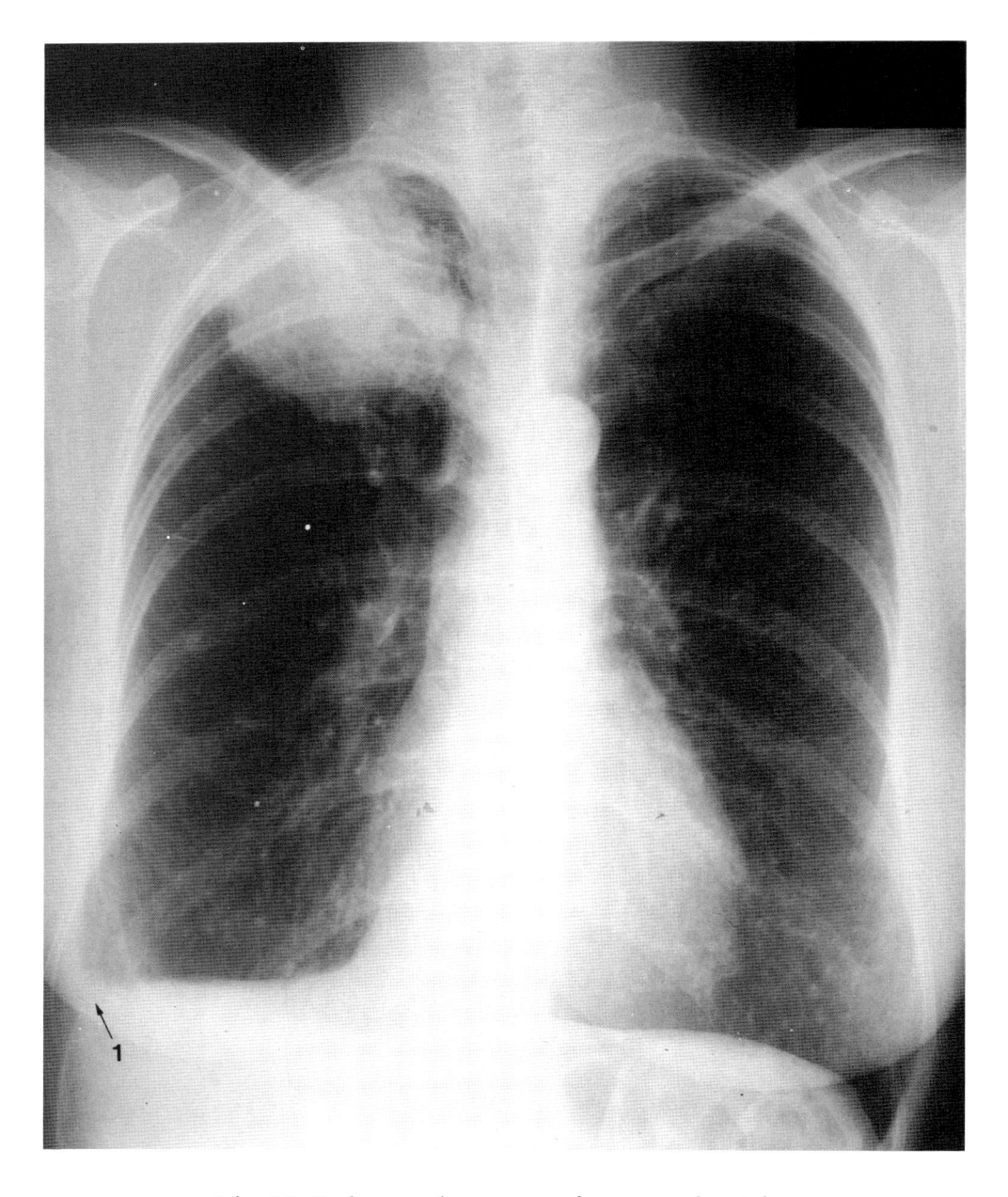

The CXR shows a large, round mass in the right upper zone. A right pleural effusion is also present (1). The likely diagnosis is carcinoma of the bronchus. (A solitary metastasis and a lung abscess are also possibilities.)

A histological diagnosis is required. The sputum should be examined for malignant cells. If this is negative then bronchoscopic or percutaneous needle biopsy should be performed. This was a primary adenocarcinoma.

Q54

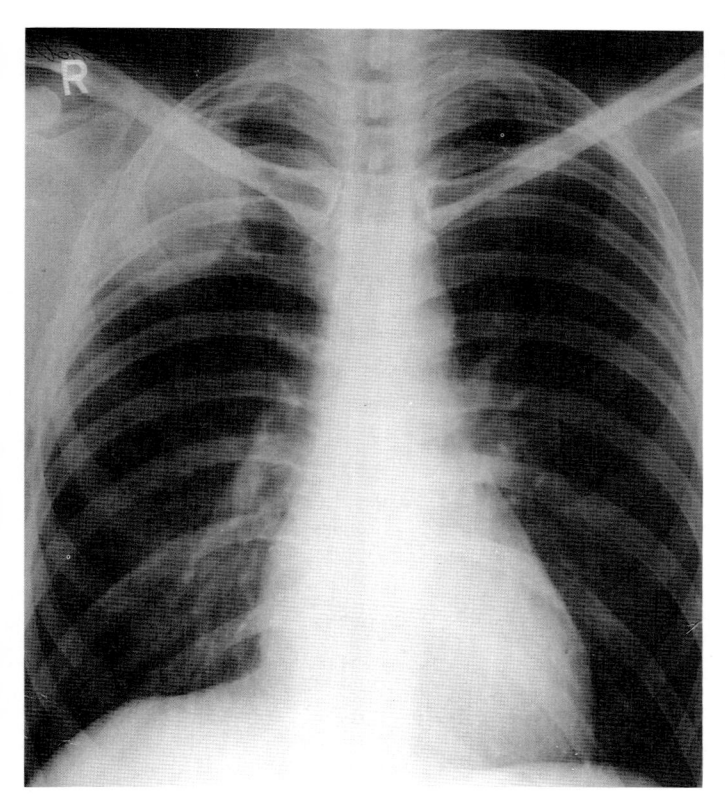

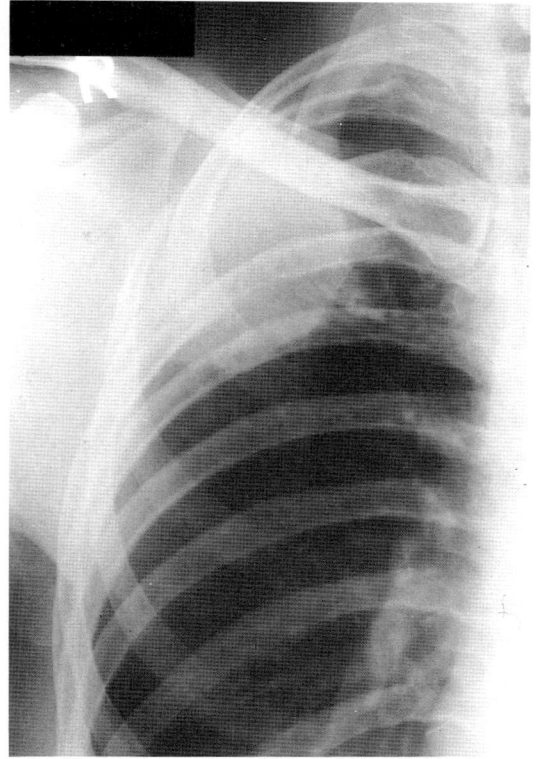

A 40-year-old male presented with right-sided chest pain. The CXR shows a right upper zone mass.
- Is the mass benign or malignant?
- What further investigation would you do?

A54

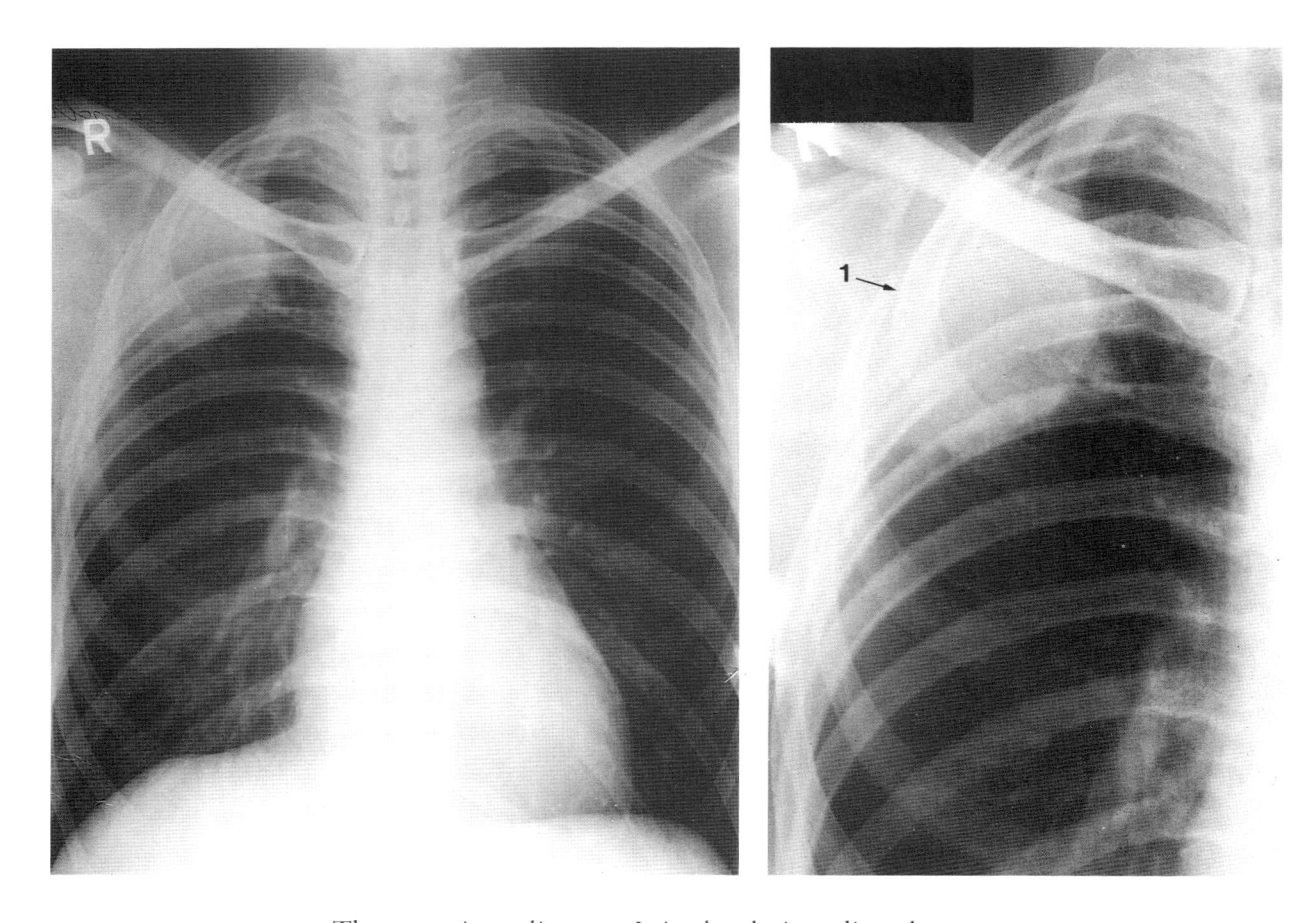

The mass is malignant. It is clearly invading the third and fourth ribs (1). Percutaneous needle biopsy is indicated. This showed adenocarcinoma.

Q55

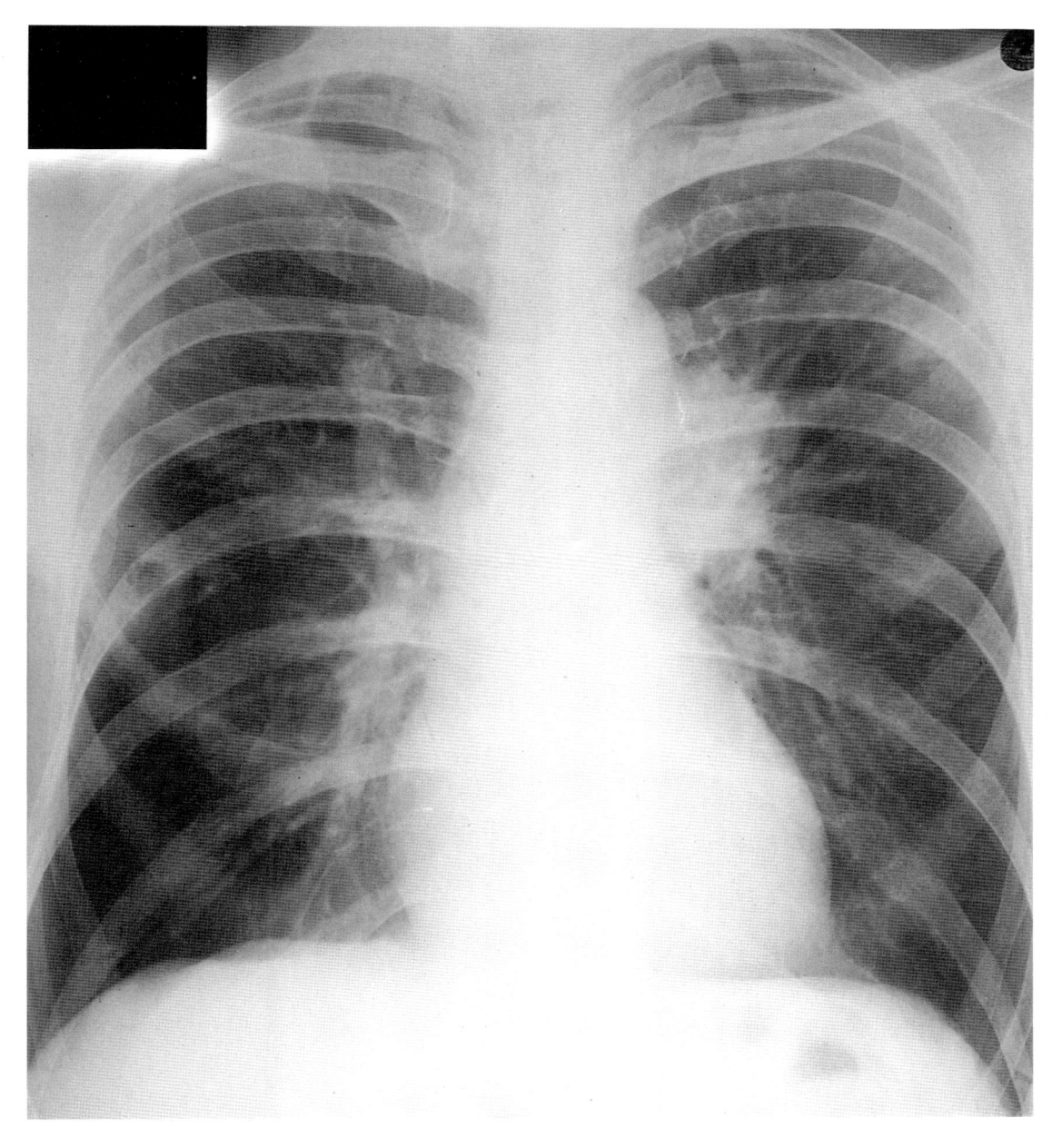

A 60-year-old man presented with a chronic cough and hoarseness of recent onset.

- Describe the CXR.
- Does this patient have benign or malignant disease?
- What is the diagnosis?
- Is the disease operable?

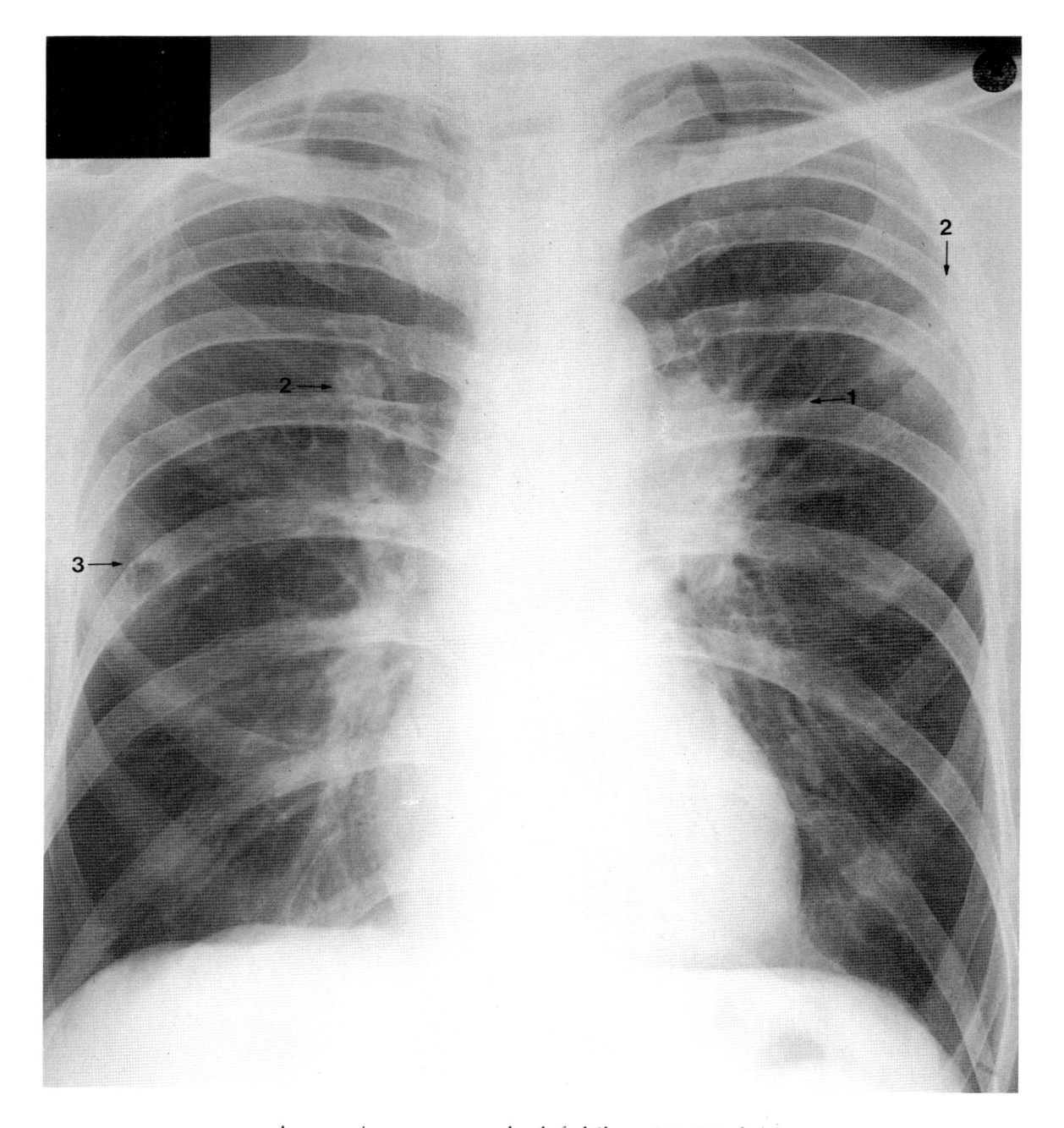

A mass is present at the left hilum (1). Nodules are also present in both lungs (2), and a destructive lesion is present in the right eighth rib (3). These features indicate a malignant process with metastatic spread. Bronchoscopy showed a poorly differentiated large cell carcinoma of the left bronchus. The tumour is clearly disseminated and therefore inoperable.

Q56

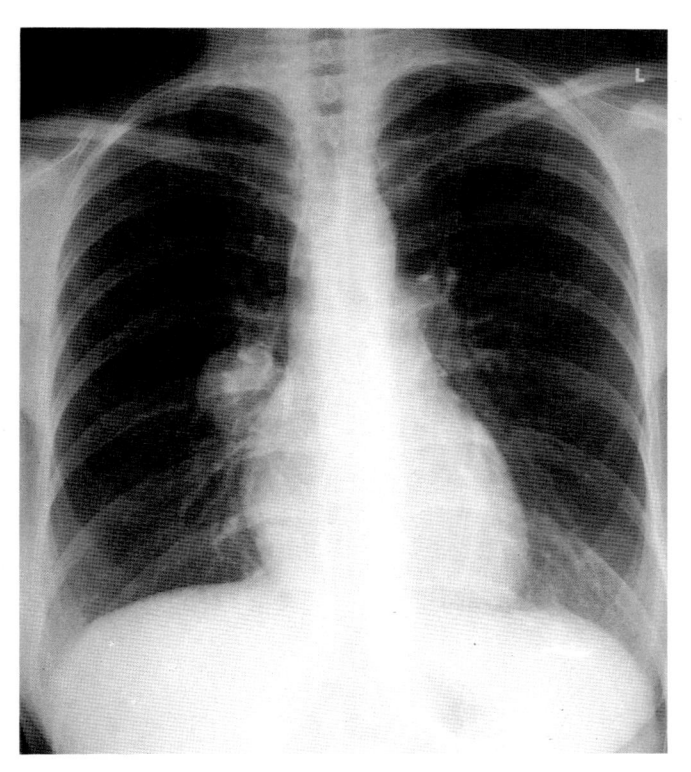

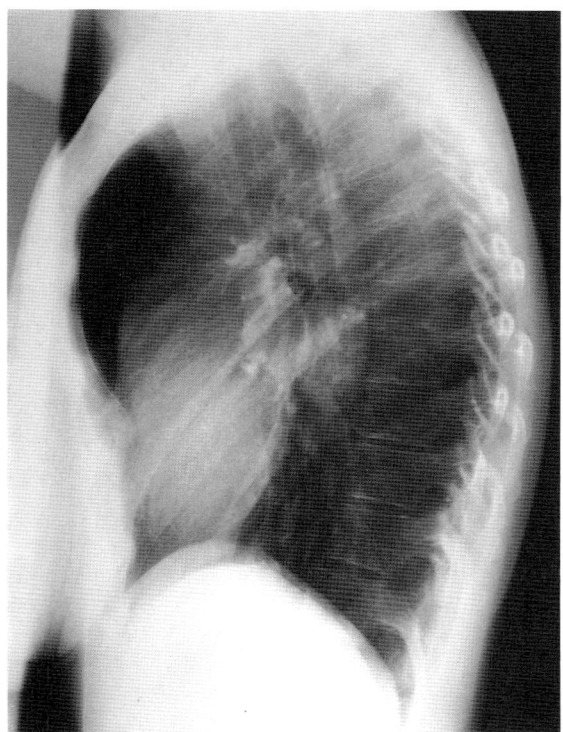

A 35-year-old female non-smoker presented with a right-sided pneumonia. This resolved with antibiotics, and these films were then taken.

- What abnormality is present on the CXR?
- What is the differential diagnosis?
- What investigation is indicated next?

A56

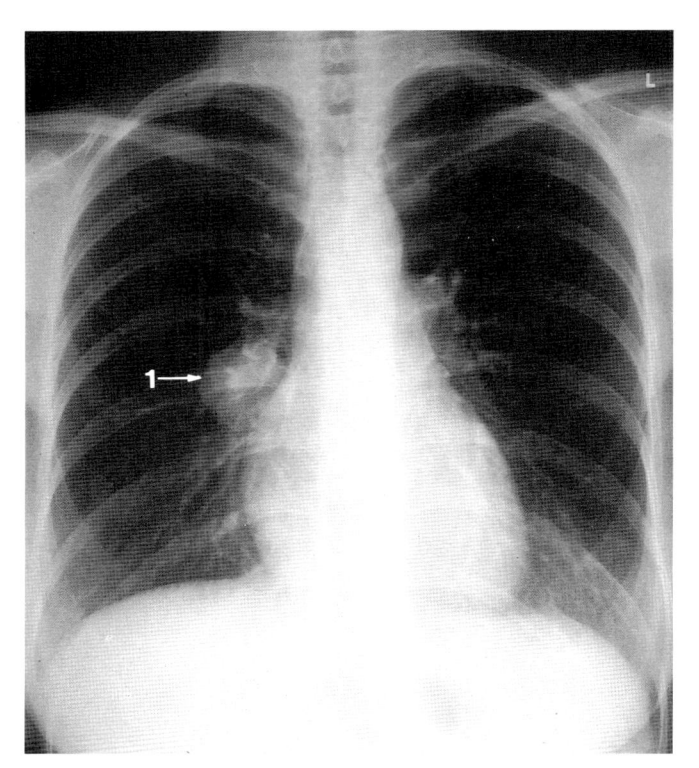

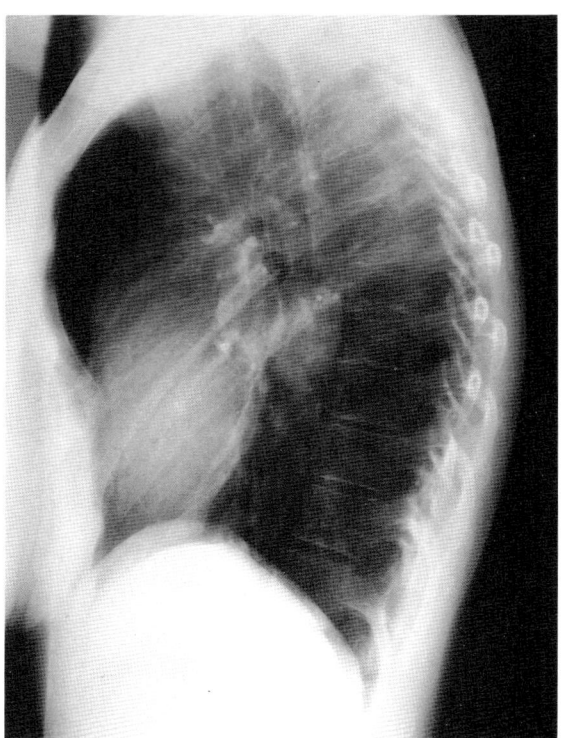

A well circumscribed mass is present at the right hilum (1). The differential diagnosis is:

a) Lymph node enlargement (due to tuberculosis, lymphoma, or possibly sarcoidosis).
b) A tumour (benign or malignant).
c) Pulmonary artery aneurysm.

Bronchoscopy is required. A tumour in the right lower lobe was biopsied, and found to be a carcinoid tumour.

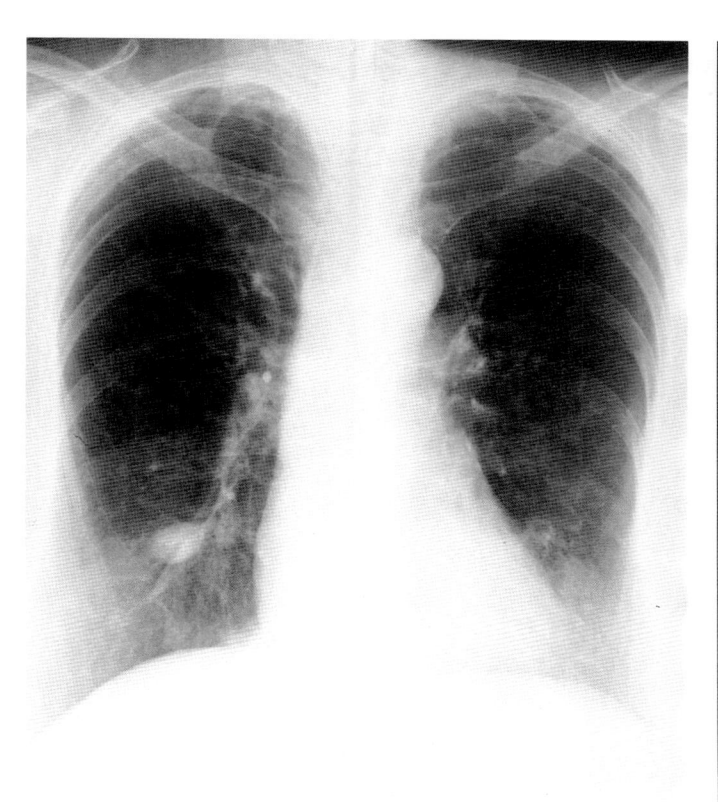

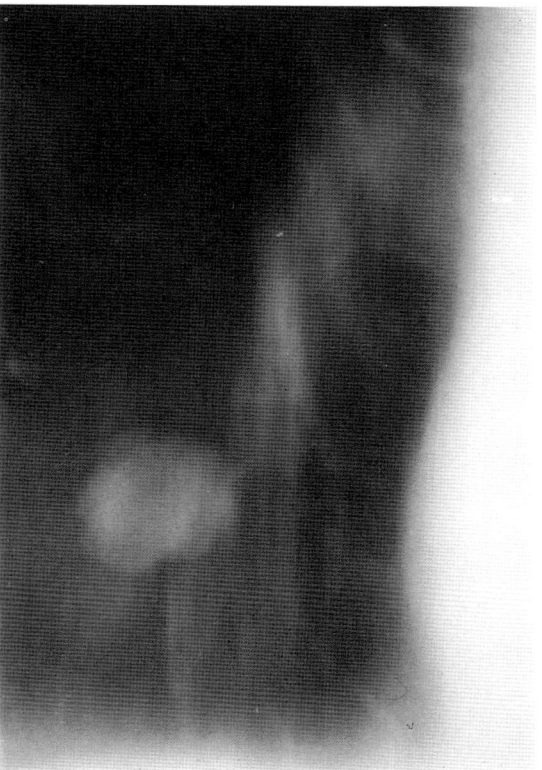

A 59-year-old female with post-menopausal bleeding had a routine pre-operative CXR prior to hysterectomy. Four years previously she had been hospitalised with a probable myocardial infarction.

- What does the CXR show?
- Is the tomogram helpful?
- What is the probable diagnosis?
- What would you do next?

A57

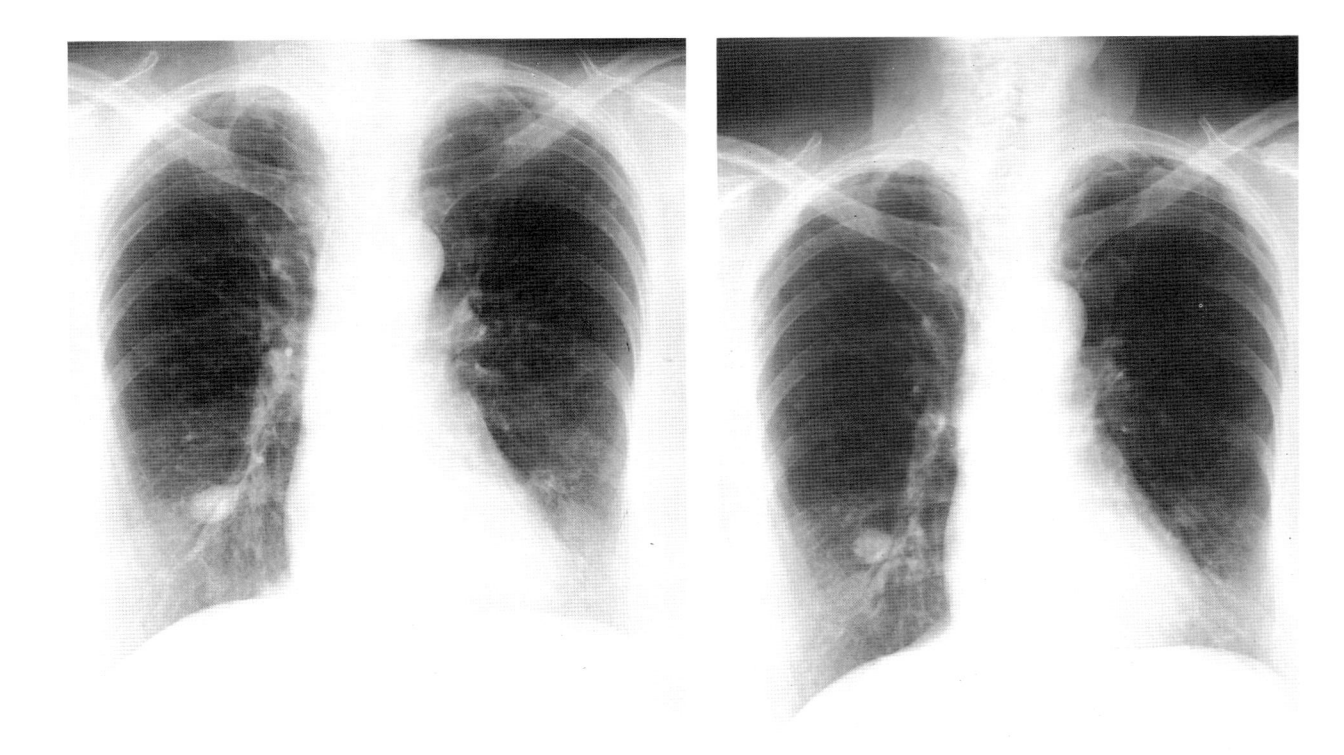

The CXR shows a solitary nodule in the right lower zone. The tomogram is helpful. It shows that the nodule has a sharp, well-defined edge, and that it is diffusely calcified. This nodule is, therefore, likely to be benign. The probable diagnosis is a granuloma due to previous infection. The next step is to try and obtain an old CXR, since if there has been no change over two years the nodule is almost certainly benign. This second CXR was taken four years earlier. The nodule is benign.

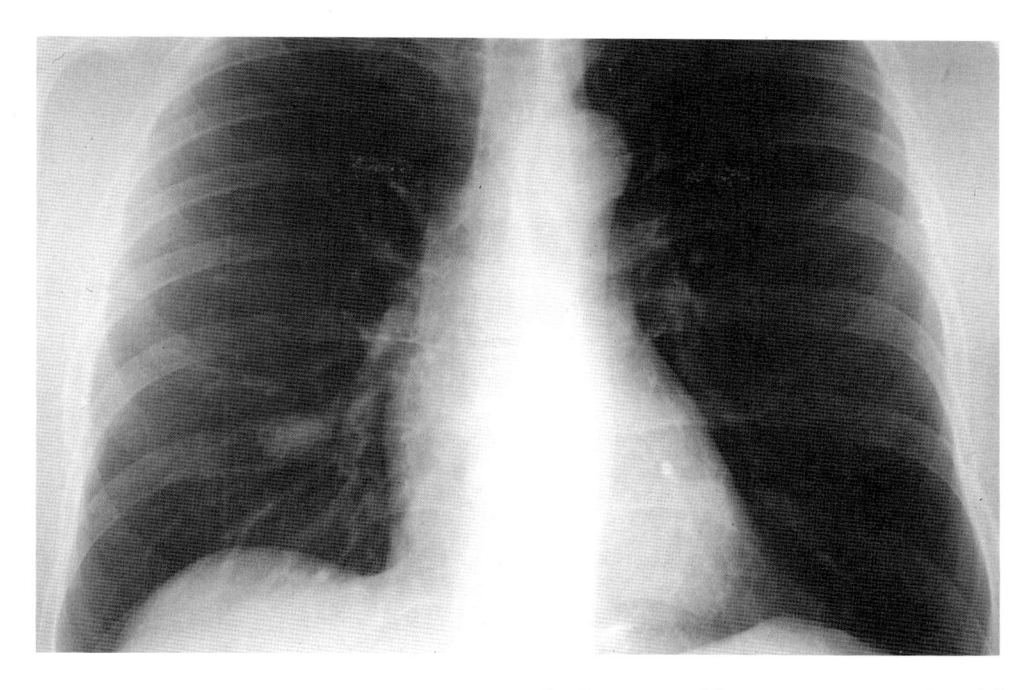

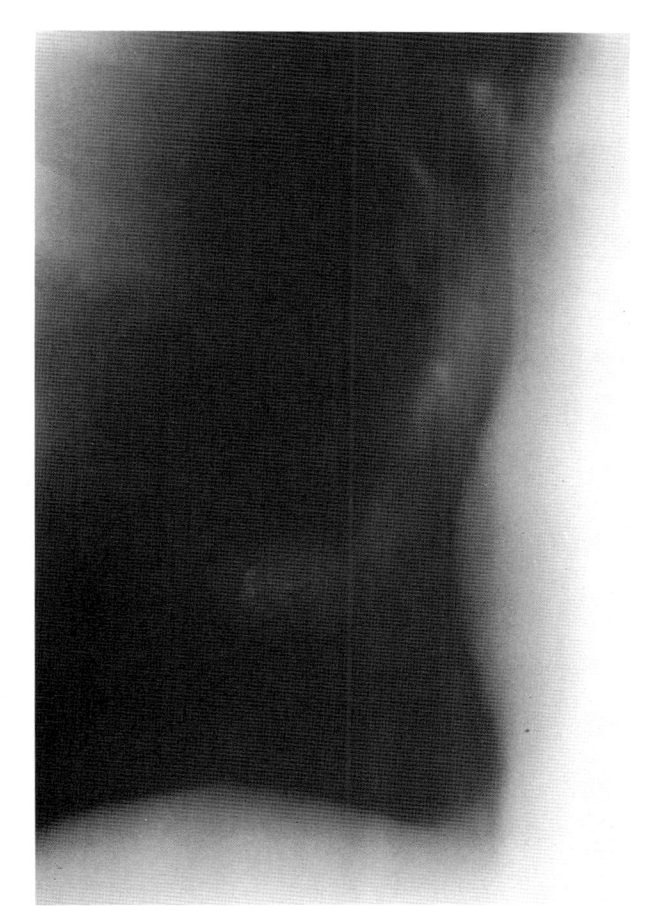

A 51-year-old man presented with testicular pain. Ten years previously a testicular cyst had been excised.

- What does the CXR show?
- What does the tomogram show?
- Is the nodule benign or malignant?
- What is the diagnosis?

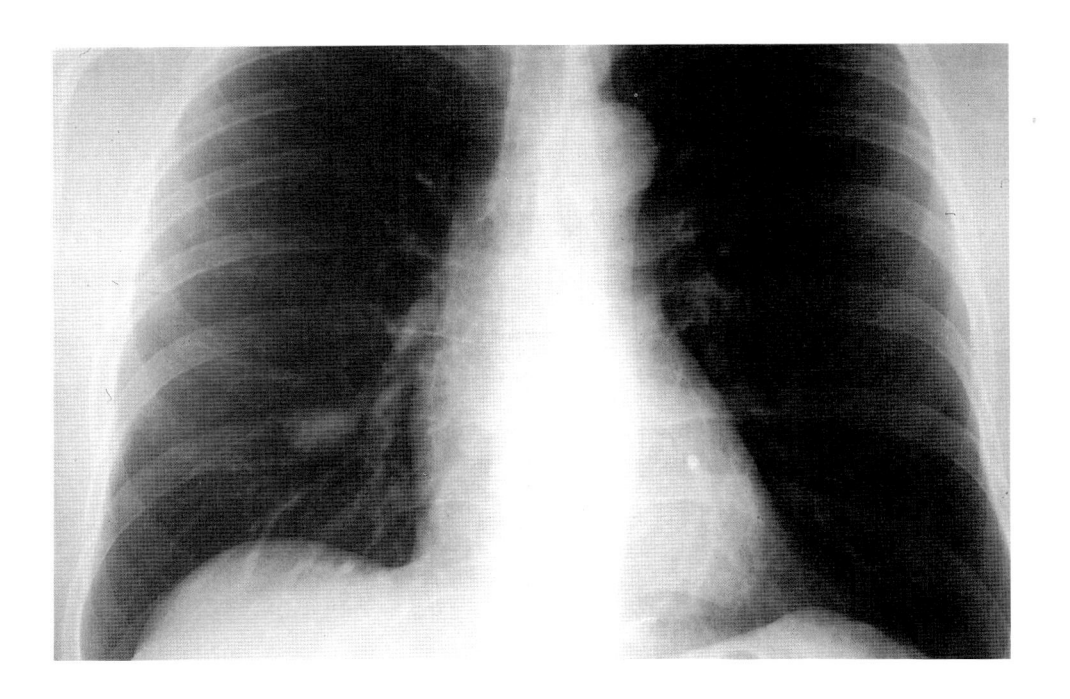

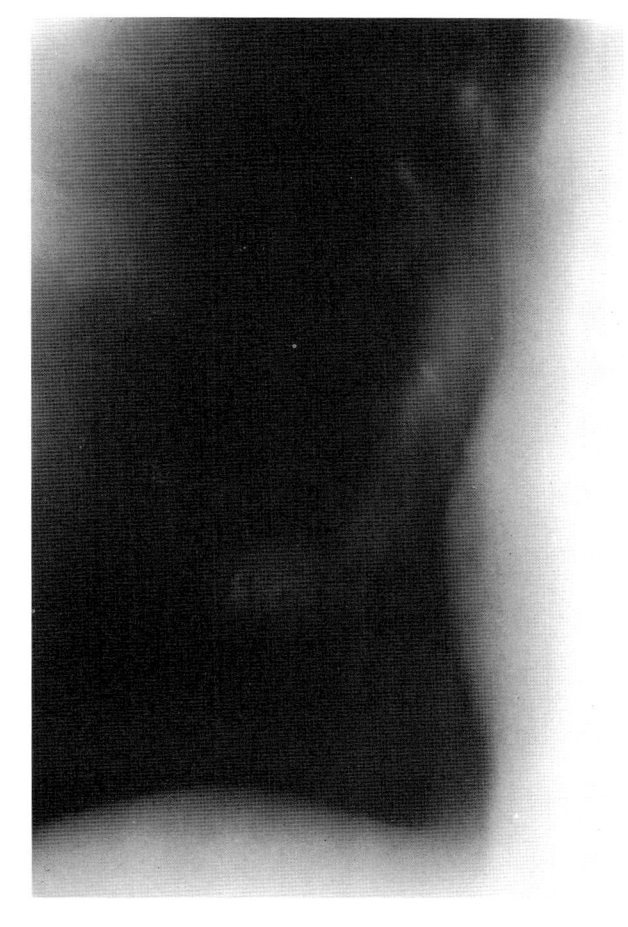

The CXR shows a solitary, sharply marginated, right lower zone opacity. The tomogram shows central popcorn calcification. The nodule is almost certainly benign, and this pattern of calcification is virtually pathognomic of a hamartoma. This was confirmed by surgery.

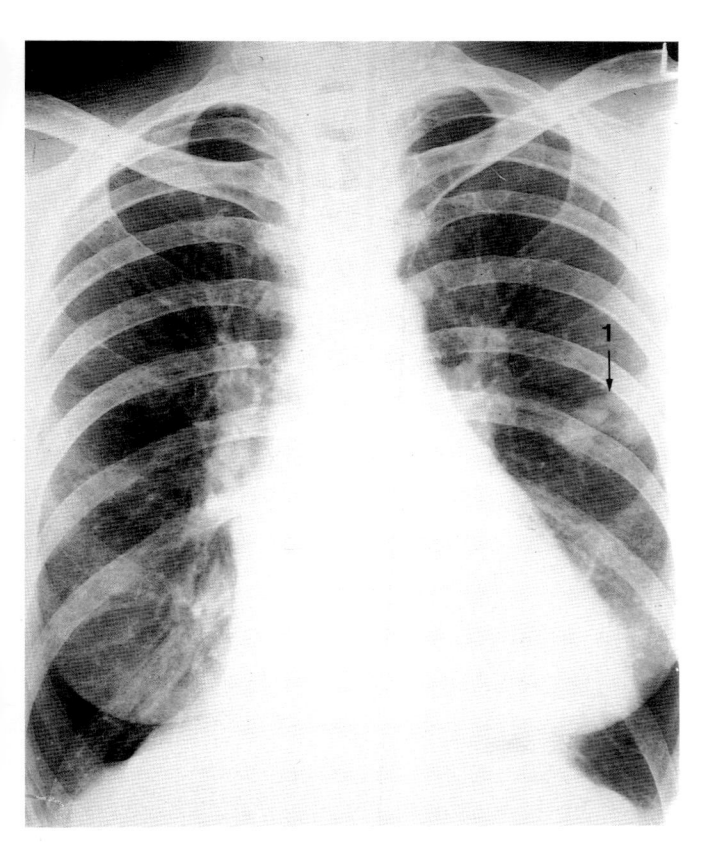

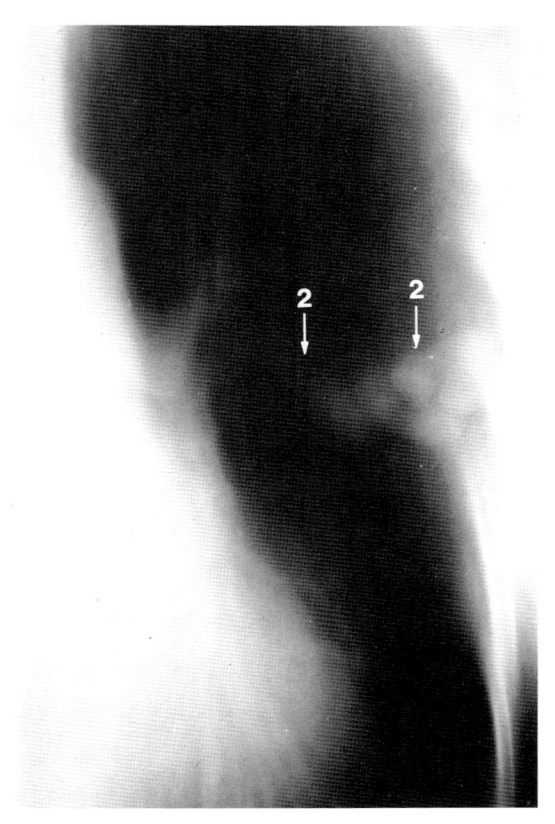

A 42-year-old female presented with haemoptysis. The CXR shows a lobulated opacity (1) in the left mid zone.

- What does the tomogram show (2)?
- Are any other lesions visible on the CXR?
- What is the diagnosis?

It is proposed to excise or embolise the left mid-zone lesion.

- What further examination would you do?

A59

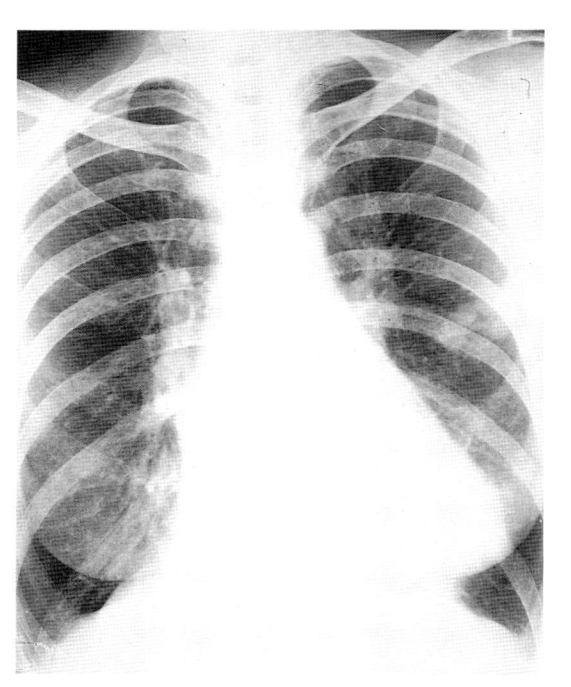

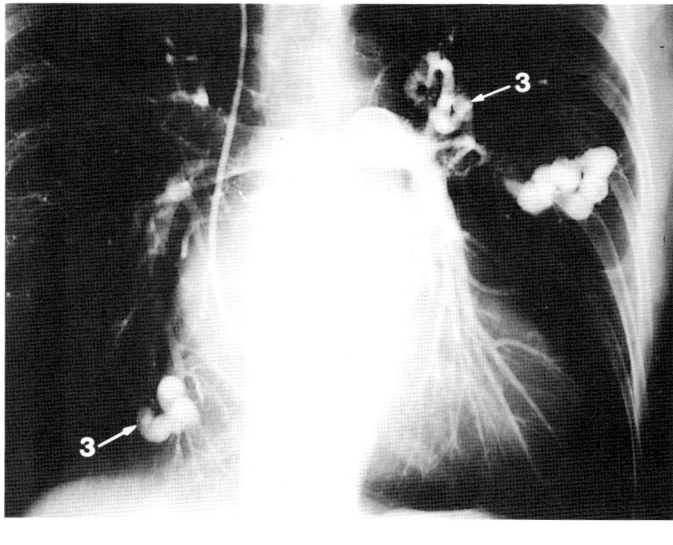

The tomogram shows that a vessel connects the lobulated structure with the hilum. No other lesions are visible on the CXR. The diagnosis is pulmonary arterio-venous malformation, or AVM.

Even though the AVM appears solitary on the CXR, approximately 30 per cent of patients have multiple AVMs. A pulmonary arteriogram should, therefore, be done. This demonstrates at least two other AVMs (3).

Q60

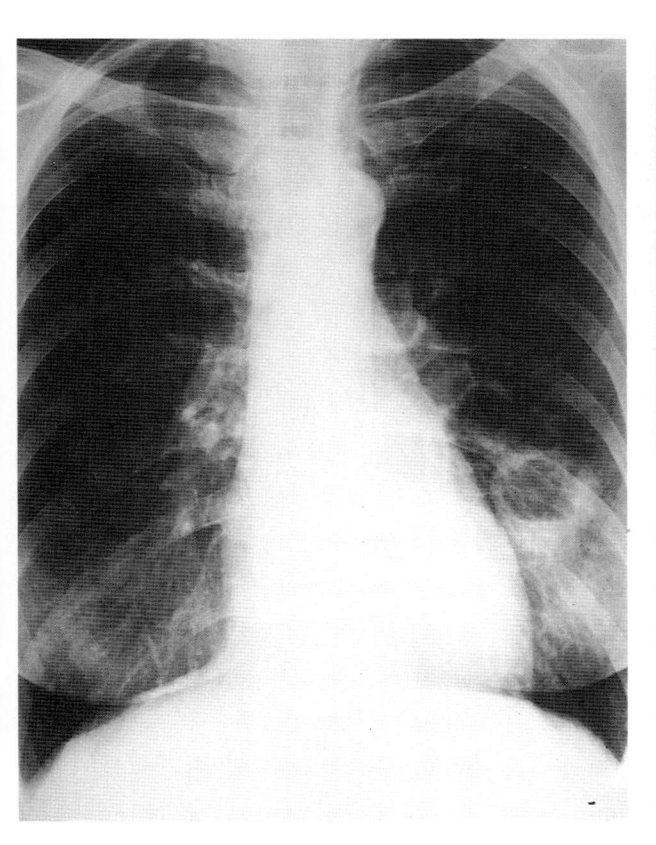

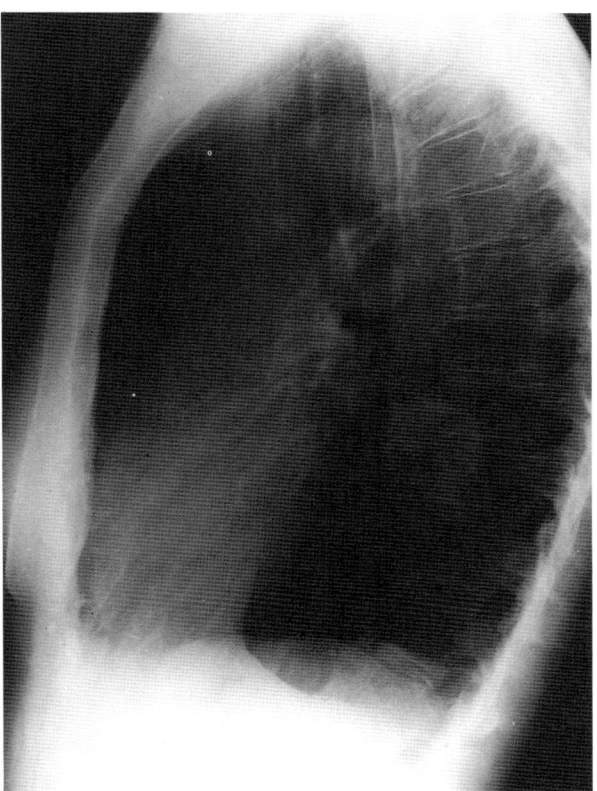

A 61-year-old female with chronic bronchitis presented with haemoptysis.

- What does the CXR show?
- What is the diagnosis?
- What further investigations would you do?

A60

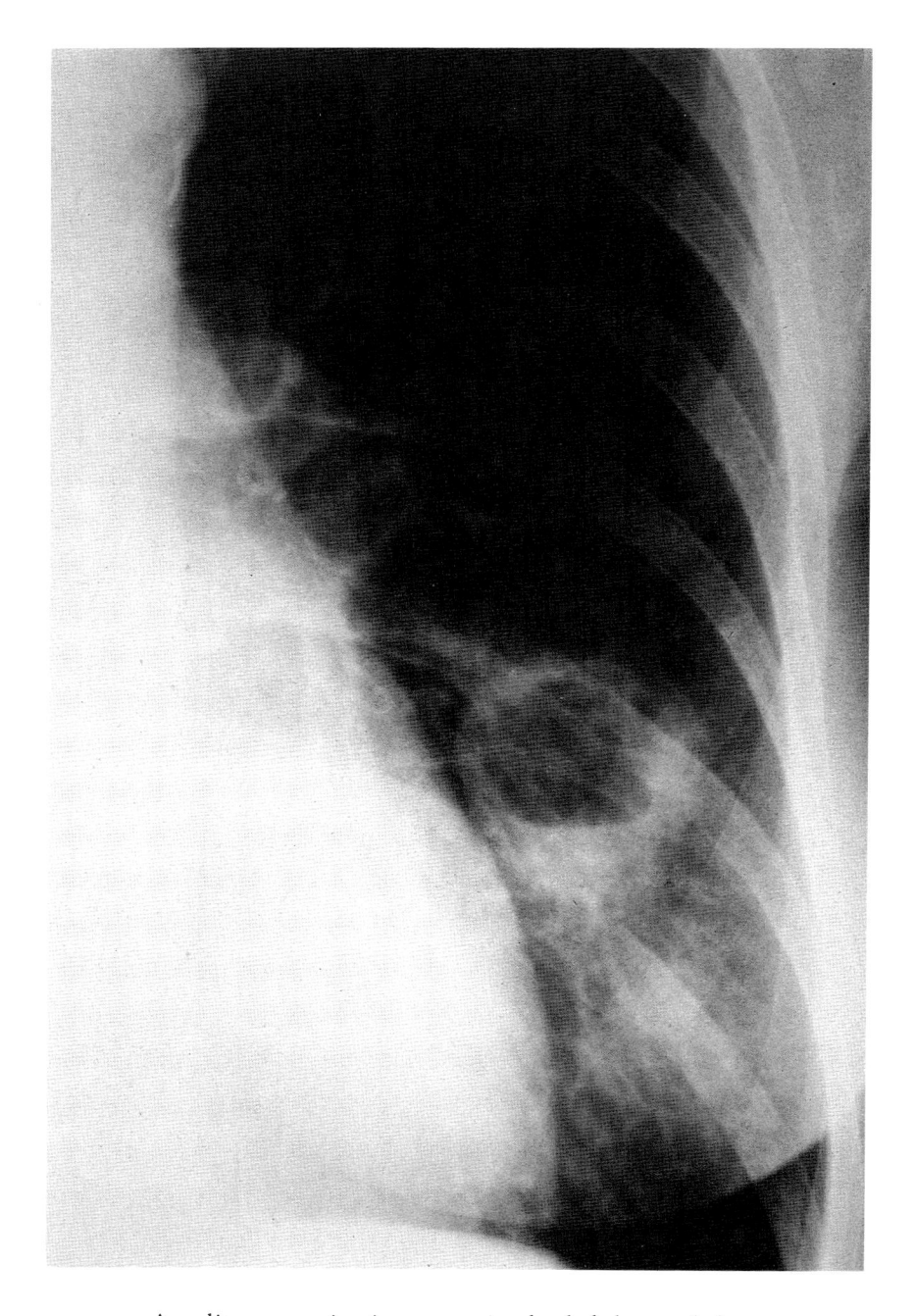

A solitary, cavitating mass in the left lower lobe is shown on the CXR. The cavity has a thick irregular wall and a fluid level. The features suggest a cavitating tumour, rather than an abscess. The sputum should be examined for pathogenic organisms and malignant cells. On bronchoscopy, a squamous cell carcinoma was found.

Q61

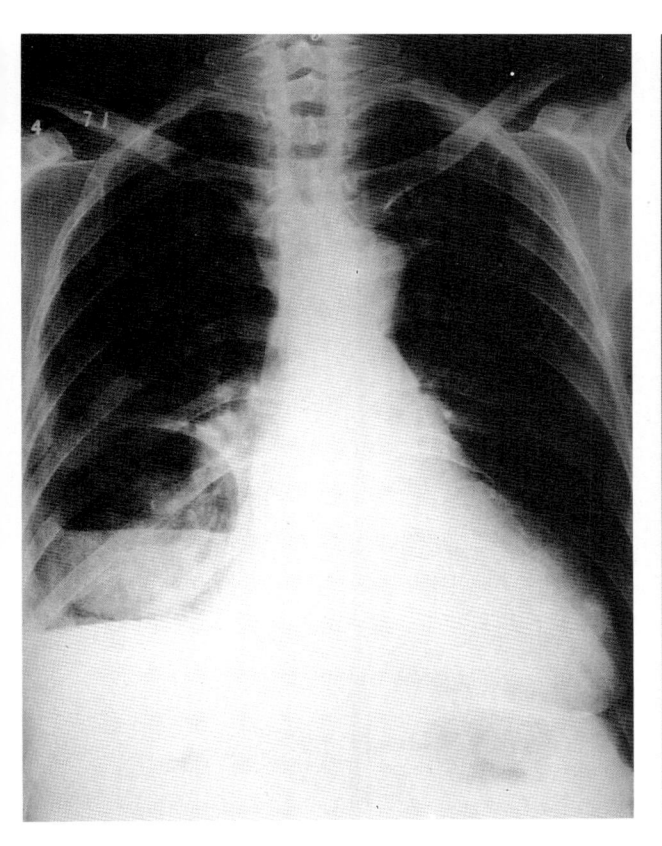

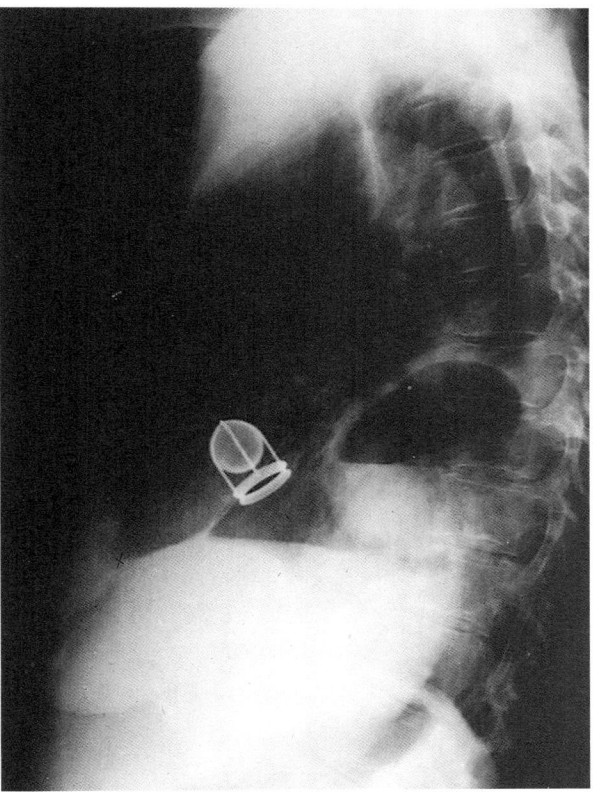

A 57-year-old woman develops fever and a cough with brown purulent sputum two weeks after major surgery.

- What operation has she had?
- Describe the right lower zone abnormality.
- What is the diagnosis?

A61

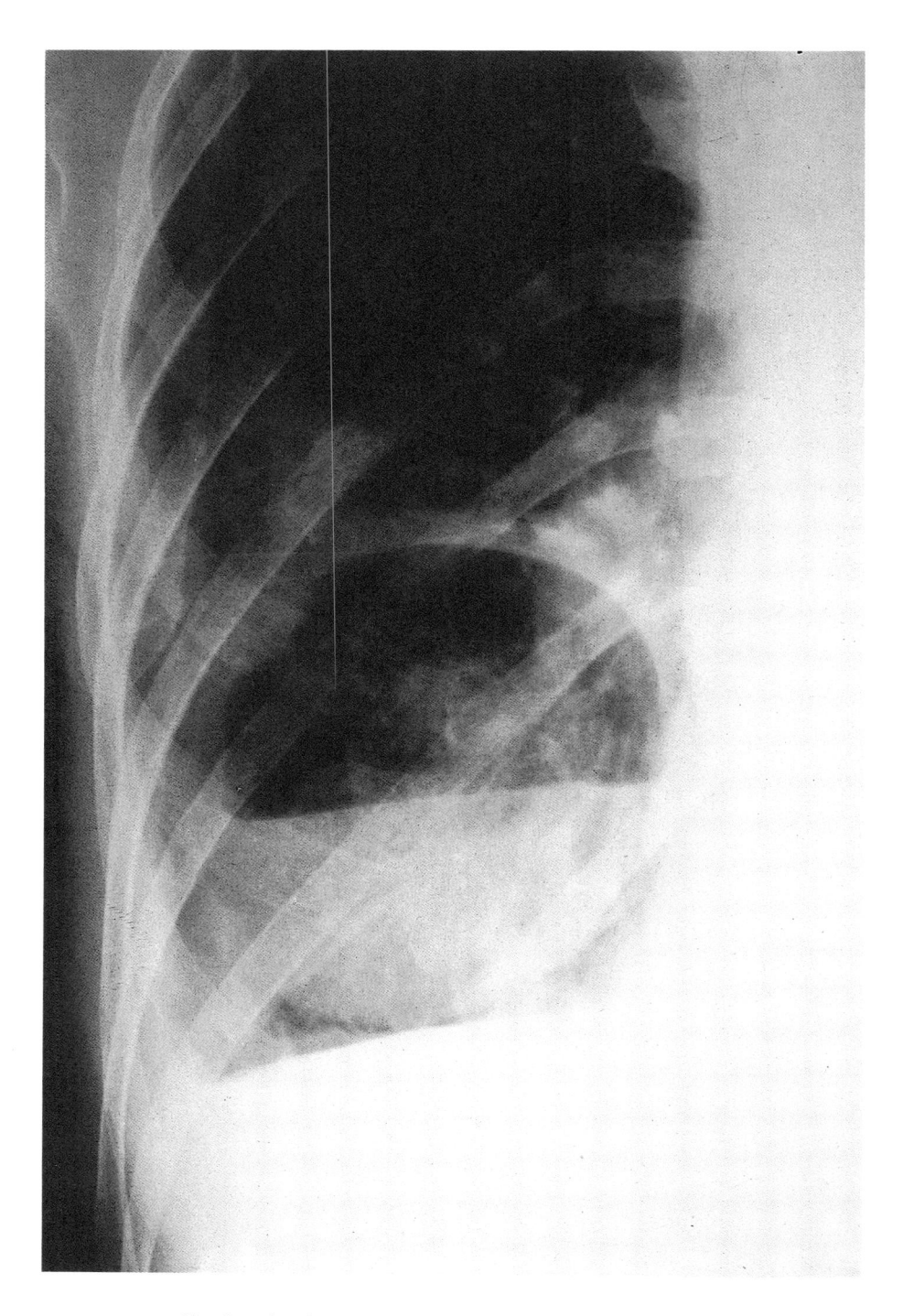

She has had an aortic valve replacement. A large cavity is present in the right lower lobe. Its wall is thick but smooth, and it contains a fluid level. The diagnosis is a lung abscess. The sputum contained *Klebsiella*.

Q62

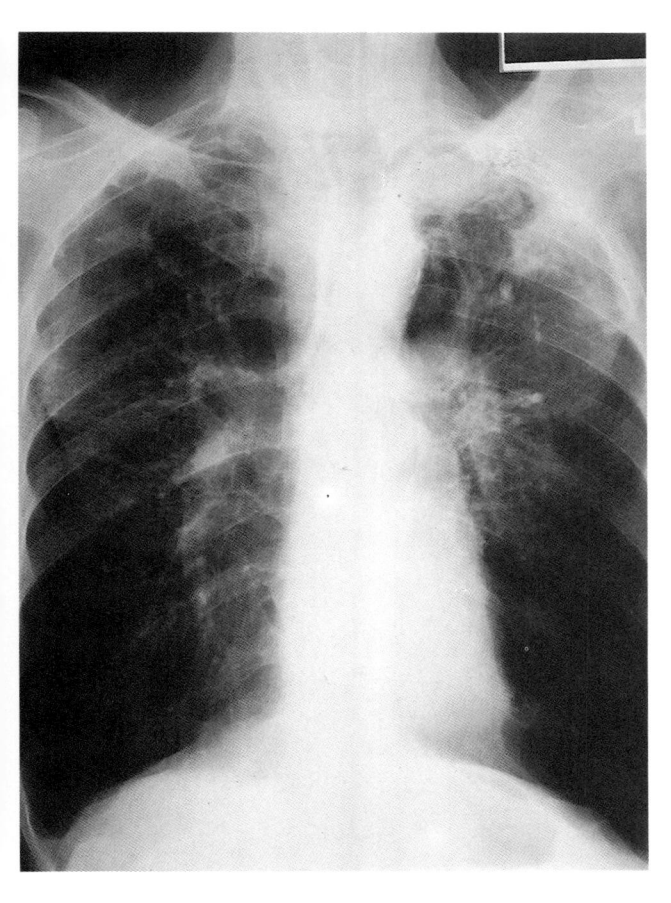

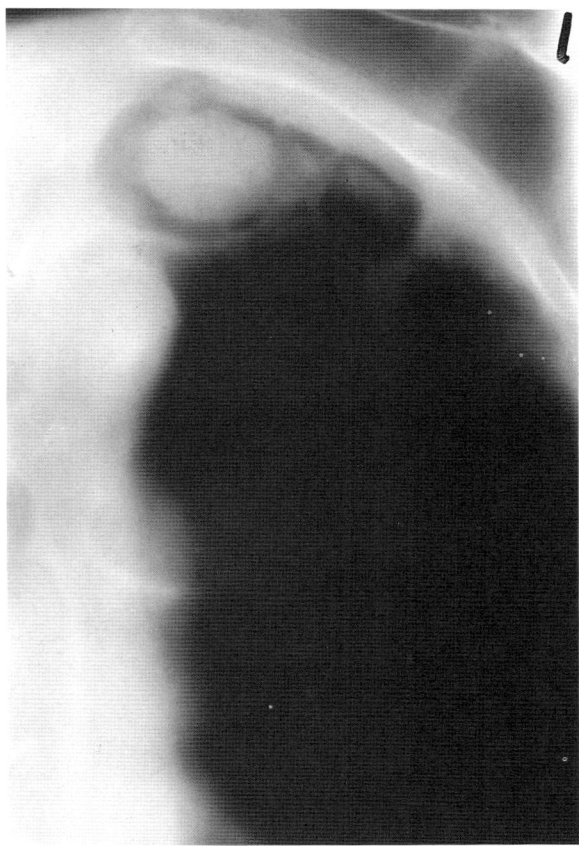

A 71-year-old man presented with chronic cough and recent haemoptysis.

- Is there any evidence of chronic obstructive airways disease?
- Is there any evidence of previous tuberculosis?
- What does the tomogram show?
- What is the diagnosis?

A62

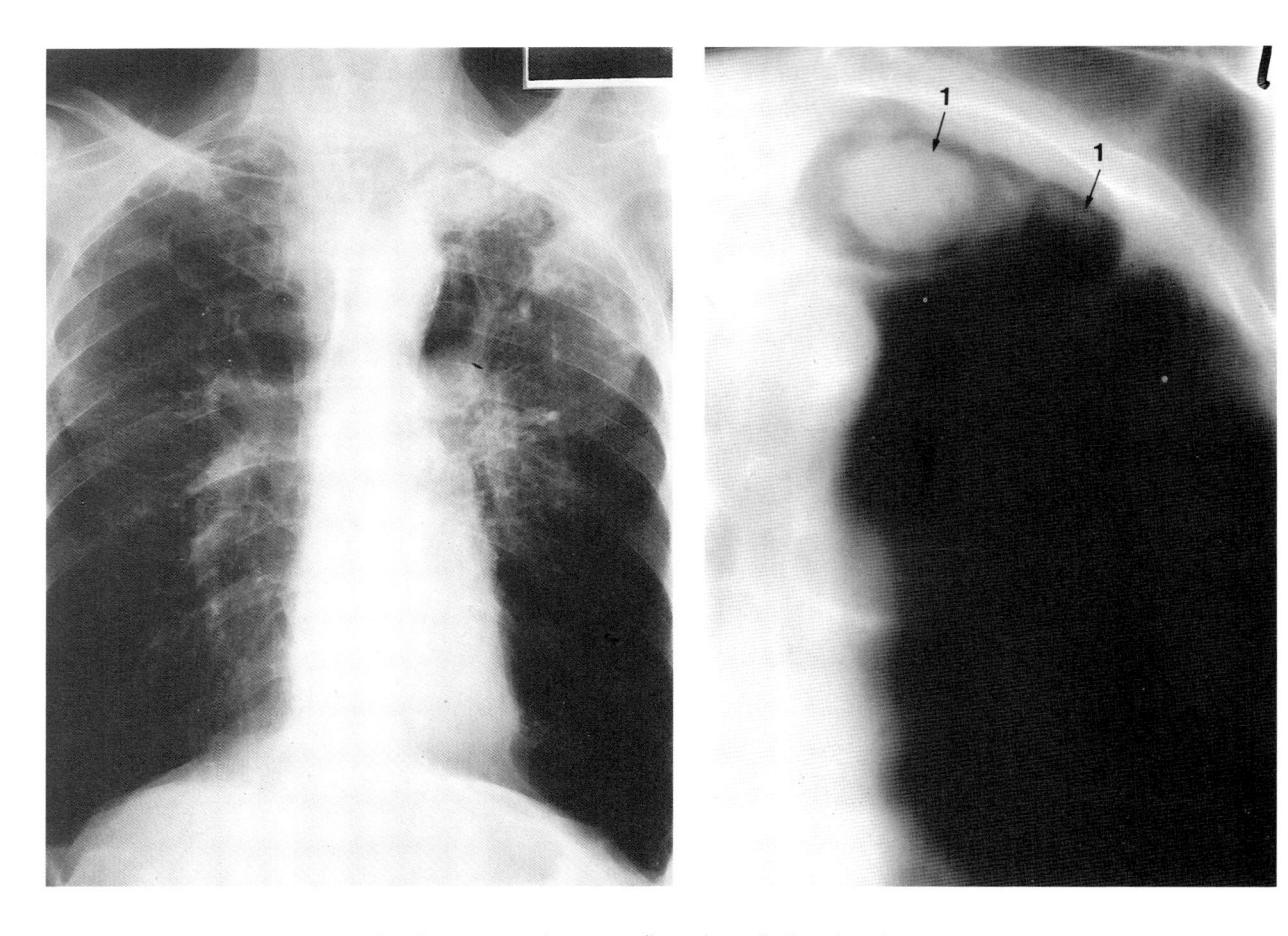

The lungs are hyperinflated and the diaphragm is low and flat. Attenuation of the vascular markings in the lower zones indicates emphysema. Enlargement of the central pulmonary arteries suggests pulmonary arterial hypertension.

There is also evidence of previous tuberculosis. The hila are elevated due to upper lobe fibrosis. The tomogram shows smooth-walled cavities at the right apex. Round masses (1) are present within these cavities. Pleural thickening is present over the lung apex. The diagnosis is mycetomas or fungus balls. They are caused by aspergillus colonising chronic pulmonary cavities.

Q63

Left heart failure may cause pulmonary venous hypertension, which on the CXR may show as:

a) Redistribution of blood flow.
b) Signs of interstitial pulmonary oedema.
c) Signs of alveolar pulmonary oedema.
d) Pleural effusion.

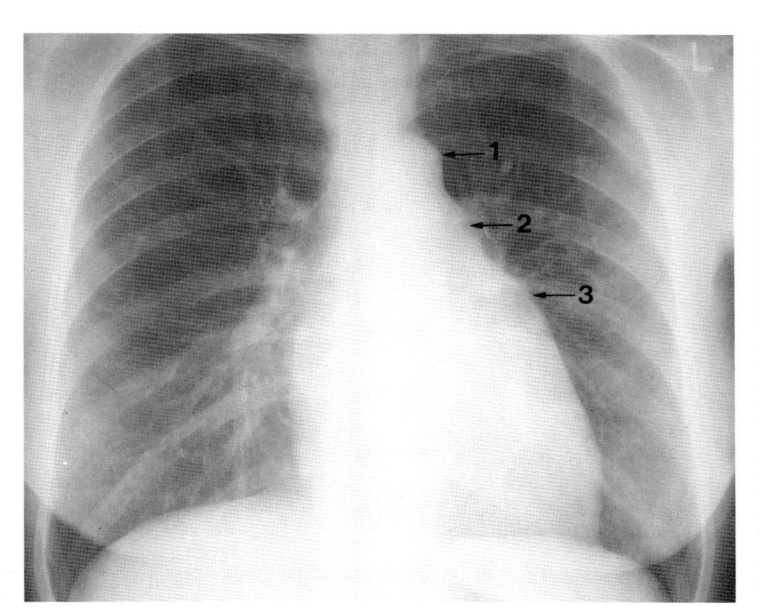

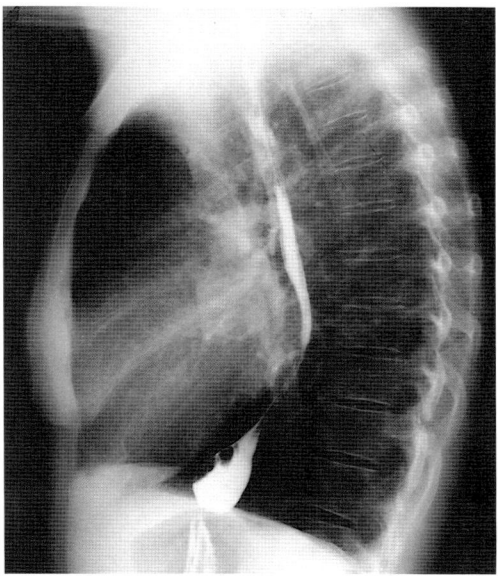

Examine the CXR of this 41-year-old woman with dyspnoea on exercise.

- Is there evidence of pulmonary venous hypertension?
- What are structures (1-3)?

The lateral film was taken with barium in the oesophagus.

- What does it show, and how else could this information be obtained?
- What is the diagnosis?

A63

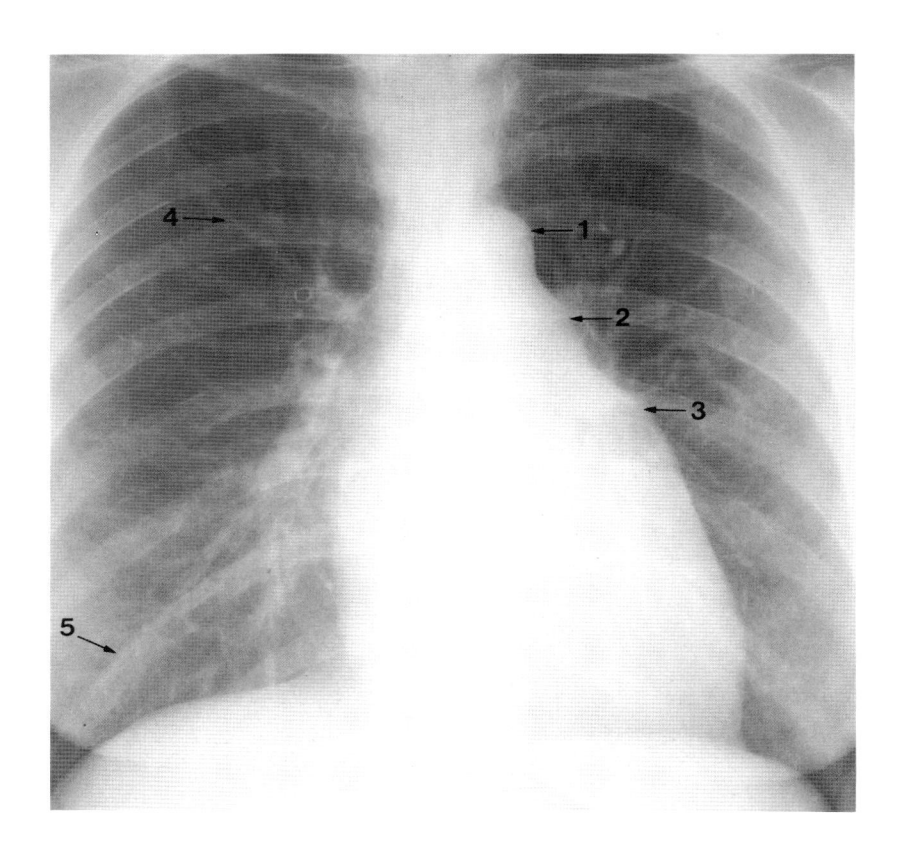

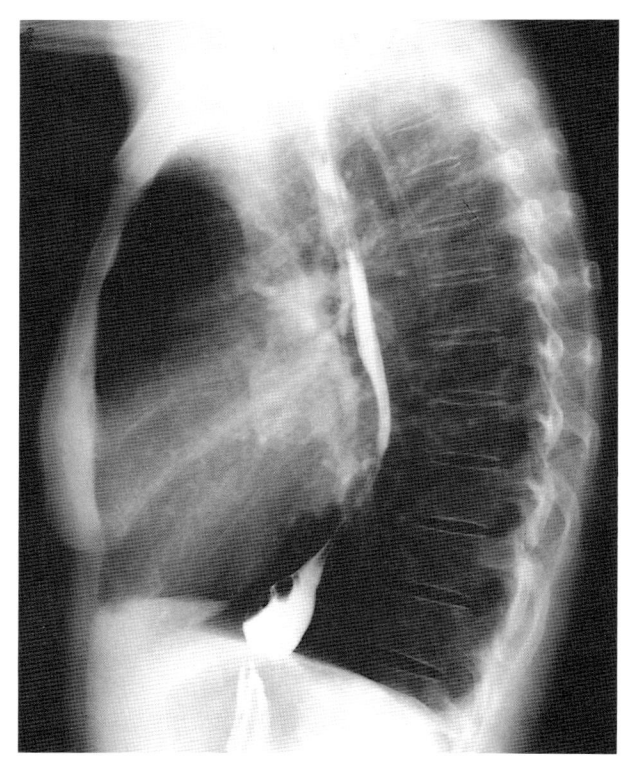

There is evidence of pulmonary venous hypertension. The upper zone vessels (4) are similar in size to lower zone vessels (5) at the same distance from the hilum. Normally the lower zone vessels are larger. There is, therefore, redistribution of blood flow. (1) = the aorta; (2) = the pulmonary trunk. It is prominent, suggesting pulmonary arterial hypertension; (3) = an enlarged left atrial appendage.

The lateral film shows that the body of the left atrium is enlarged and is displacing the oesophagus posteriorly. An ultrasound scan would show left atrial enlargement more accurately. The diagnosis is rheumatic mitral valve disease.

Q64

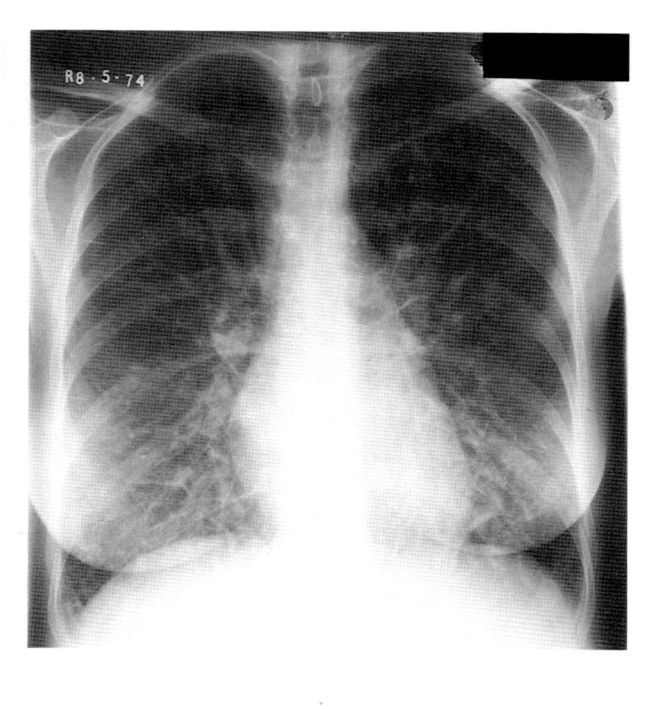

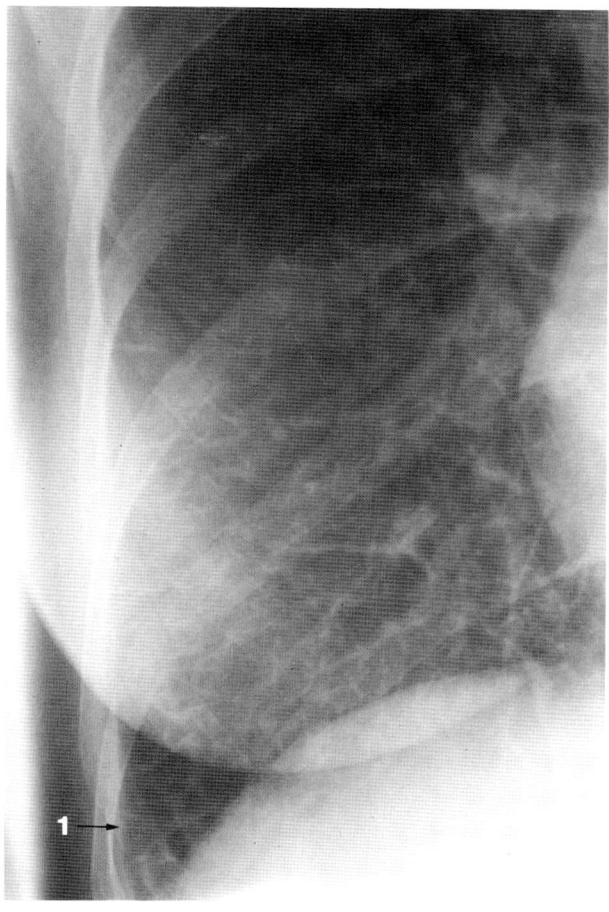

A 33-year-old woman presented with a history of rheumatic fever and recent, progressive dyspnoea.

- What are the linear densities (1) in the periphery of the lower zones?
- What may cause these densities?
- What is the diagnosis in this case?

A64

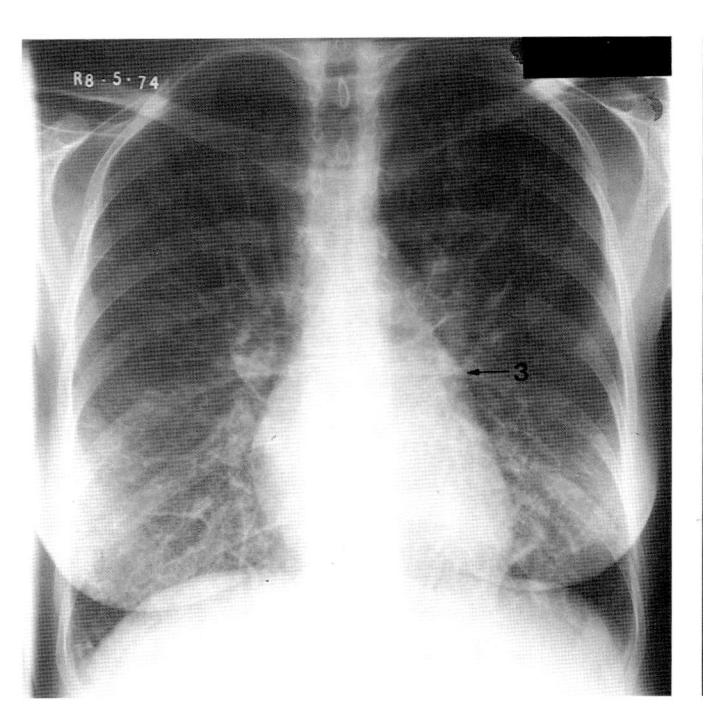

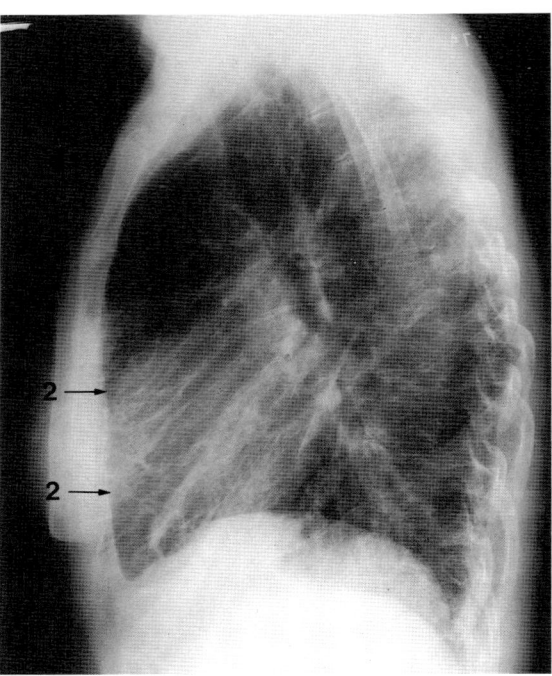

The linear densities in the periphery of the lower zones are interstitial or Kerley B lines. They are also seen retrosternally (2). They are most often seen in interstitial pulmonary oedema, when they are due to fluid collecting in the interlobular septa. Other causes are lymphangitis carcinomatosa, sarcoidosis, and silicosis. The diagnosis in this case is mitral stenosis. Note the enlarged left atrial appendage (3).

Q65

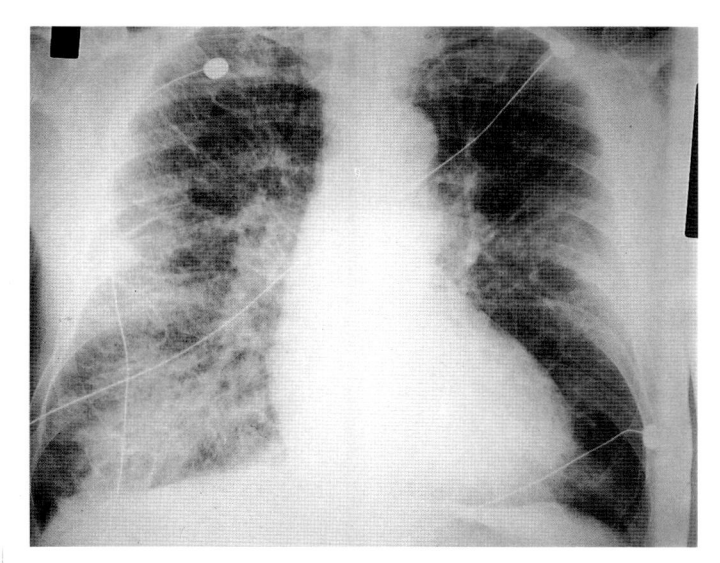

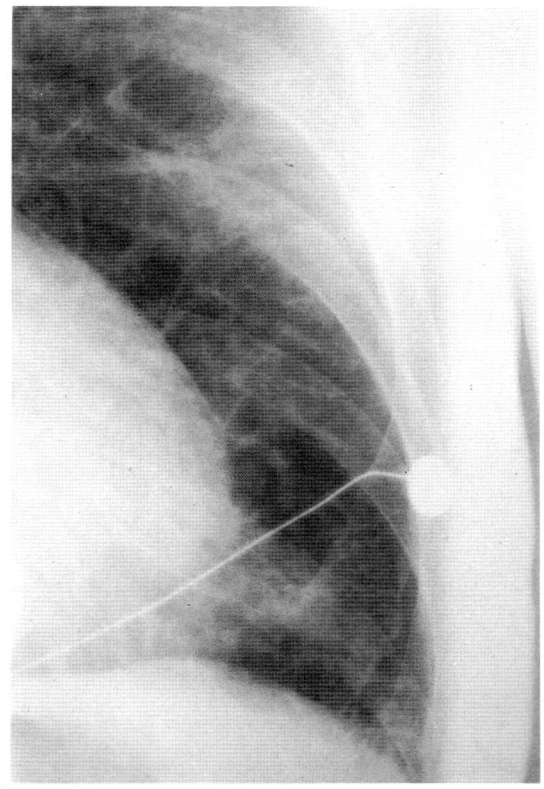

A 76-year-old man presented with acute myocardial infarction.

- Is there any radiological evidence of heart failure?

A65

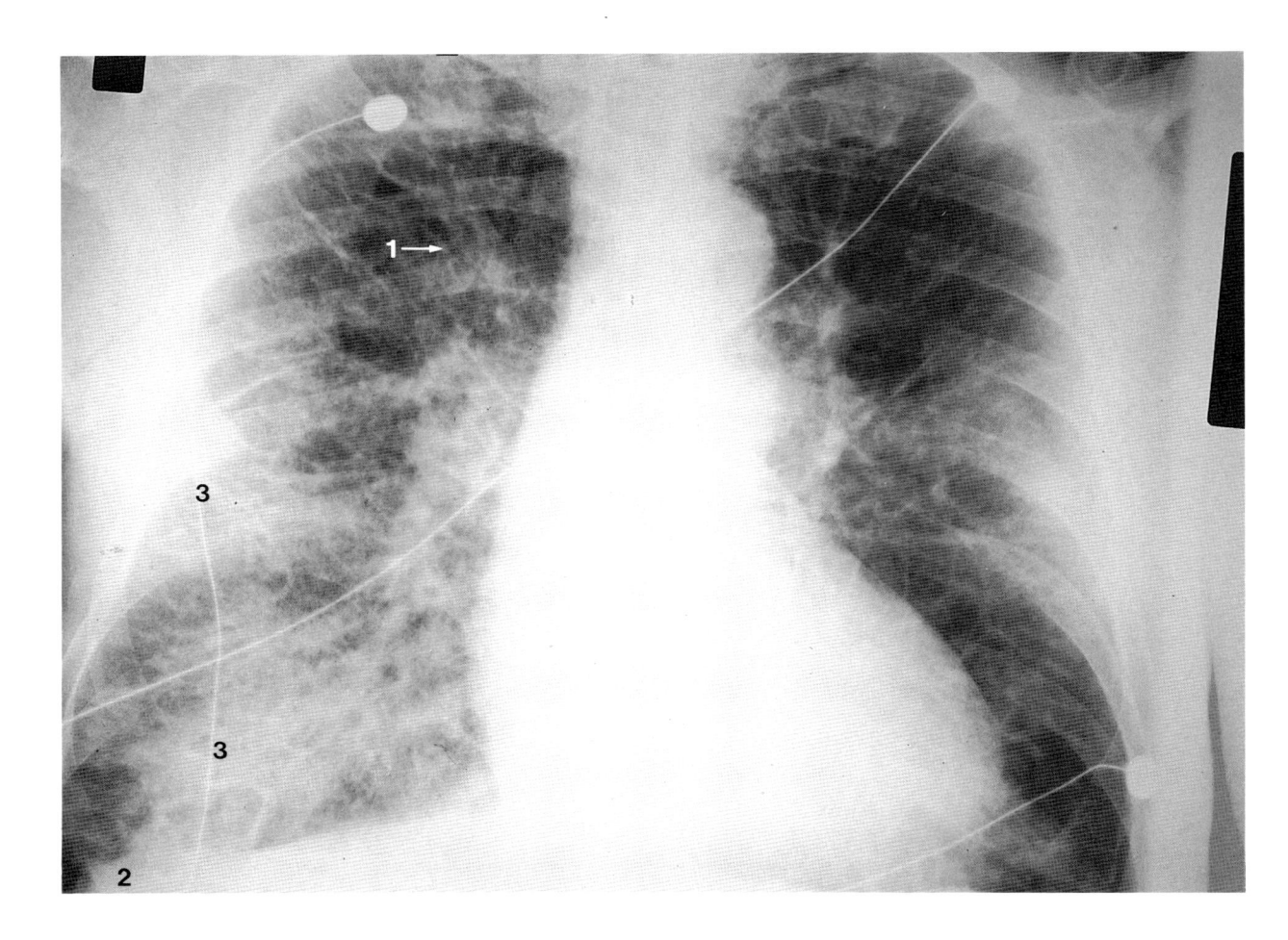

There is evidence of severe pulmonary venous hypertension:

a) The upper zone vessels are distended (1).
b) Interstitial lines are present at both bases (2).
c) Areas of consolidation (3) indicate alveolar pulmonary oedema.

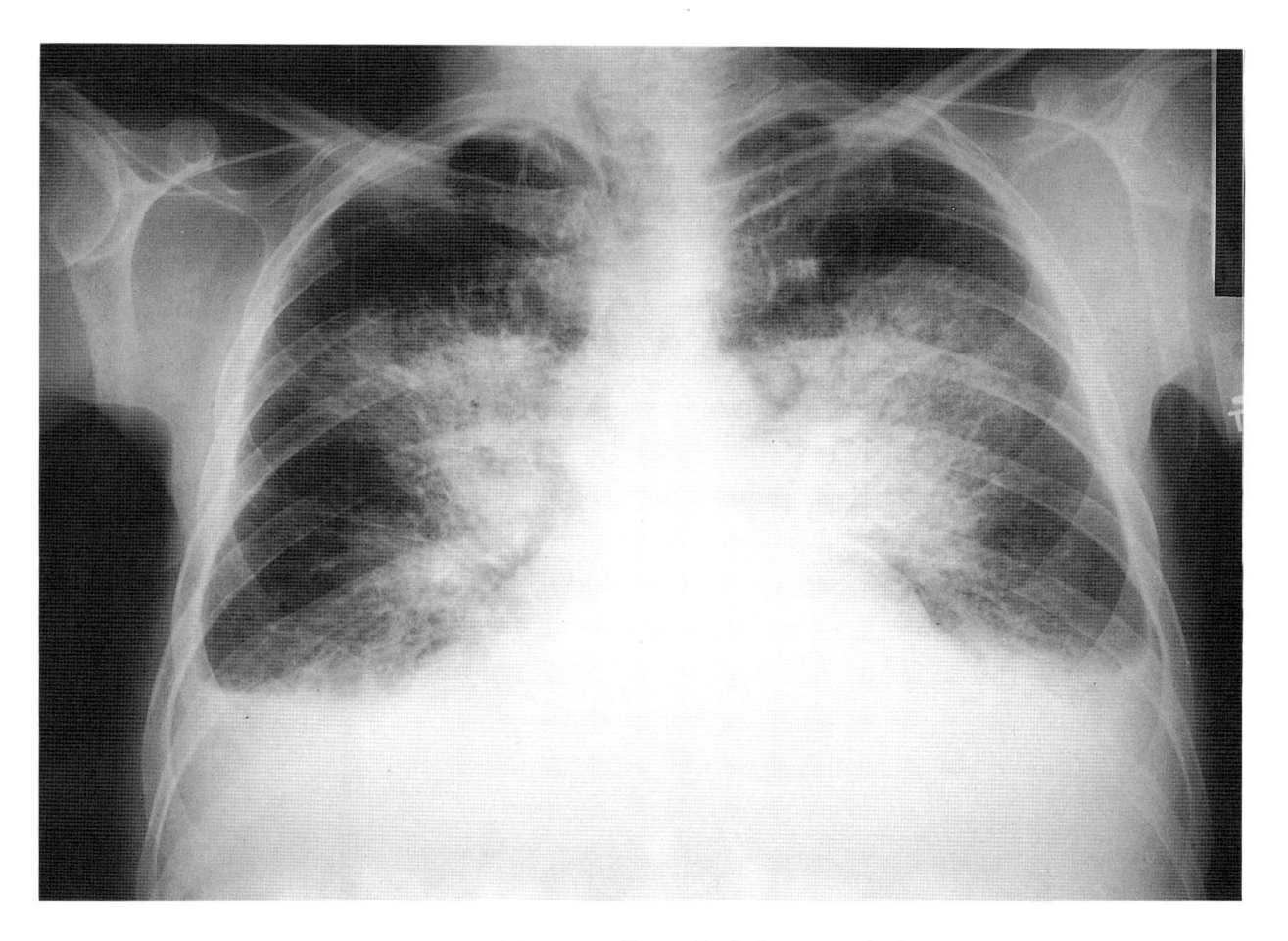

A 51-year-old man collapsed while at work, having complained of acute chest pain.

- What abnormalities are seen in the lungs?
- Is the heart size normal?
- What is the diagnosis?

A66

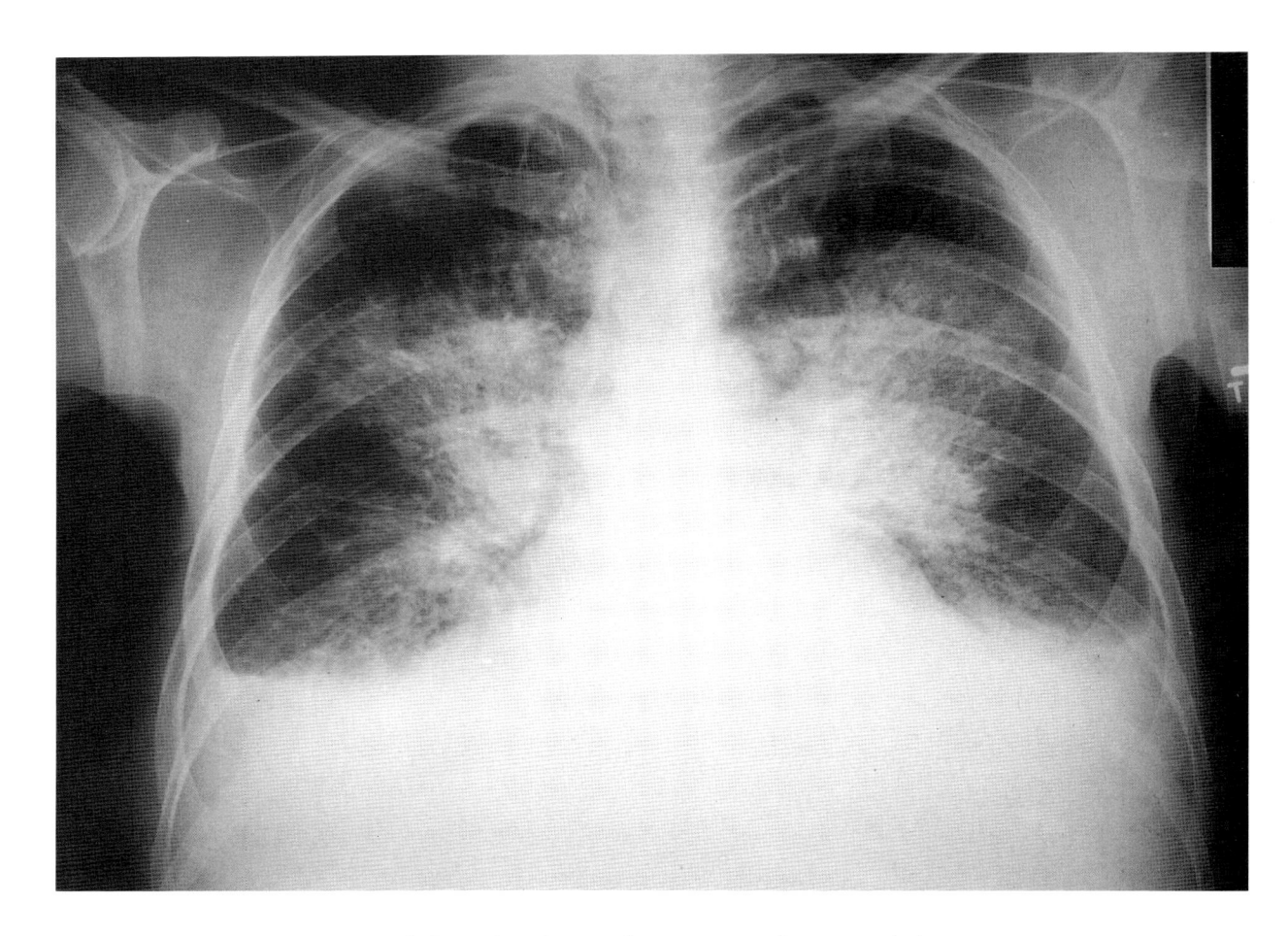

Perihilar alveolar pulmonary oedema and bilateral pleural effusions are seen. The heart size is normal. The diagnosis is acute myocardial infarction. The combination of severe pulmonary oedema and normal heart size suggests either an acute cardiac event or non-cardiogenic pulmonary oedema.

Q67

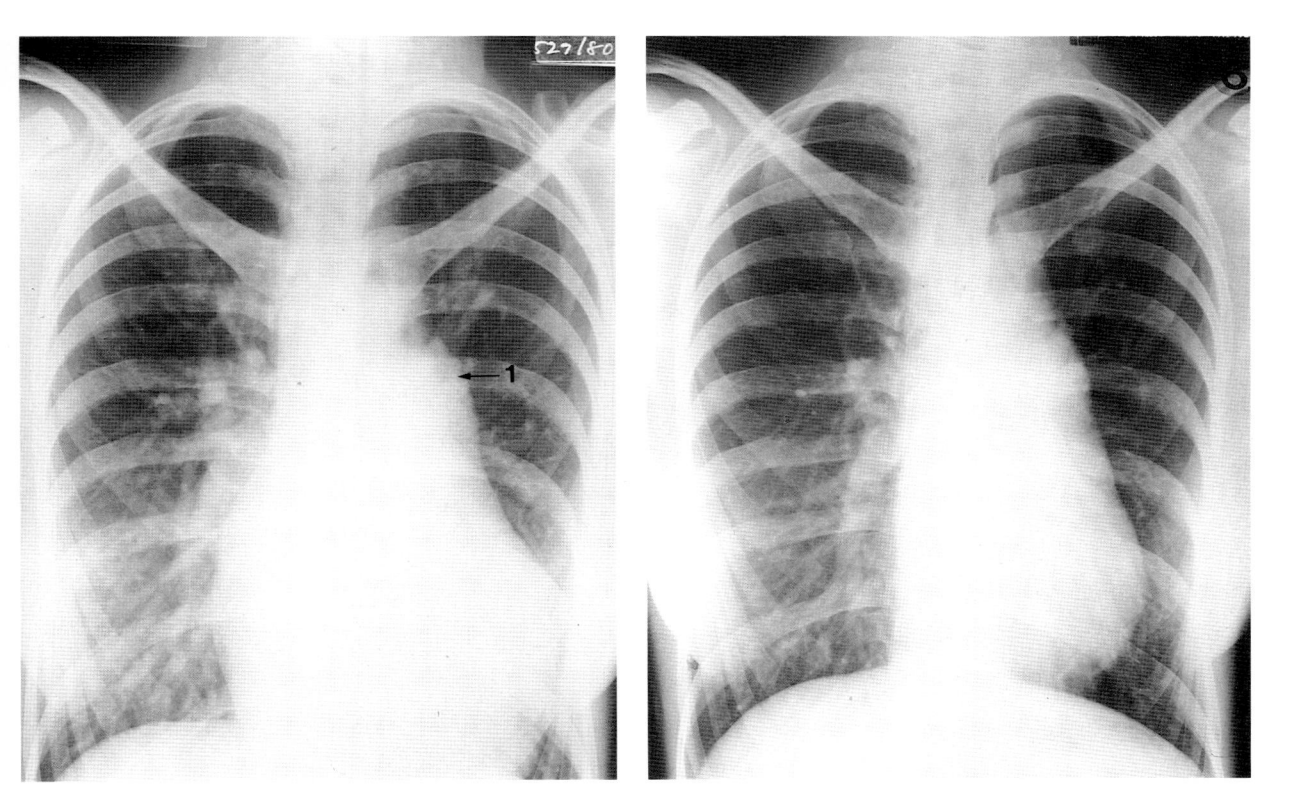

A 22-year-old female was asymptomatic. At a routine medical examination, a systolic murmur was heard at the left sternal edge. There was no evidence of cyanosis. Compare the CXRs taken before and after surgery. On the pre-operative film:

- Is the pulmonary vascular pattern normal?
- What is this structure (1)?
- Is the heart size normal?
- What was the operation?

A67

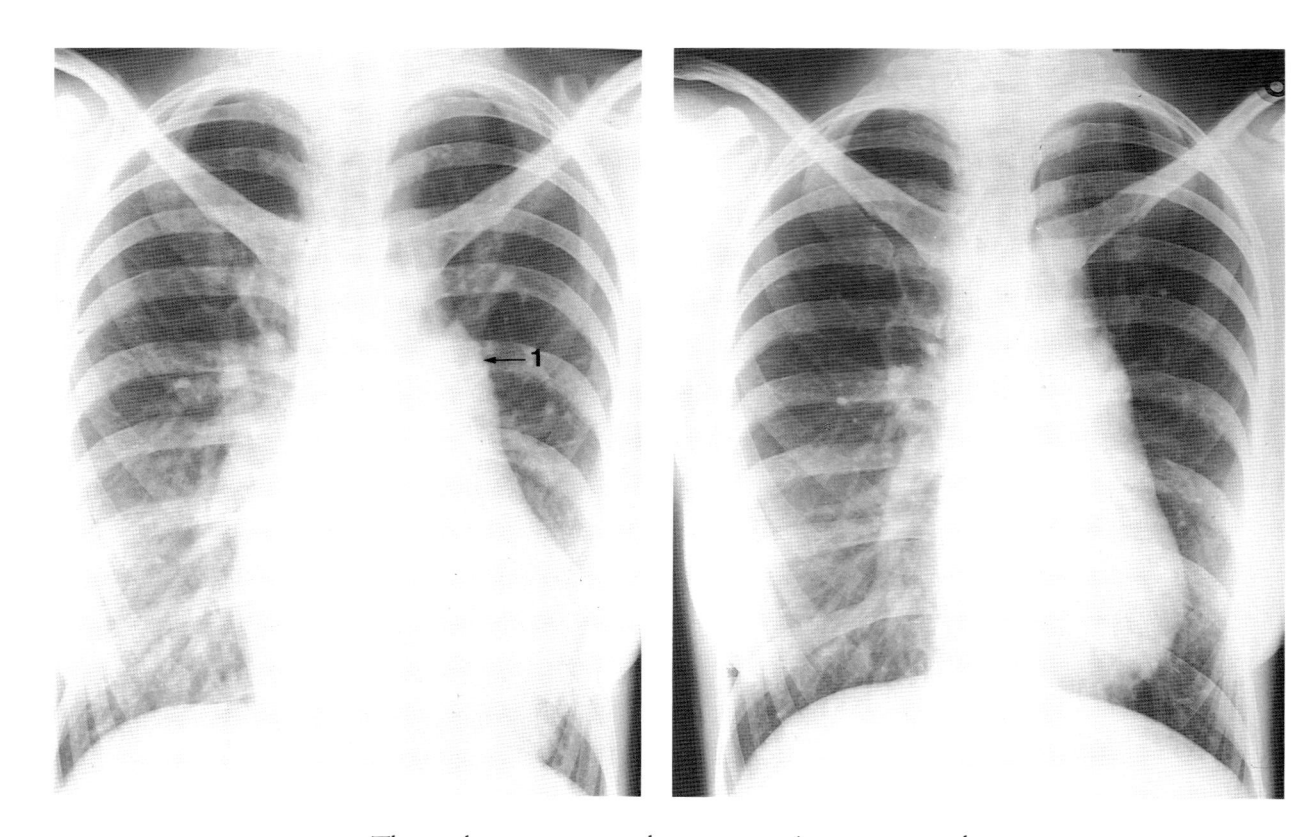

The pulmonary vascular pattern is not normal. There is pulmonary plethora, indicating increased blood flow through the lungs. (1) = the pulmonary trunk. It is enlarged due to increased flow. The heart is enlarged. The operation was closure of an atrial septal defect. On the post-operative film the pulmonary plethora has diminished, and the heart size has decreased.

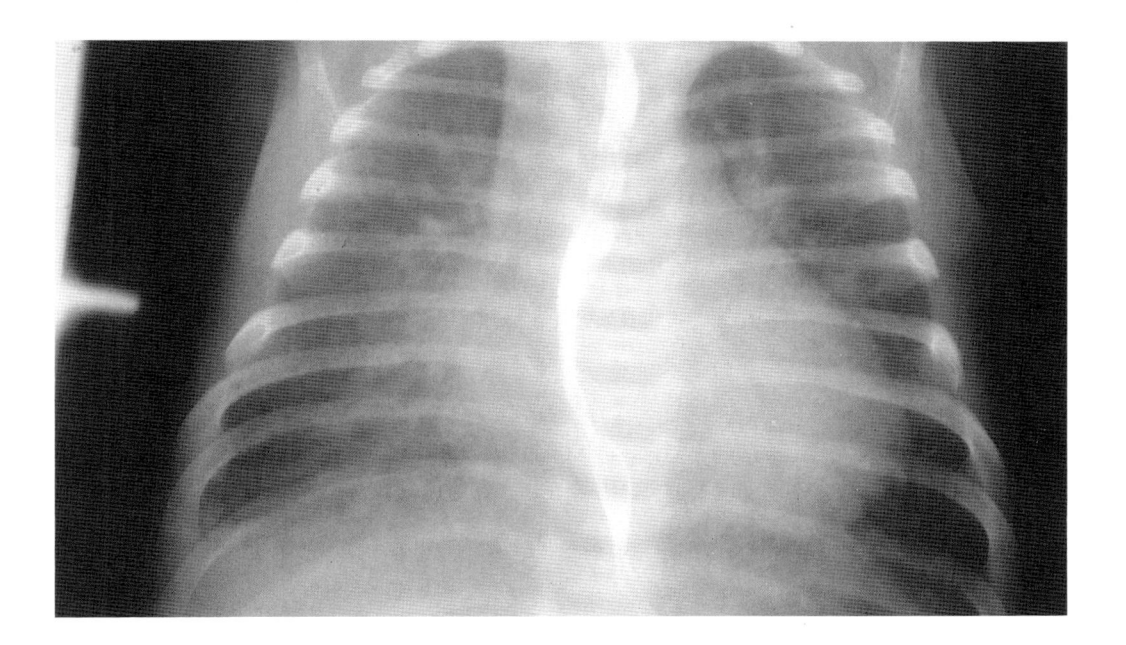

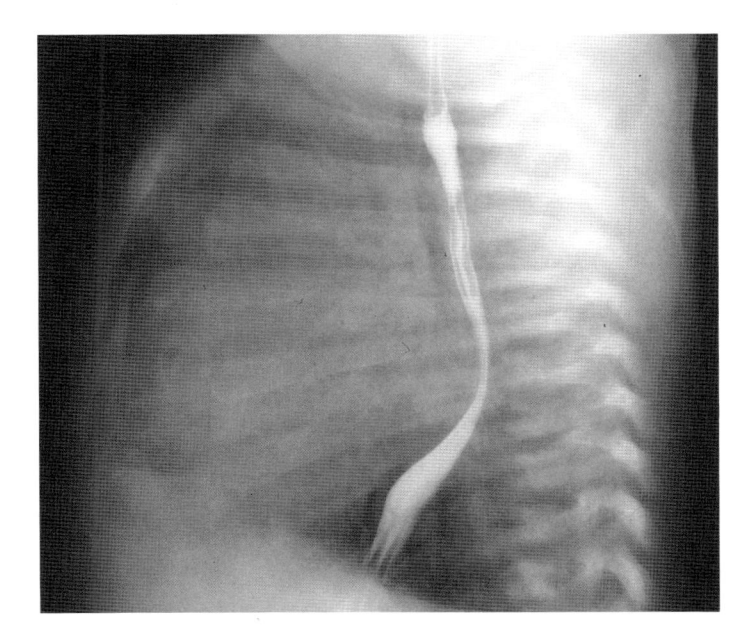

A two-and-a-half-month-old child presented with a pan-systolic murmur. The child was not cyanosed.

- Is there an intracardiac shunt?
- Barium is present in the oesophagus. What does it show?
- What is the diagnosis?

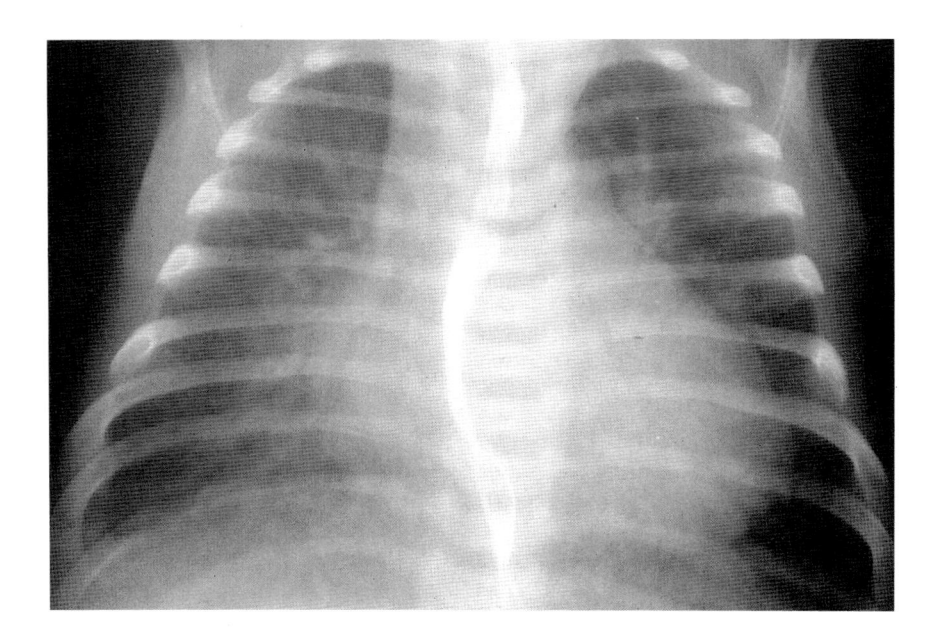

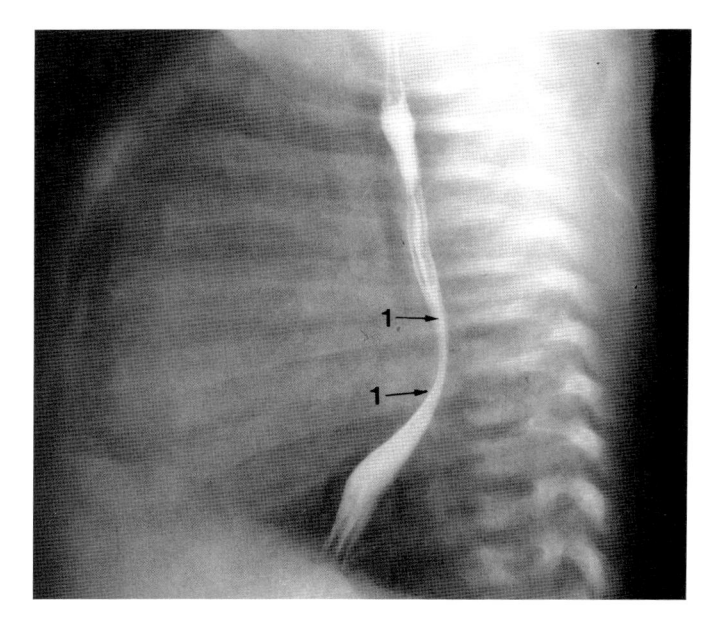

Pulmonary plethora is present and indicates increased flow through the lungs. Since the child is not cyanosed this must be due to a left-to-right shunt. Enlargement of the left atrium (1) is causing posterior displacement of the barium-filled oesophagus. In the presence of a left-to-right shunt, left atrial enlargement indicates that the atrial septum is intact. The diagnosis is ventricular septal defect.

Q69

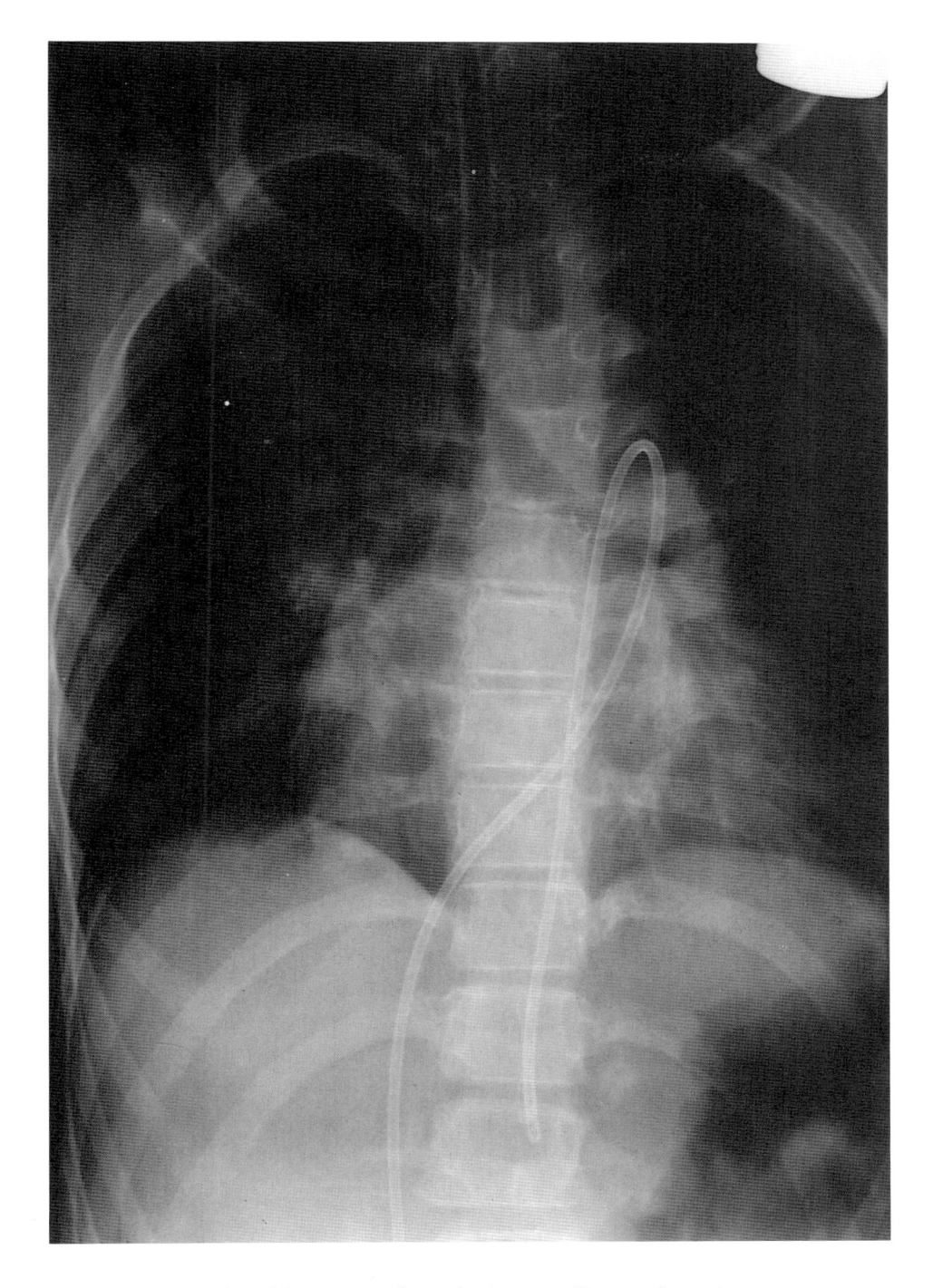

This film was taken during cardiac catheterisation.

- What route is the catheter taking?
- What is the diagnosis?

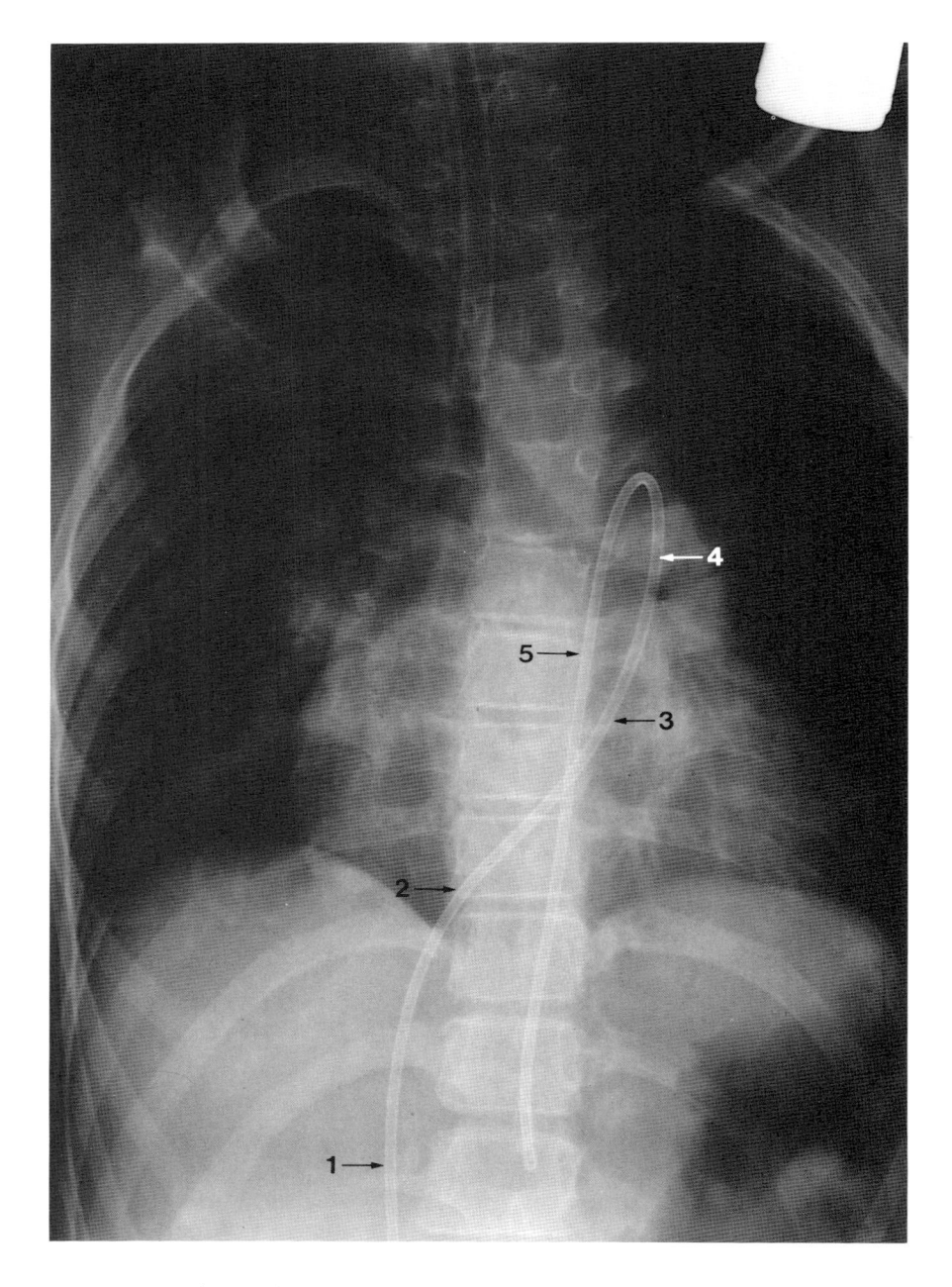

The catheter has been introduced via a femoral vein. It is passing from inferior vena cava (1), through the right atrium (2) and tricuspid valve, and into the right ventricle (3), and then into the pulmonary trunk (4), and finally into the descending aorta (5). The diagnosis is patent ductus arteriosus. If the ductus arteriosus were not patent, the catheter could not have passed from pulmonary artery to descending aorta.

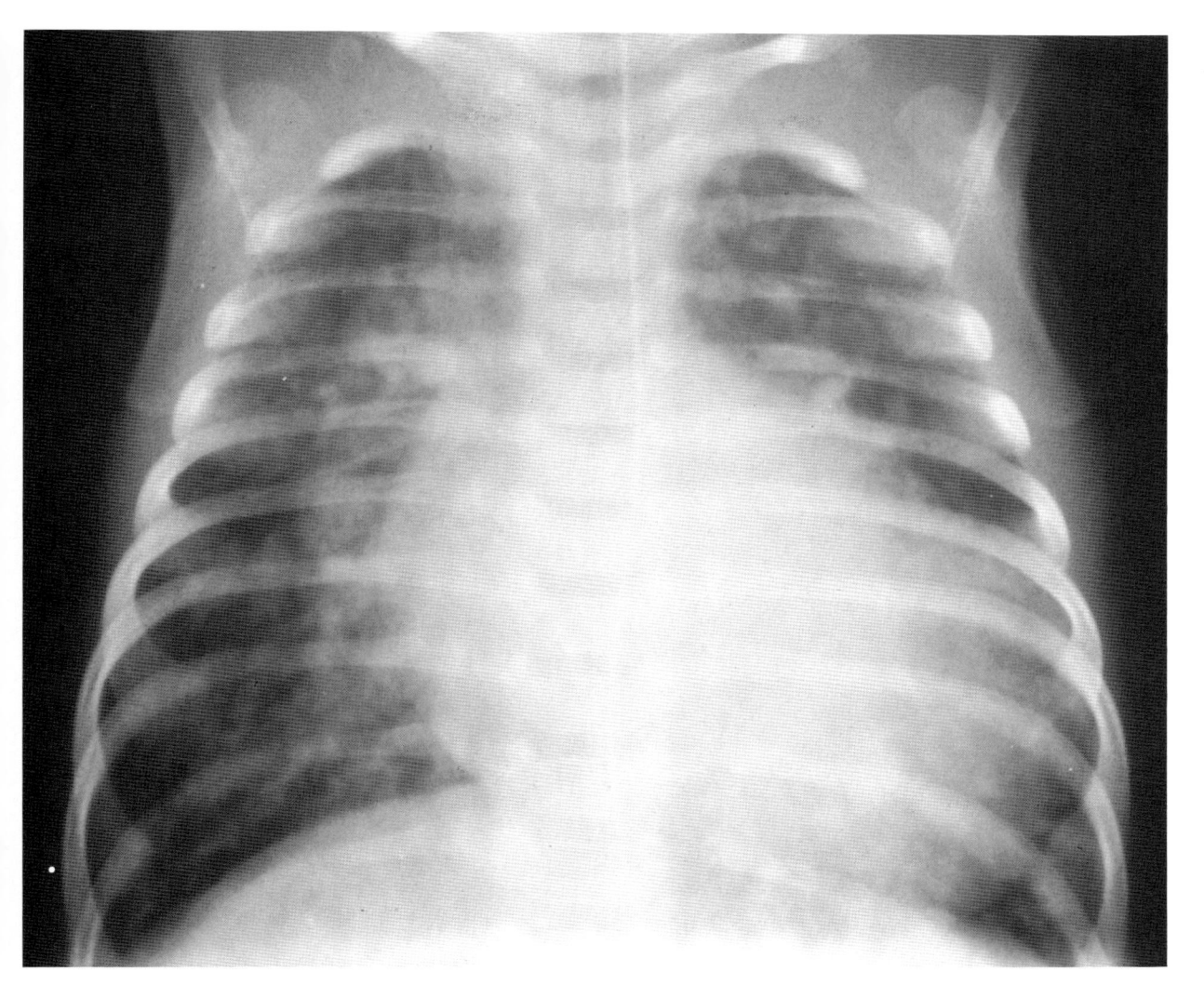

A 2-day old child presented with cyanosis and tachypnoea.

- Is the pulmonary blood flow normal?
- Why is the child cyanosed?
- Comment on the pulmonary trunk.
- What is the diagnosis?

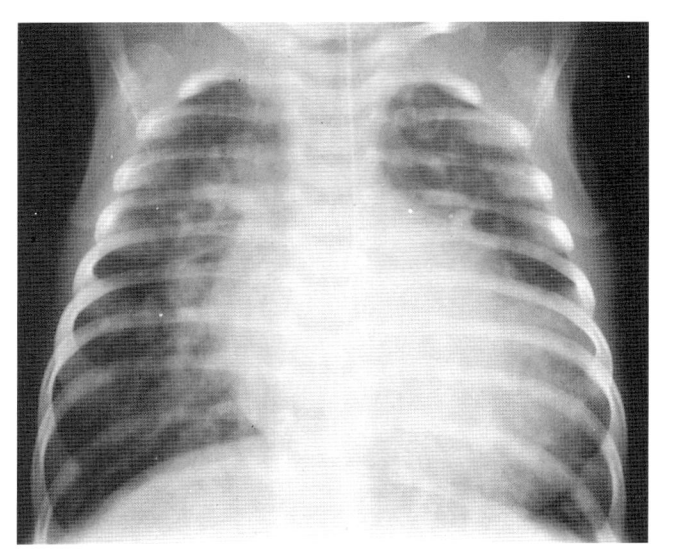

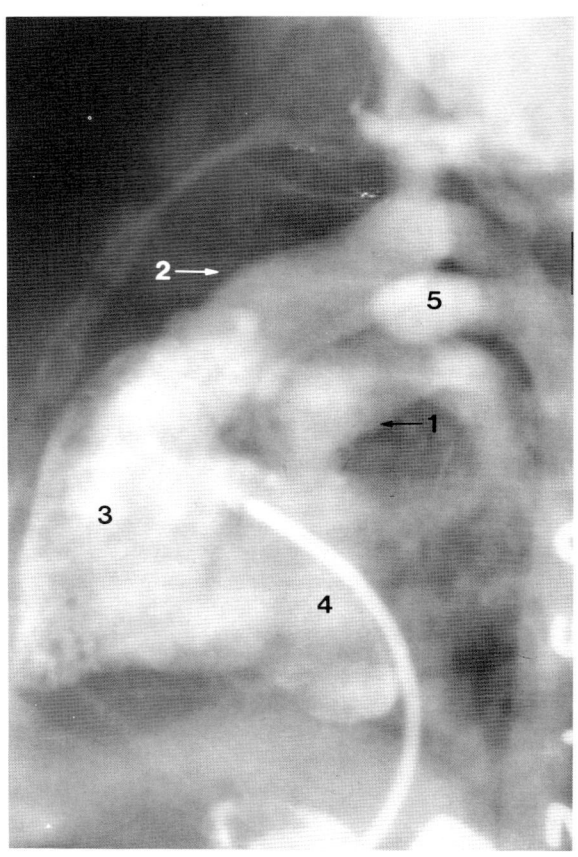

There is pulmonary plethora. The combination of pulmonary plethora and cyanosis means that there is mixing of venous and arterial blood and bi-directional shunting. The pulmonary trunk is not visible. The angiogram shows that the pulmonary trunk (1) is immediately posterior to the aorta (2).

The diagnosis is transposition of the great arteries. The aorta (2) arises anteriorly from the right ventricle (3), and the pulmonary trunk (1) arises from the left ventricle (4). A ventricular septal defect is present, and there is also a patent ductus arteriosus (5).

Q71

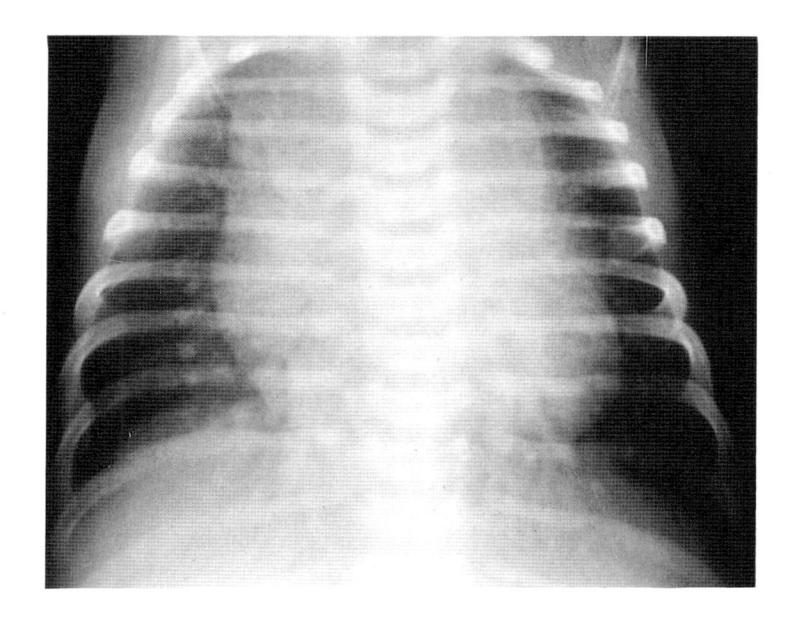

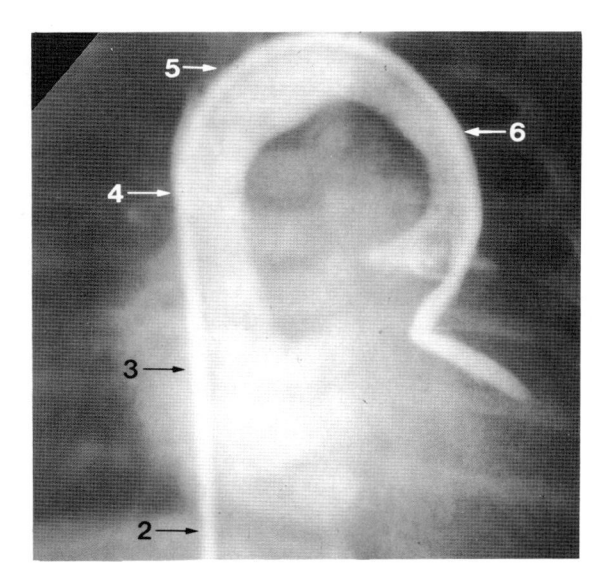

A 6-month-old child presented with failure to thrive and cyanosis.

- Is the pulmonary vascularity normal?
- Comment on the cardiovascular silhouette.
- Describe the route of the catheter in the angiogram.
- Are the systemic veins normal?
- What is the diagnosis?

A71

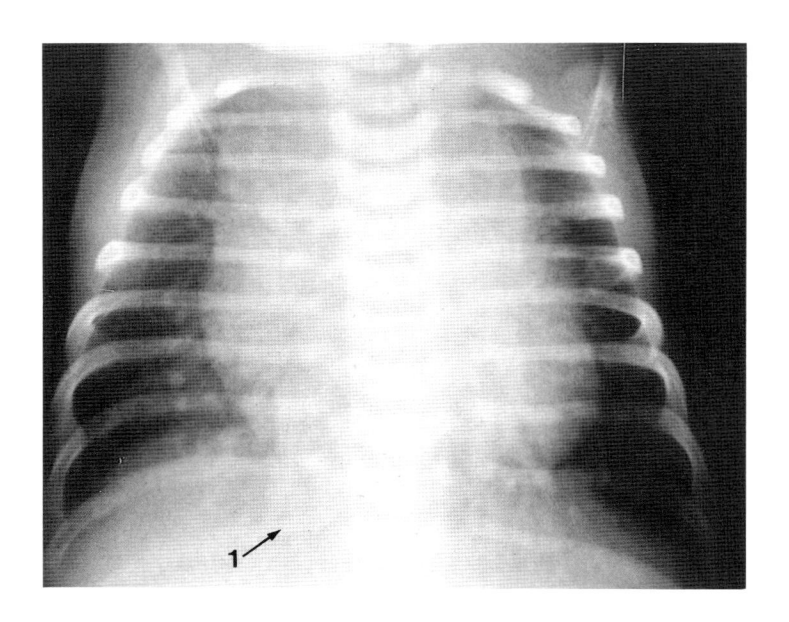

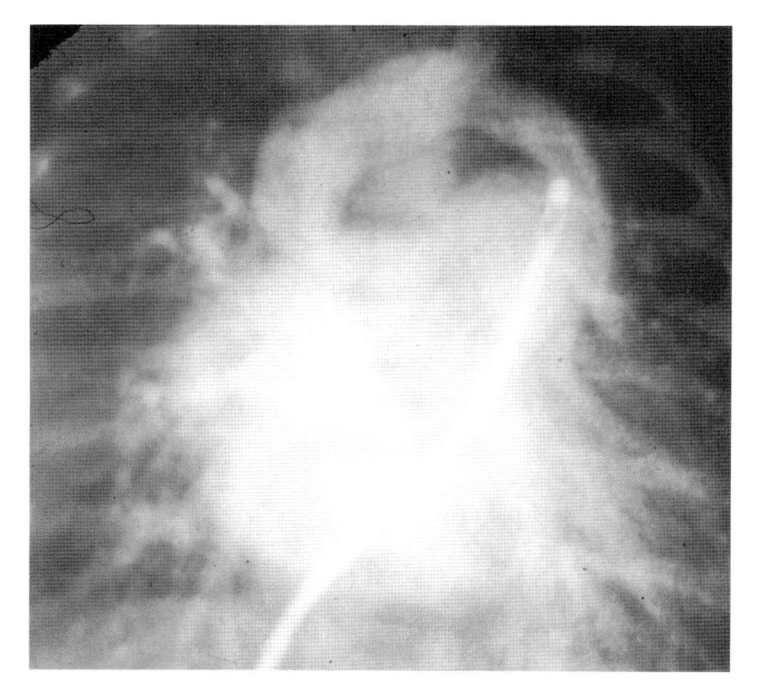

There is pulmonary plethora. The lower lobe vessels (1) are enlarged. The superior mediastinum is widened.

The catheter has been introduced from a femoral vein. It passes from inferior vena cava (2), through the right atrium (3), into the superior vena cava (4), innominate vein (5), and into a persistent left superior vena cava (6).

The systemic veins are dilated, accounting for the widening of the superior mediastinum. The angiogram on this page is the venous phase of the pulmonary arteriogram. It shows the venous return of both lungs into the persistent left SVC and then to innominate vein, right SVC and right atrium. The diagnosis is total anomalous pulmonary venous return.

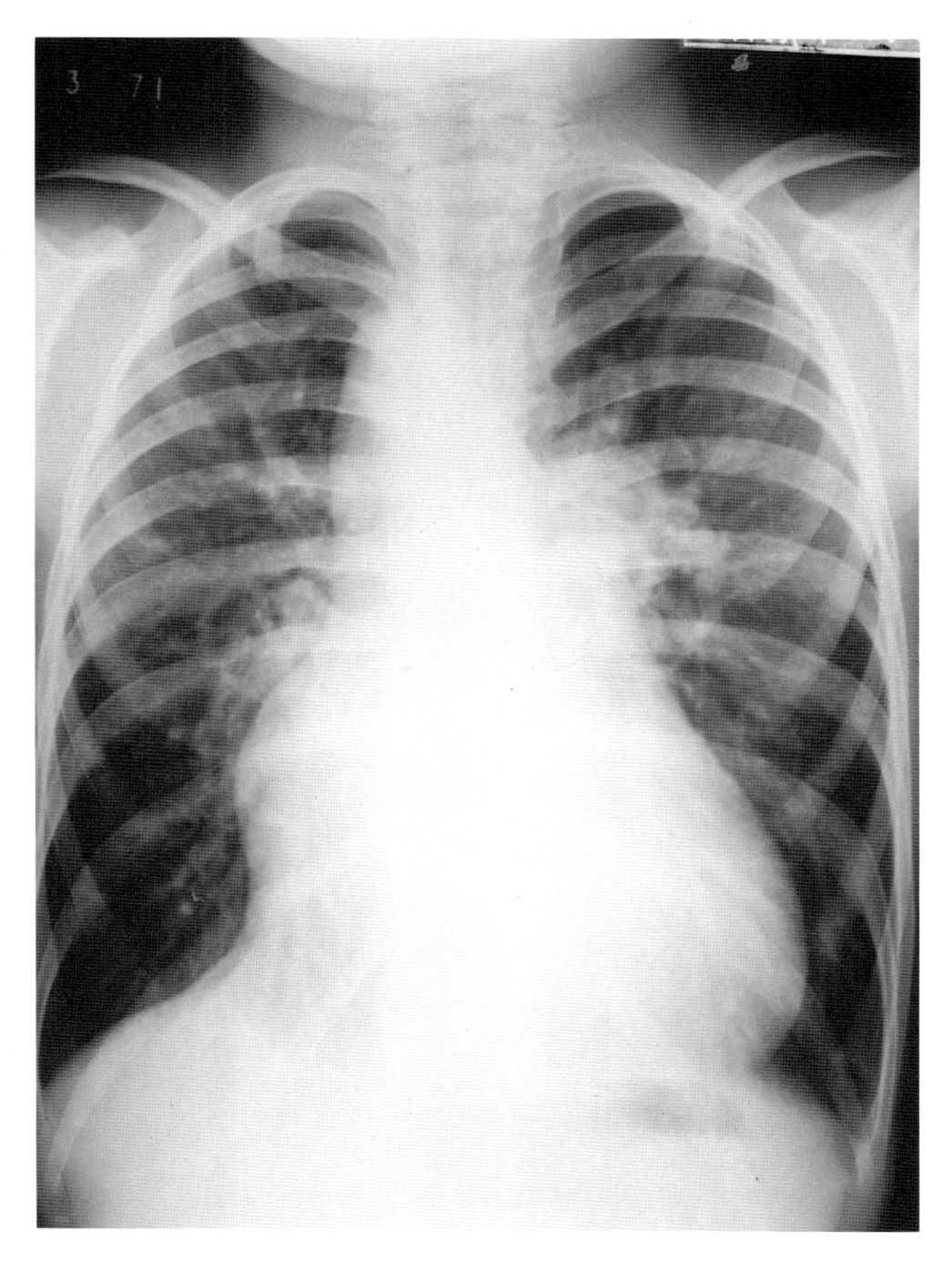

A 9-year-old male was cyanosed since birth.

- Describe the pulmonary vascularity.
- Is the aortic arch normal?
- What is the diagnosis?

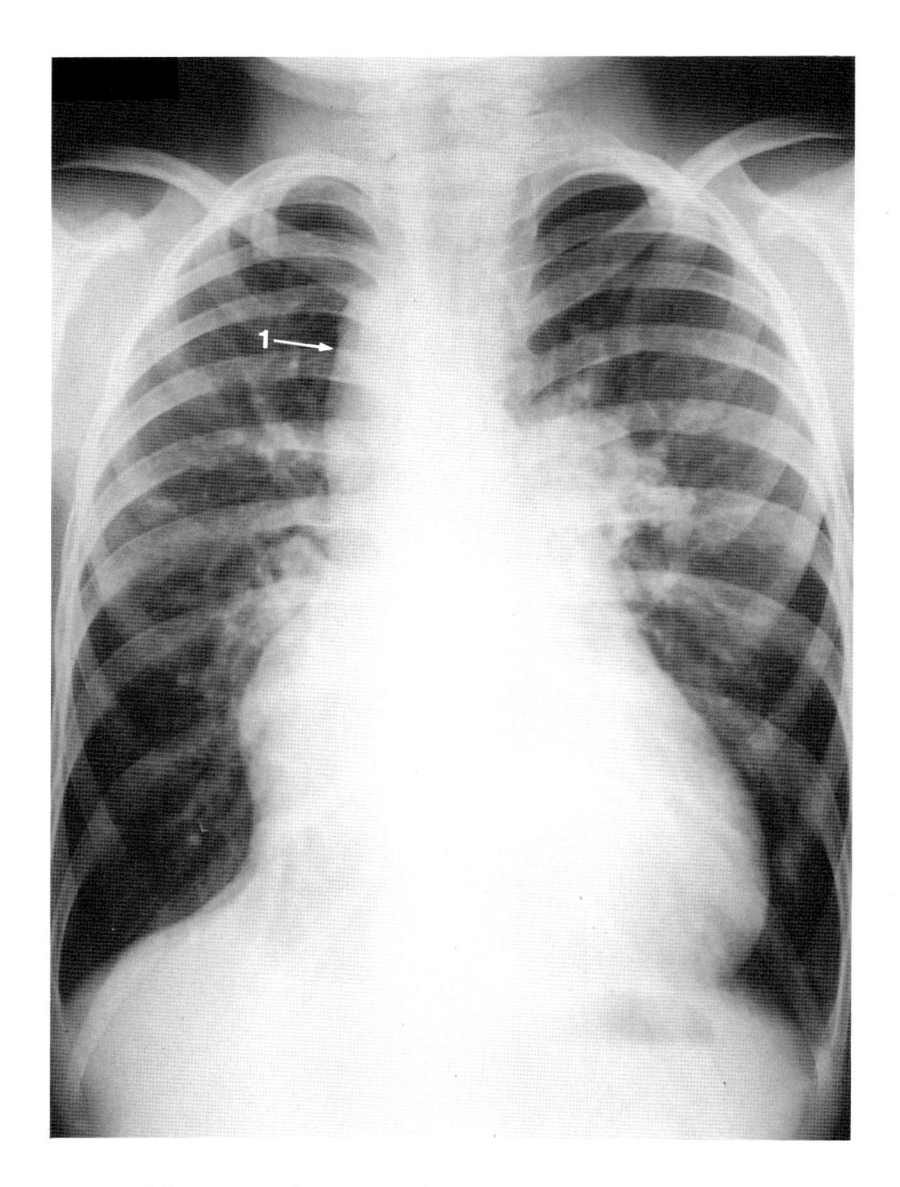

There is pulmonary plethora. The aortic arch is right-sided (1). The diagnosis is truncus arteriosus. Fifty per cent of cases of truncus arteriosus have a right-sided aortic arch.

Right-sided aortic arch may occur without heart disease. It is also seen in:

a) Tetralogy of Fallot (25 per cent of cases).
b) Pulmonary atresia (25 per cent of cases).
c) Ventricular septal defect (3 per cent of cases).
d) Truncus arteriosus (50 per cent of cases).

The combination of pulmonary plethora, cyanosis and right arch only occurs in (d).

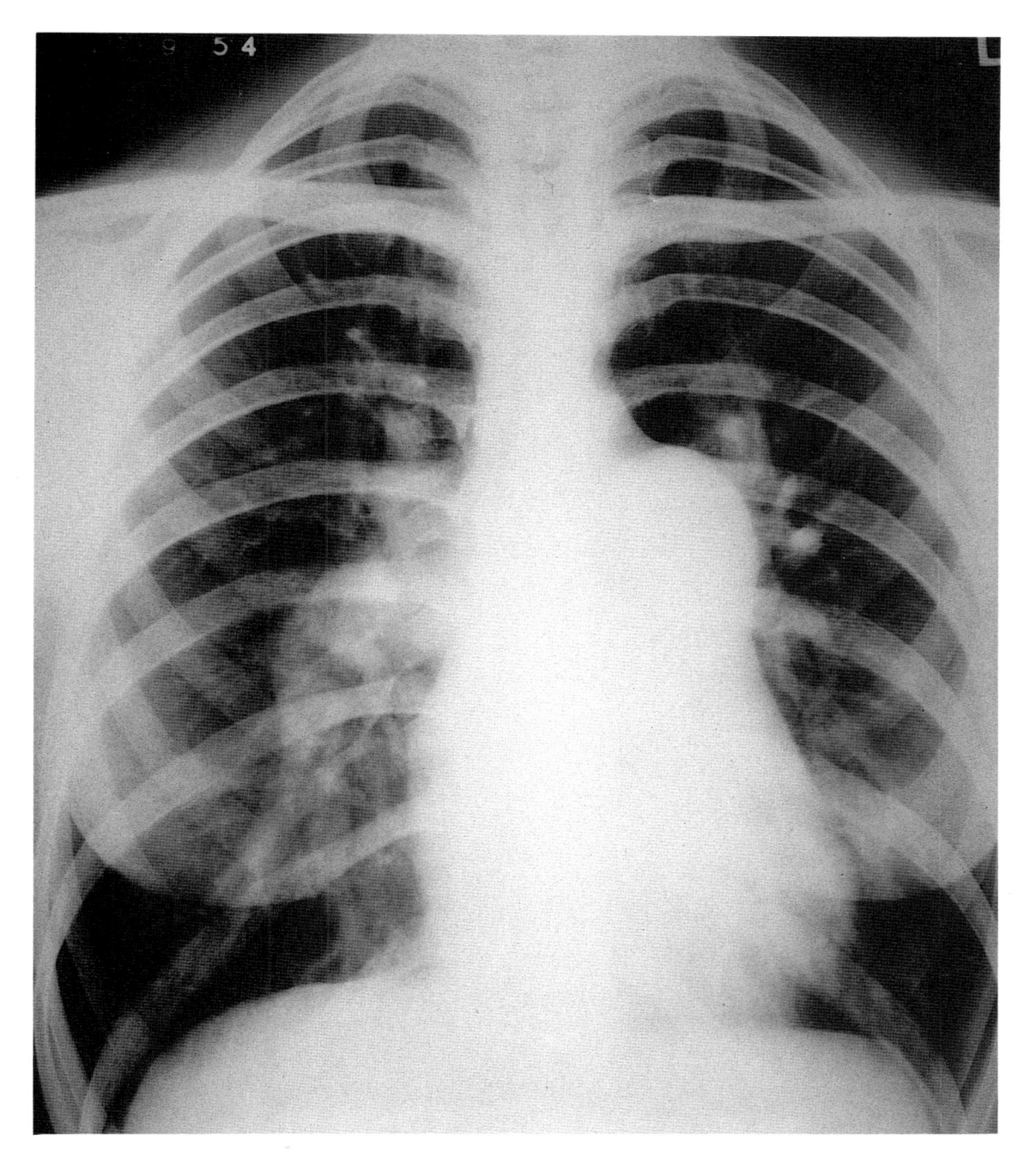

A 28-year-old female presented with progressive dyspnoea, central cyanosis and finger clubbing.

- Comment on the pulmonary vascularity.
- What are its significance and possible causes?
- What is the diagnosis in this case?

A73

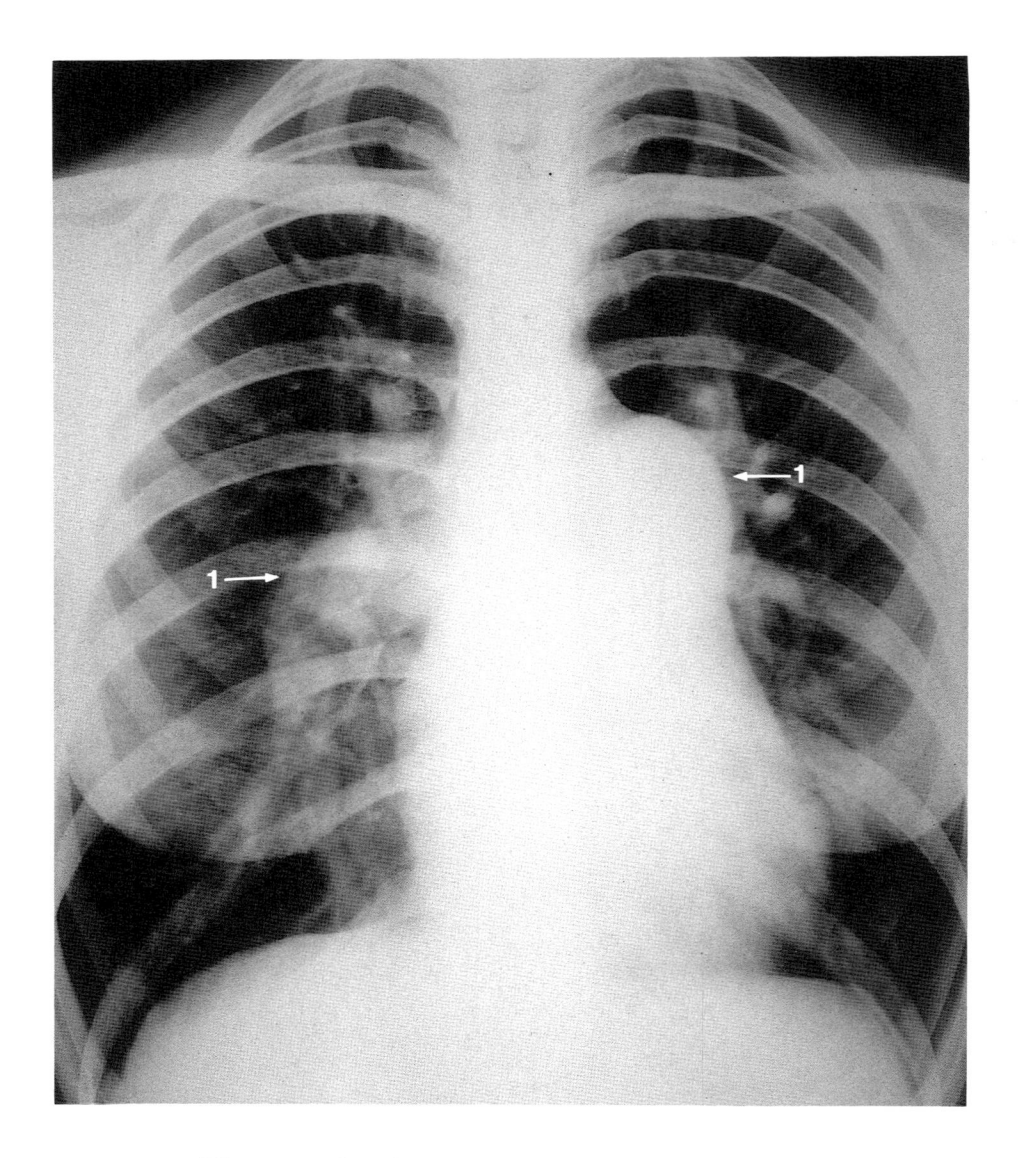

The central pulmonary arteries (1) are dilated, but the peripheral vascular pattern is attenuated. This pattern indicates pulmonary arterial hypertension, which may be due to:

a) Pulmonary venous hypertension.
b) Chronic respiratory disease.
c) Intracardiac shunt.
d) Pulmonary embolism (or other pulmonary arterial occlusive disease).
e) High altitude.
f) Drugs and poisons.

The diagnosis is Eisenmenger atrial septal defect.

Q74

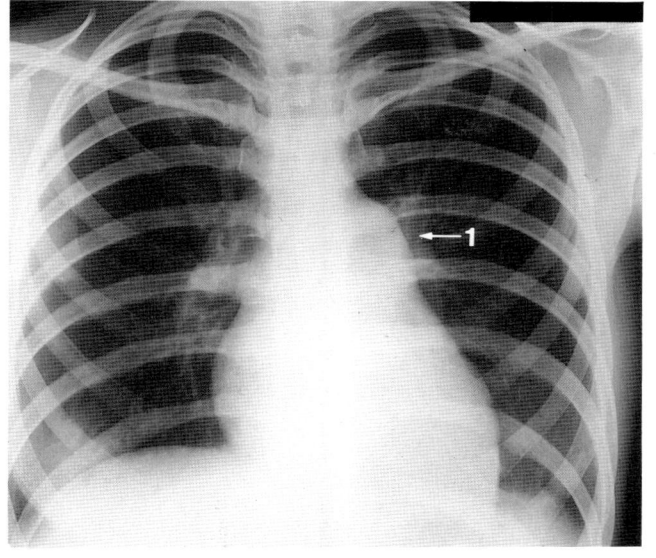

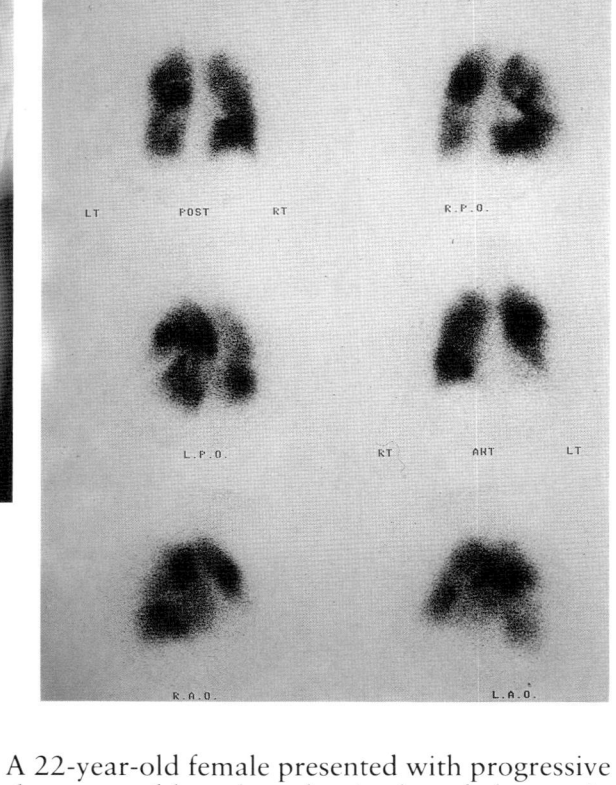

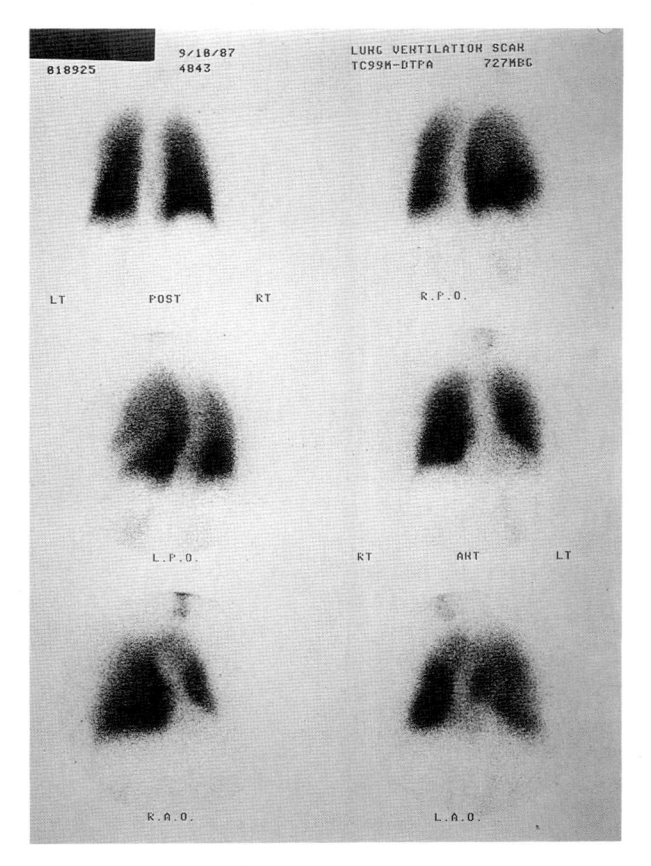

A 22-year-old female presented with progressive shortness of breath and episodes of chest pain and haemoptysis.
Examine the CXR.

- Do the lungs look normal?
- What is this structure (1)? Is it normal?

Now examine the isotope lung scans.

- Why are there two sets of lung scans?
- What do they show?
- What is the diagnosis?

A74

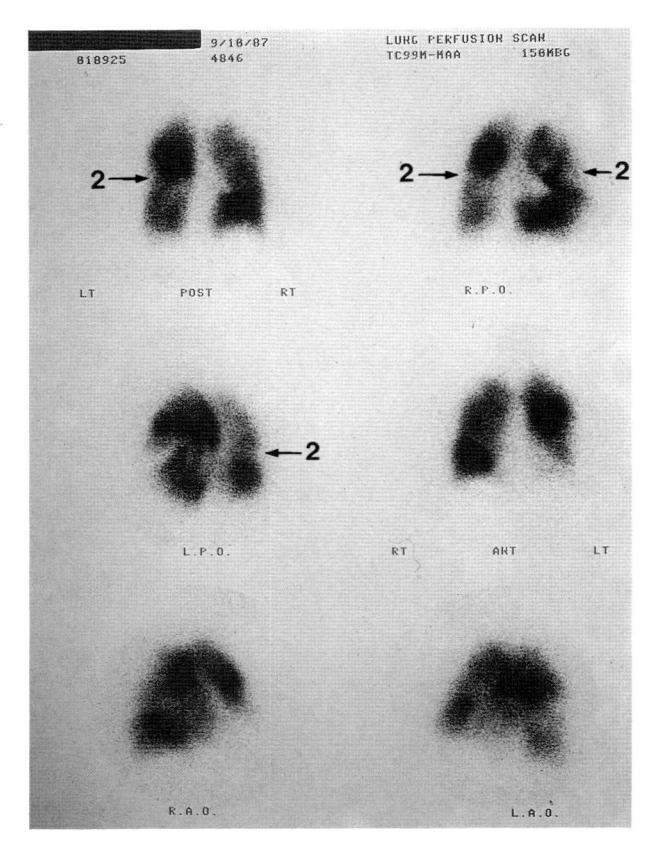

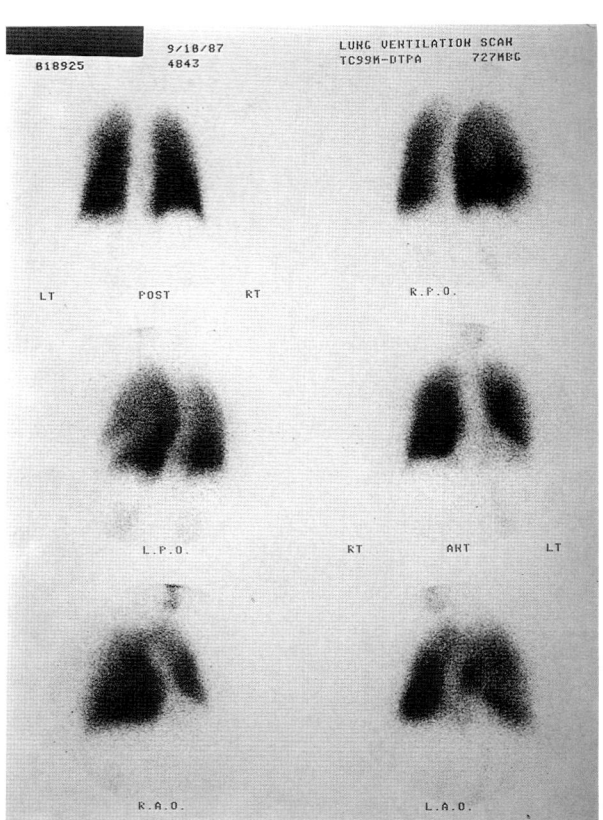

The peripheral pulmonary vascular pattern is uneven. (1) = the pulmonary trunk. It is enlarged, raising the possibility of pulmonary arterial hypertension.

The first set of lung scans is a perfusion study, and the second set is a ventilation scan. Perfusion defects may be produced by both thromboembolic disease and parenchymal lung disease. In parenchymal lung disease, however, there are usually matching ventilation defects, but in thromboembolic disease ventilation usually appears normal.

The lung scans show multiple pleural-based segmental defects (2) on the perfusion scan, but the ventilation scan is normal. The diagnosis is recurrent pulmonary emboli.

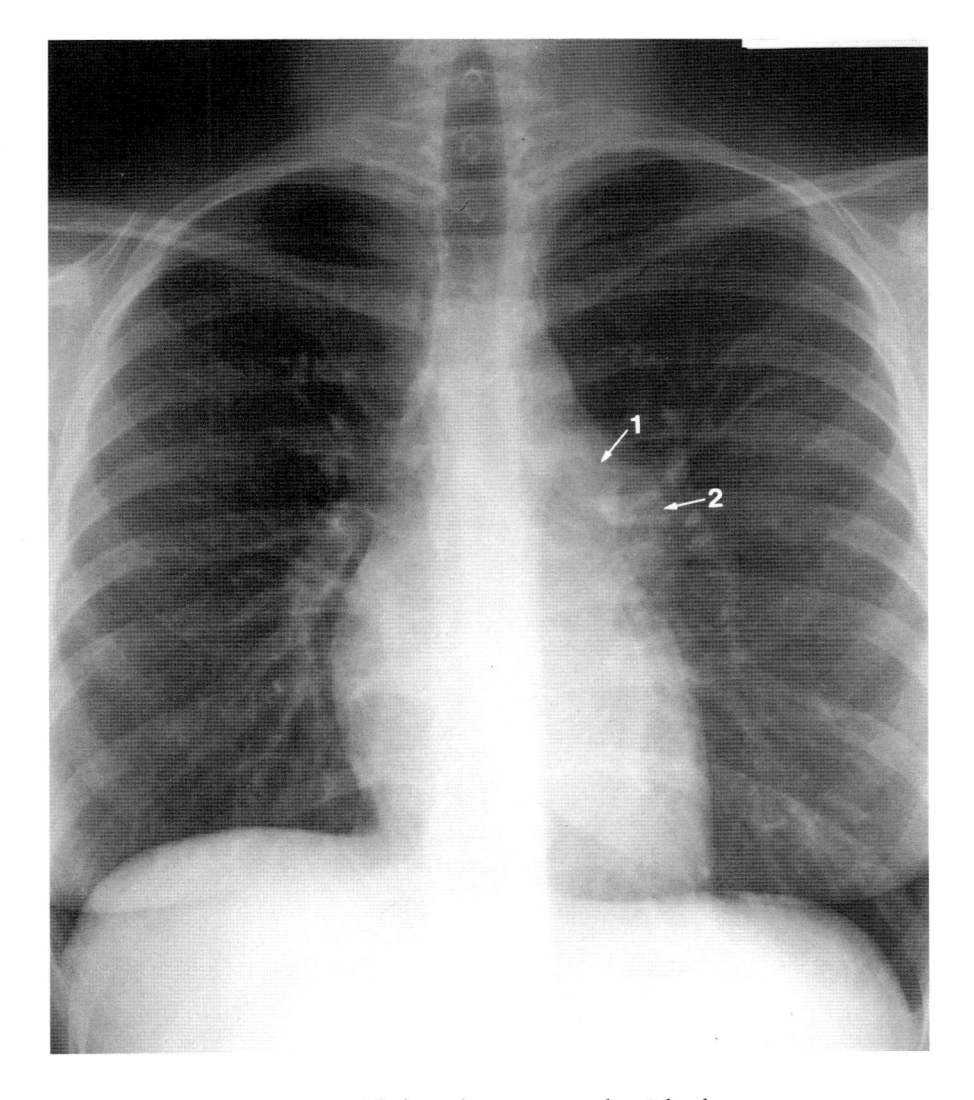

A 19-year-old female presented with dyspnoea on exercise. The electrocardiogram showed evidence of right ventricular hypertrophy.

The CXR shows enlargement of the pulmonary trunk (1). This may be due to:

a) Increased flow through the pulmonary arteries.
b) Increased pressure in pulmonary arteries.
c) Post-stenotic dilatation.

- What is structure (2)?

- Comment on the peripheral pulmonary vasculature.

- What is the diagnosis?

A75

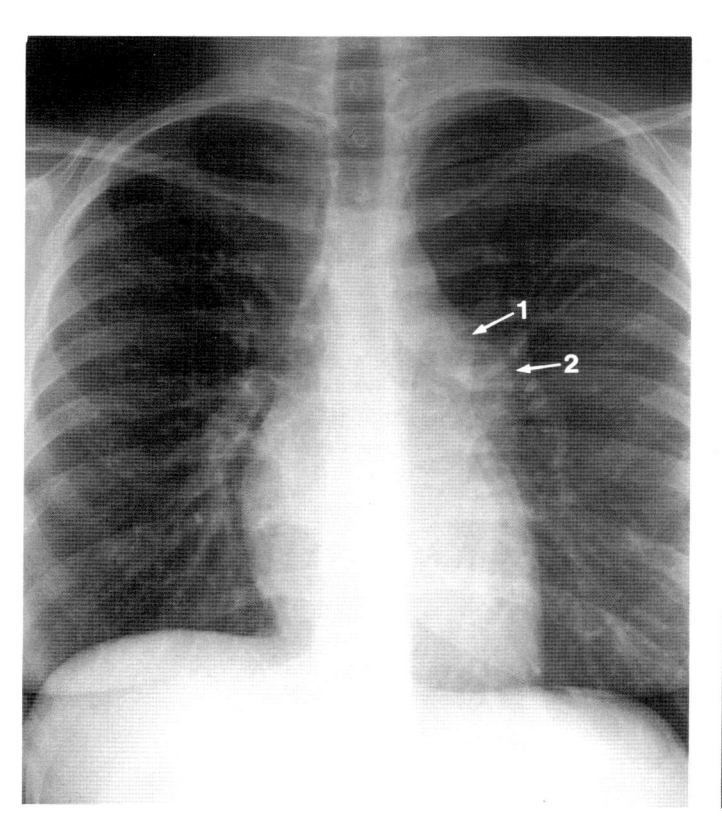

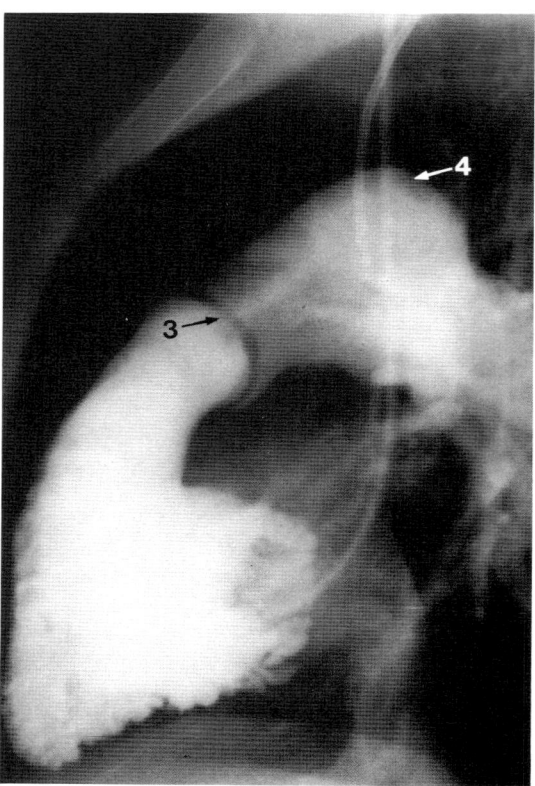

(2) = the left pulmonary artery. The peripheral pulmonary vasculature looks normal. The diagnosis is pulmonary valve stenosis. Typically, post-stenotic dilatation involves the pulmonary trunk and the left pulmonary artery. The lateral projection of the right ventriculogram demonstrates doming pulmonary valve leaflets (3), and post-stenotic dilatation of the pulmonary trunk (4).

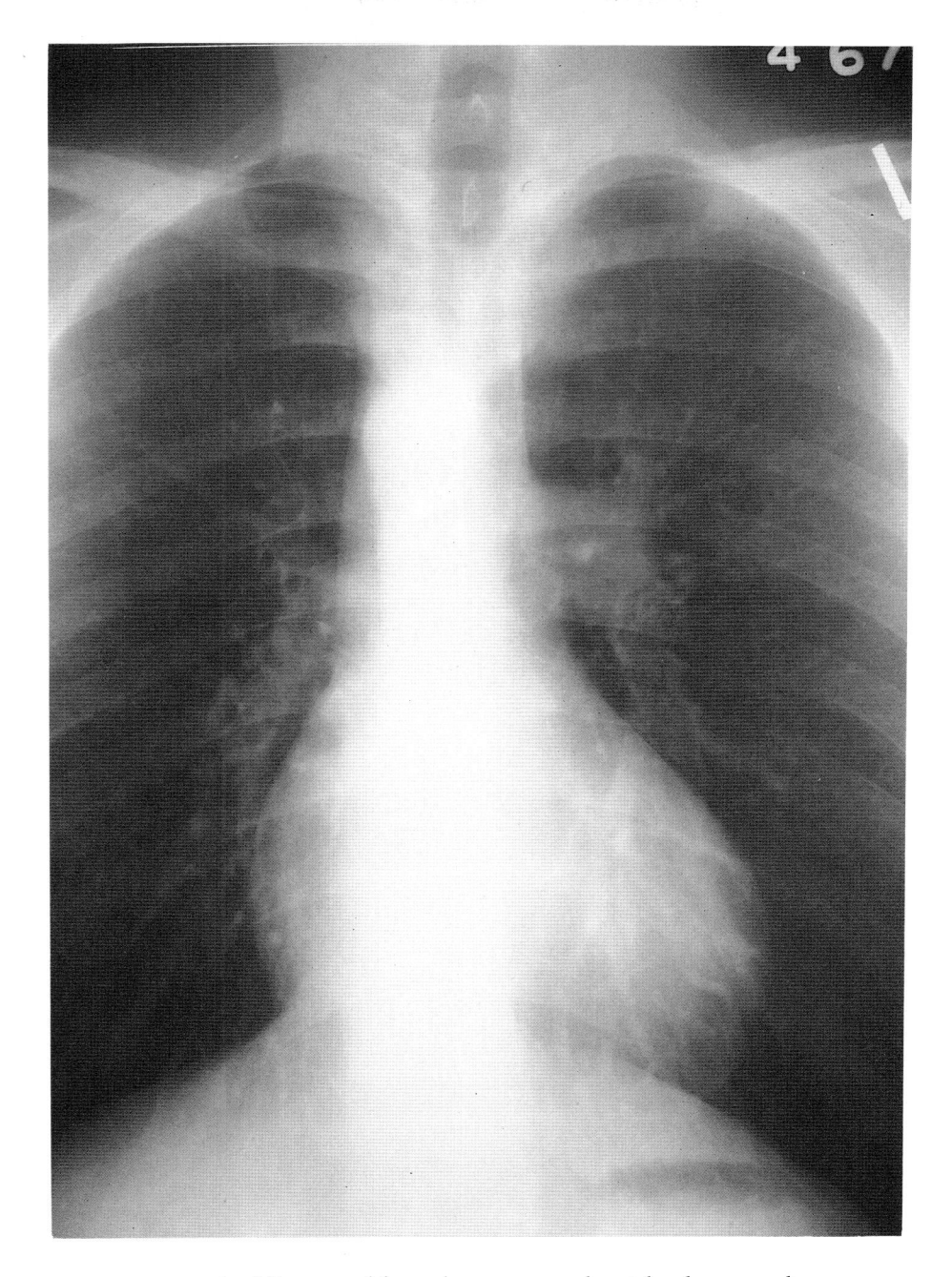

A 20-year-old male presented with decreased exercise tolerance. He had been cyanosed since birth.

- Is the aorta normal?
- Is pulmonary perfusion normal?
- What is the diagnosis?

A76

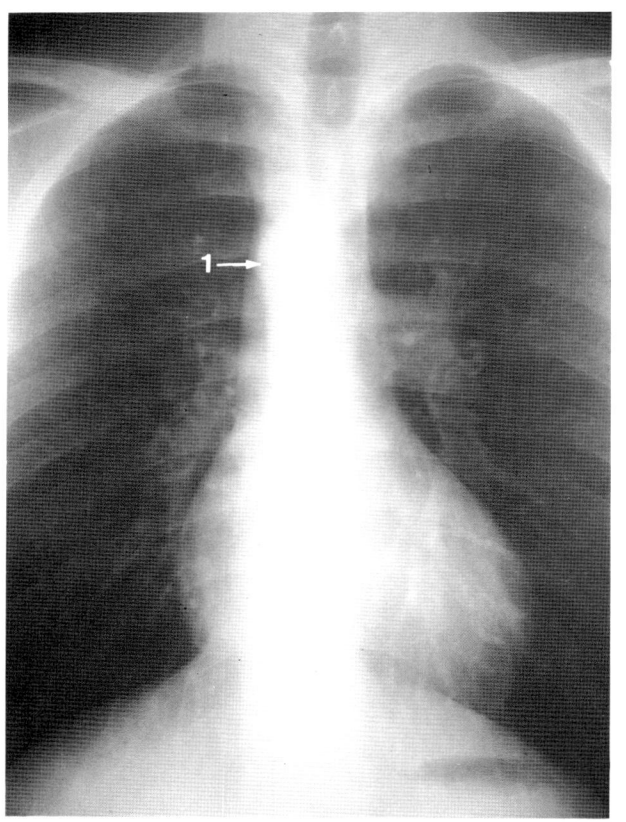

The aortic arch is right-sided (1), and the lungs are oligaemic. The diagnosis is tetralogy of Fallot. The right anterior oblique and left anterior oblique right ventriculograms demonstrate right ventricular hypertrophy, pulmonary infundibular stenosis (2), a sub-aortic ventricular septal defect (3), and aorta (4) overriding the ventricular septum (5). LV = left ventricle, RV = right ventricle.

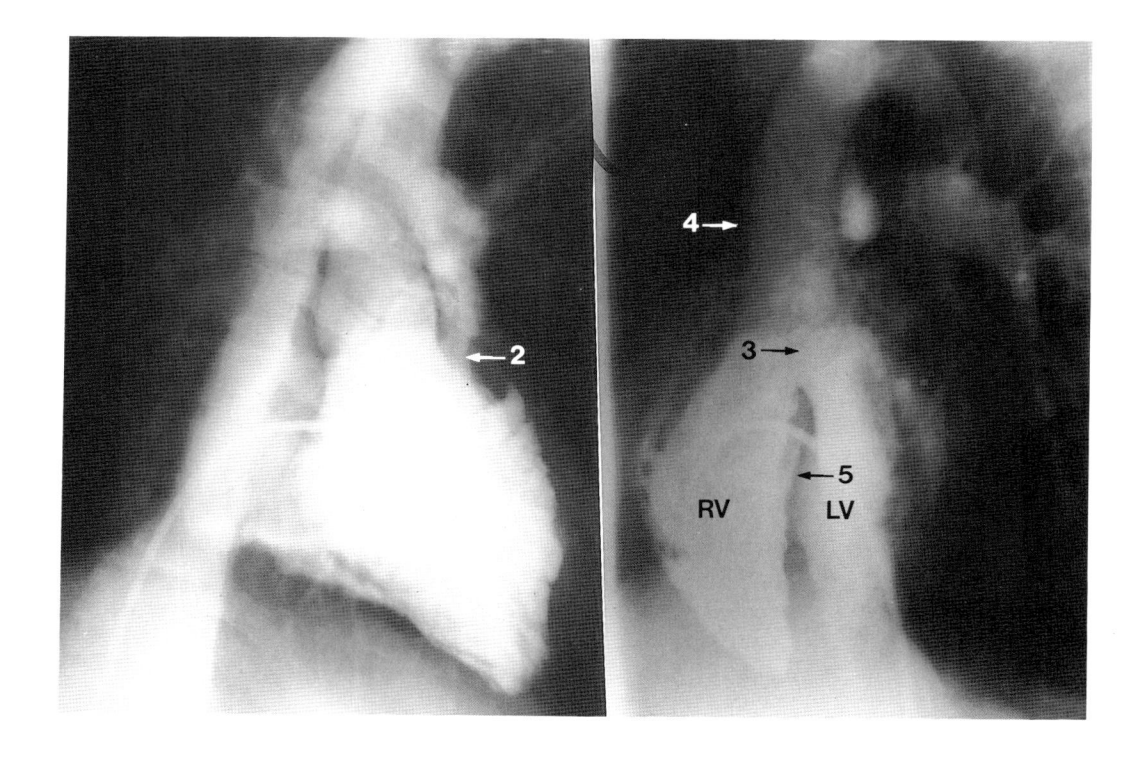

Q77

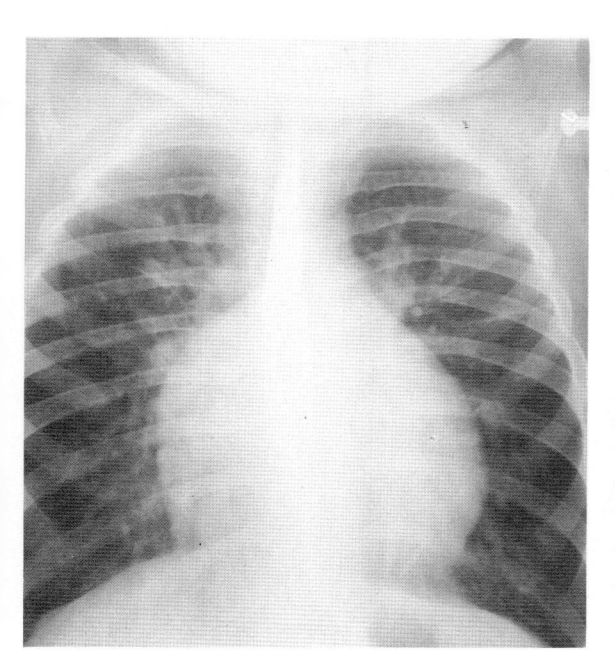

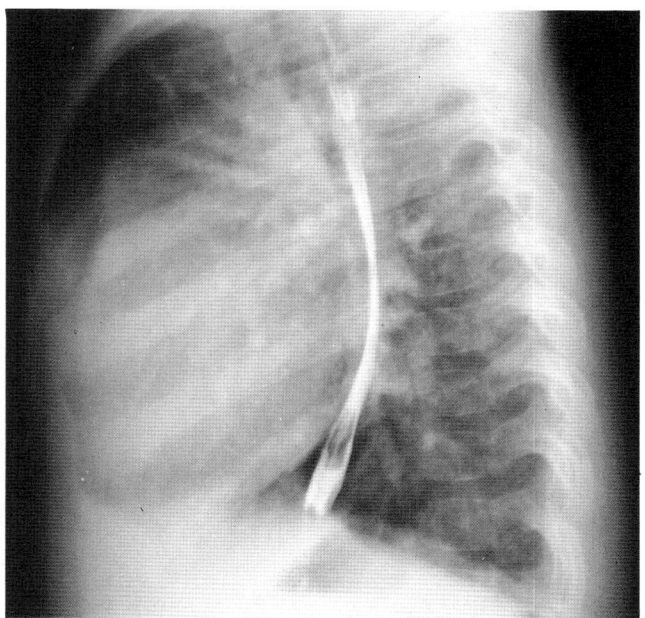

A child with Down's Syndrome presented with frequent chest infections. Clinically there was no evidence of cyanosis.

- Comment on the pulmonary vascularity.
- Which cardiac chamber is enlarged?
- What is the diagnosis?
- Have you noticed any skeletal abnormality?

A77

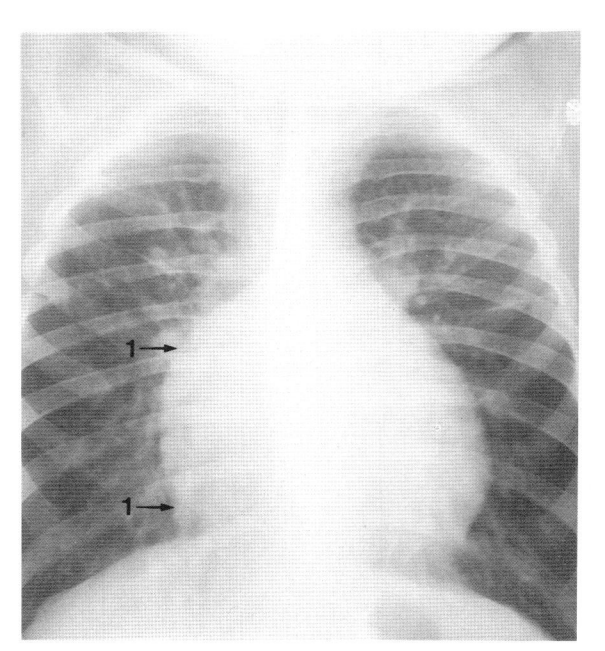

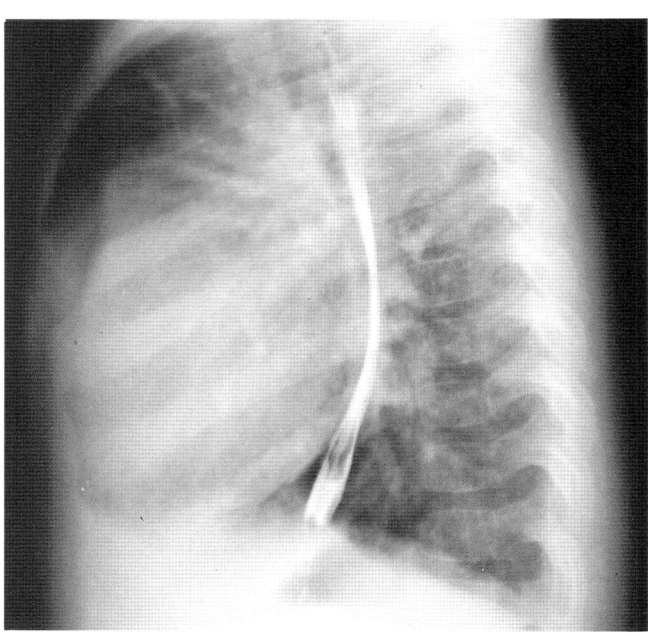

There is pulmonary plethora. The right atrium (1) is enlarged. The diagnosis is atrioventricular septal defect, which is associated with Down's Syndrome. This child has an ostium primum atrial septal defect. There are only 11 pairs of ribs, which may also be a feature of Down's Syndrome.

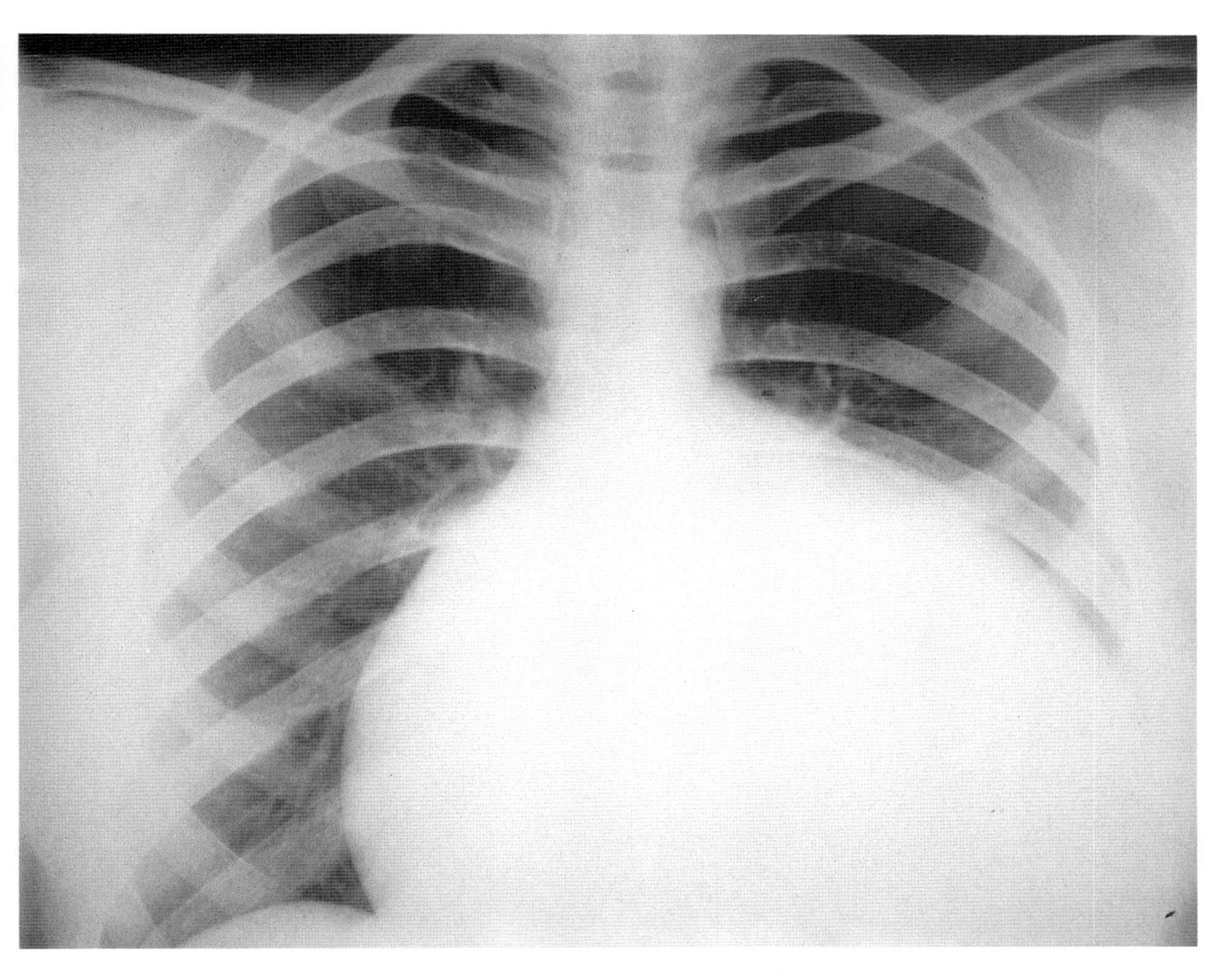

A 40-year-old male presented with poor exercise tolerance and frequent palpitations. On examination there was mild central cyanosis.

- Comment on the pulmonary vascularity.
- What part of the heart is enlarged?
- What is the diagnosis?

A78

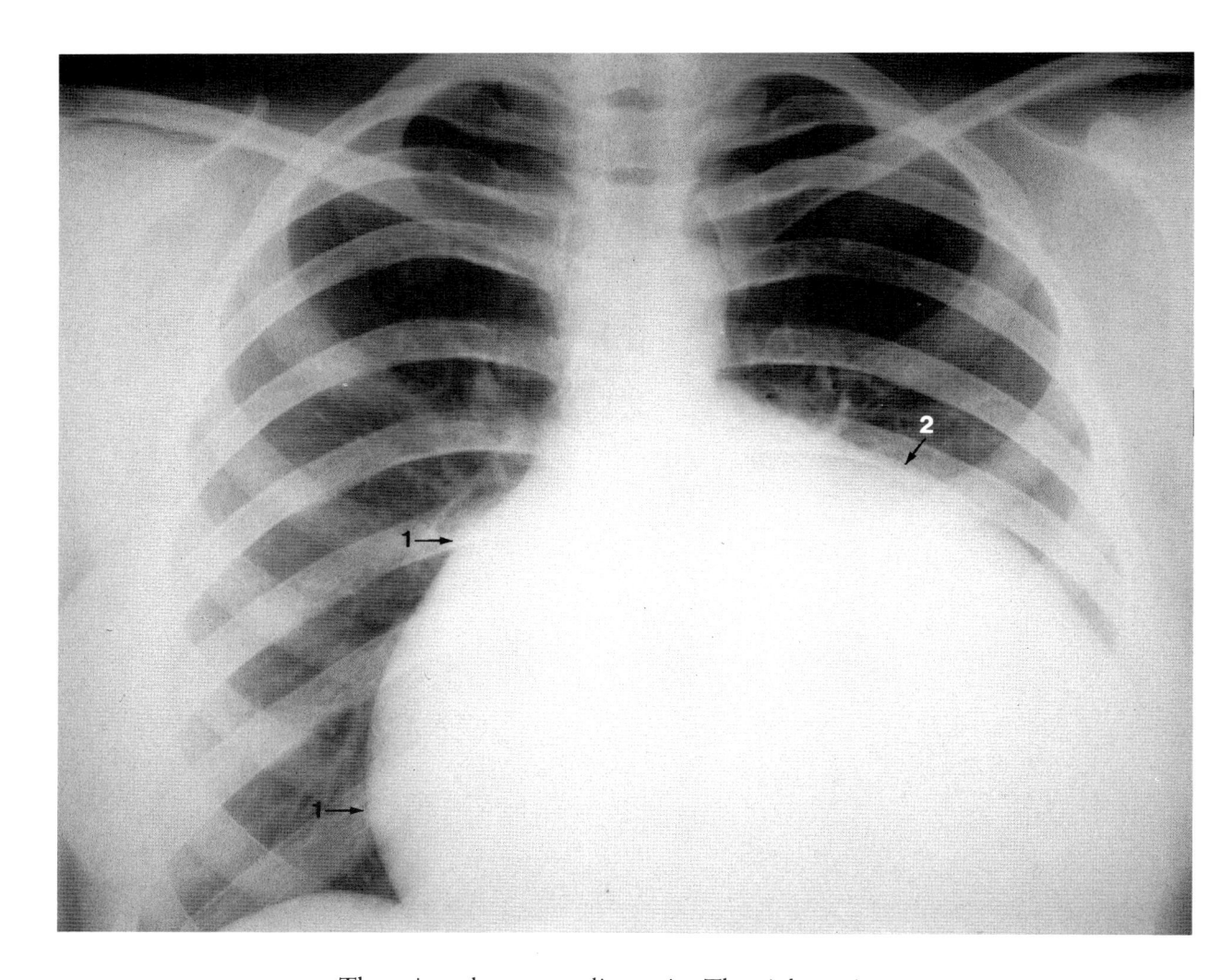

There is pulmonary oligaemia. The right atrium is enlarged (1). In addition, the increased convexity of the left heart border (2) is due to dilatation of the right ventricular outflow tract. The diagnosis is Ebstein's anomaly of the tricuspid valve. The central cyanosis is due to right-to-left shunting across the foramen ovale.

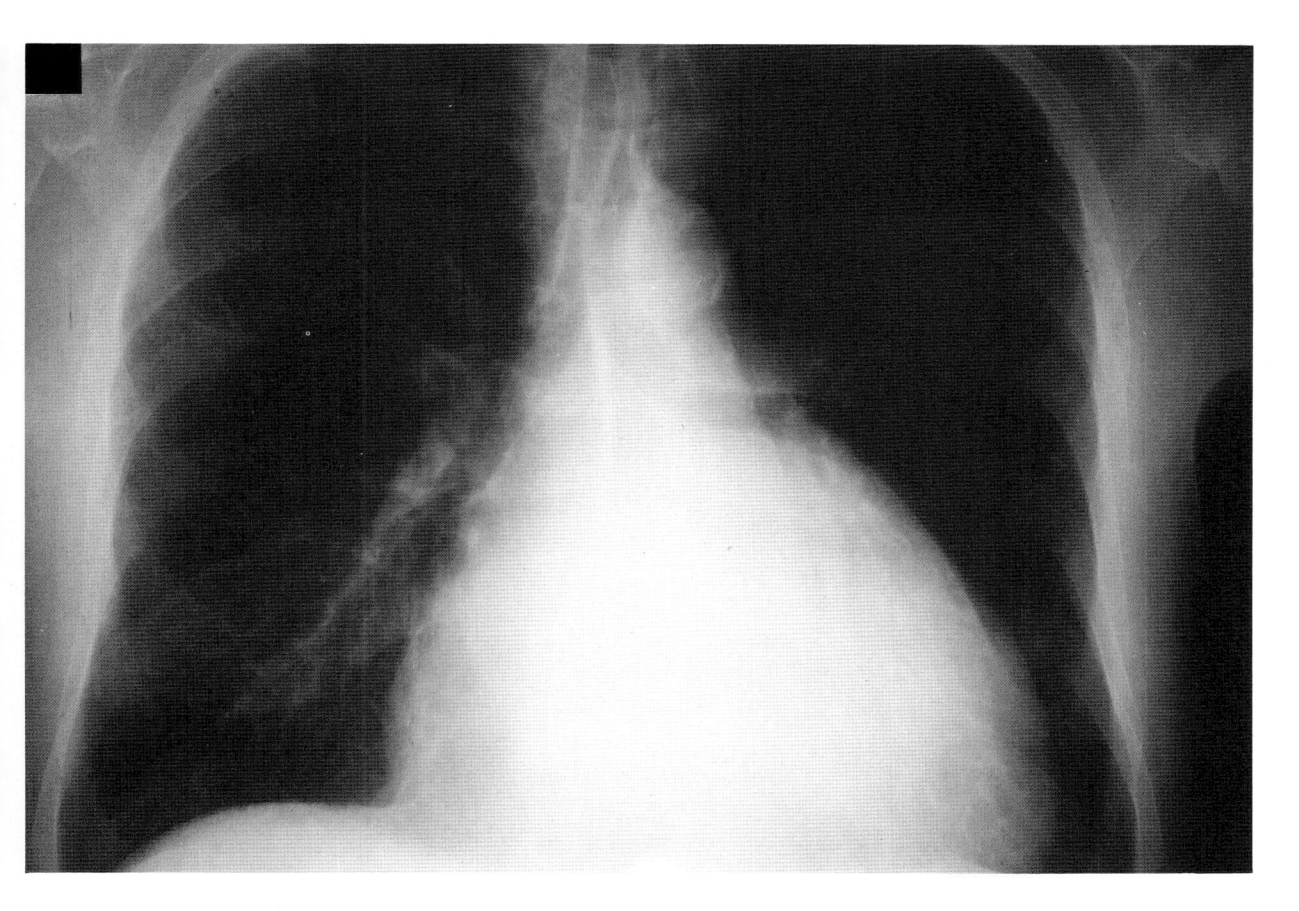

A 42-year-old man presented with dyspnoea on exertion. On examination there was atrial fibrillation, and a loud apical pan-systolic murmur was heard.

- What is the diagnosis?
- The heart is enlarged. Is there any evidence of specific chamber enlargement?
- How could this be confirmed?

A79

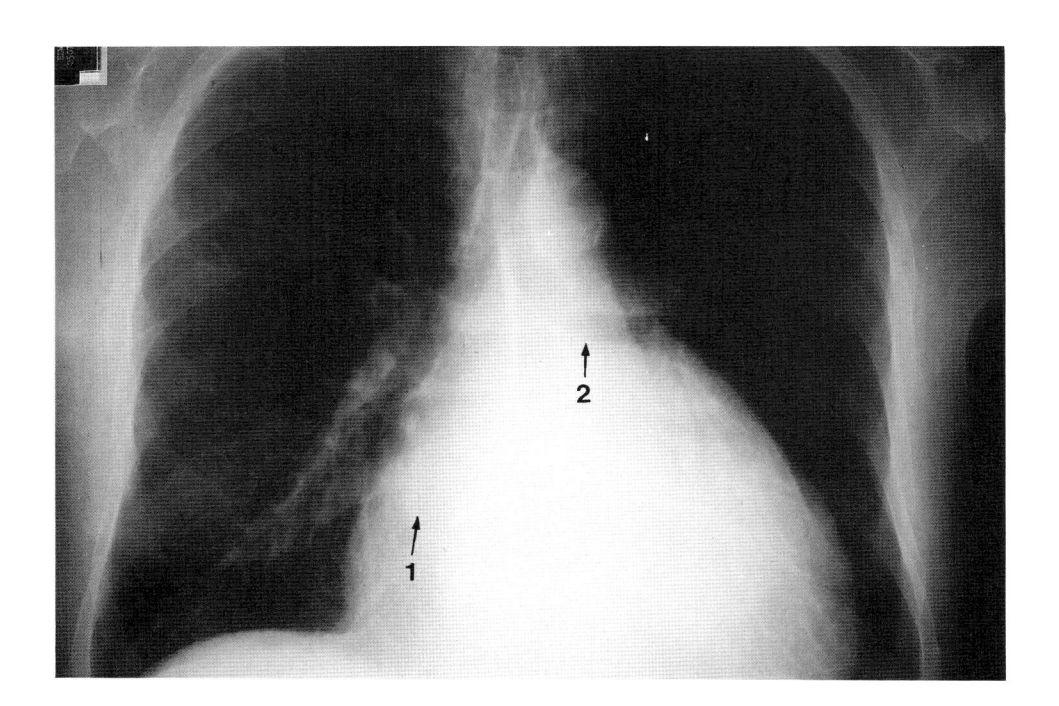

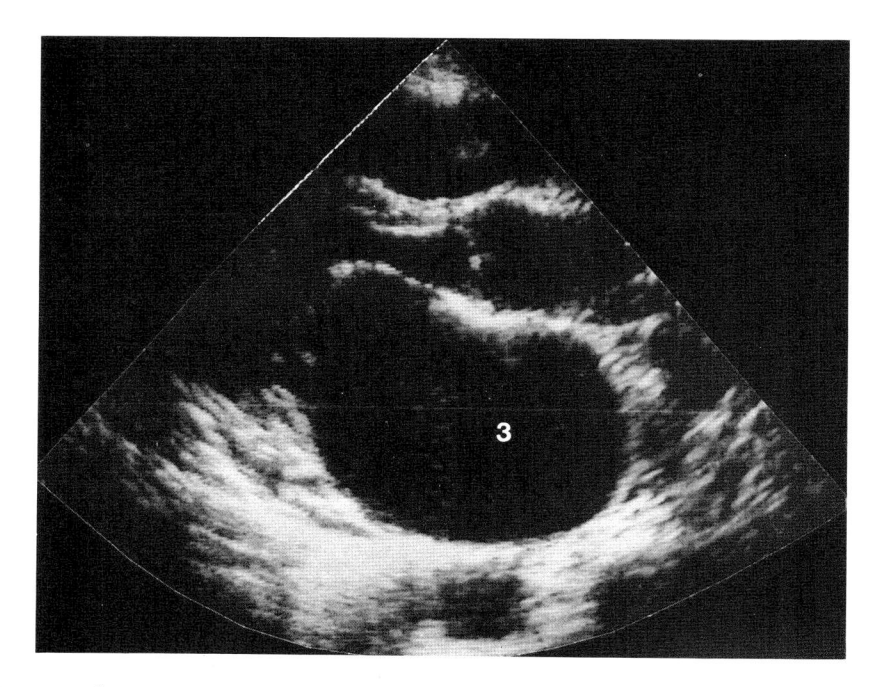

The diagnosis is mitral regurgitation. A double density (1) visible over the right side of the heart and elevation of the left bronchus (2) indicate left atrial enlargement. Prominence of the right heart border suggests right atrial enlargement, and prominence of the left heart border suggests left ventricular enlargement. Ultrasound scan of the heart confirmed multiple chamber enlargement. The slice illustrated demonstrates enlargement of the body of the left atrium (3). The mitral valve cusps were thickened and calcified. The aortic valve was normal.

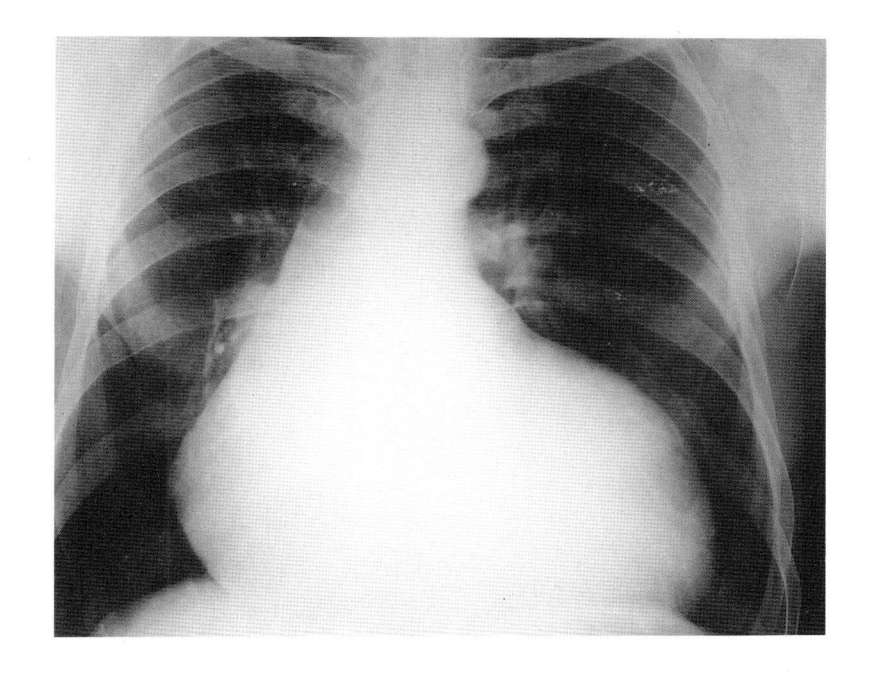

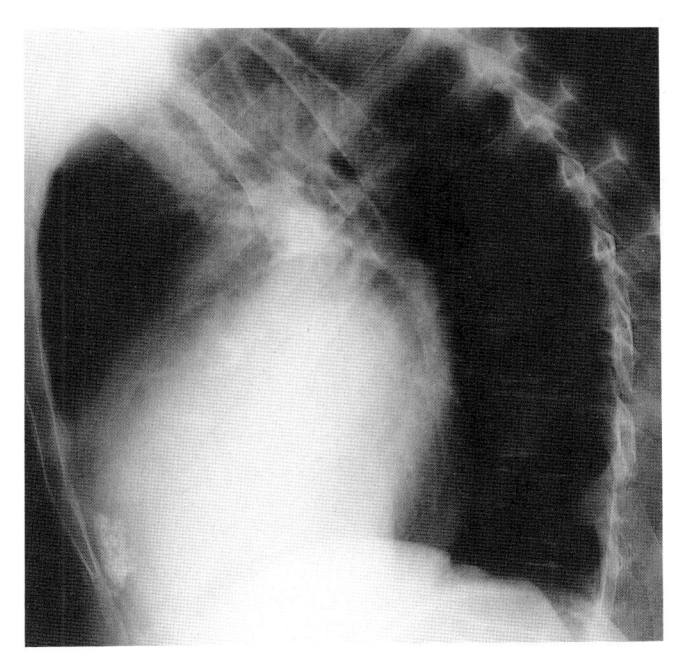

A 53-year-old presented with exertional dyspnoea and an early diastolic murmur.

- Which cardiac chamber is enlarged?
- Is it hypertrophied or dilated?
- What is the diagnosis?

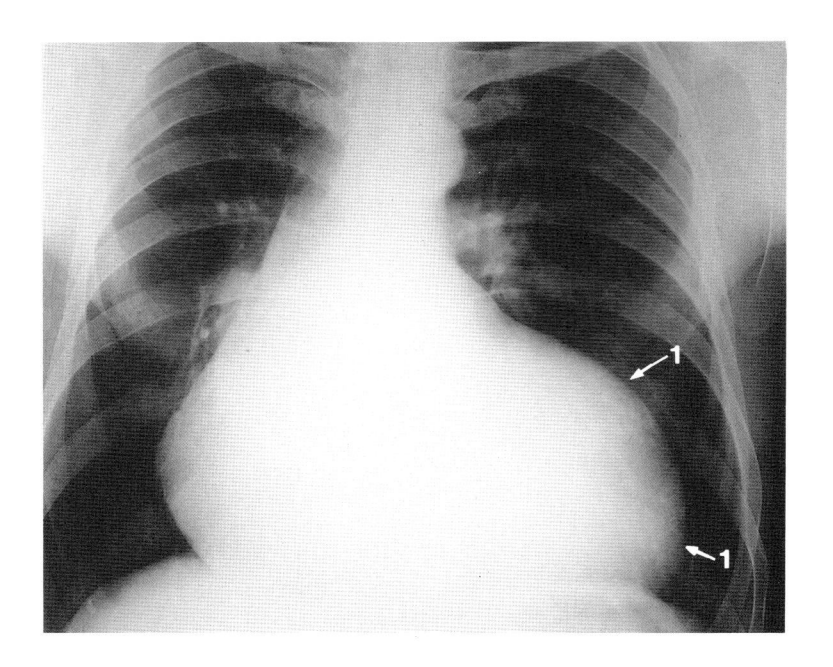

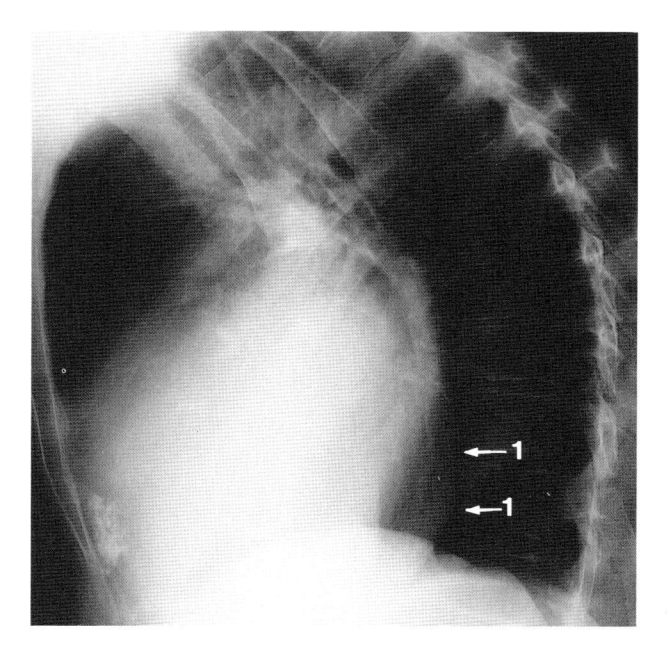

The left ventricle (1) is enlarged and shows features of both hypertrophy and dilatation. Left ventricular hypertrophy alters the shape of the heart, making the left heart border more convex than normal. However, hypertrophy alone does not increase the size of the heart. Enlargement therefore indicates dilatation of the ventricle. The diagnosis is aortic regurgitation.

Q81

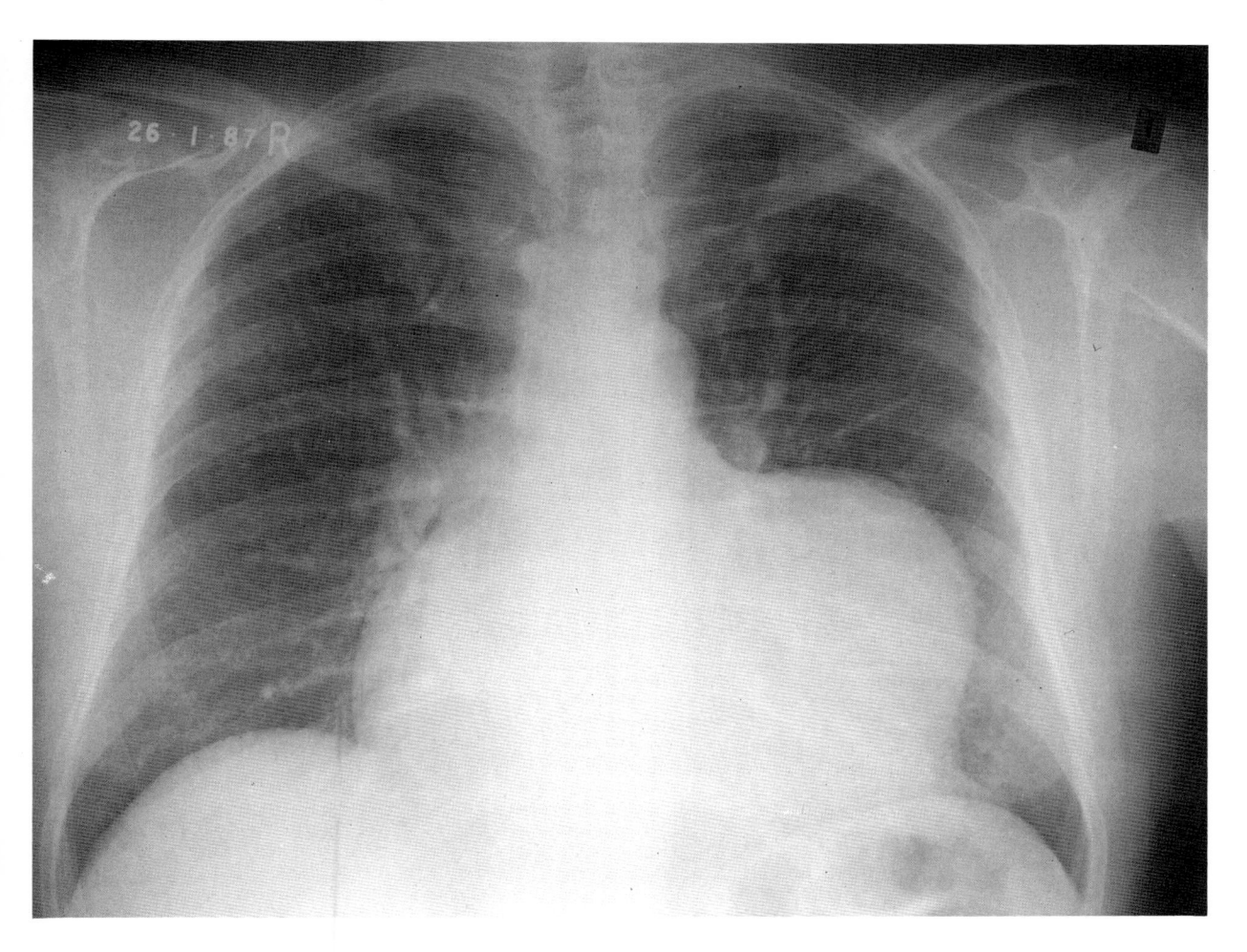

A 42-year-old male presented with a history of myocardial infarction, and now complained of dyspnoea on minimal exertion.

- Are the lungs normal?
- Comment on the cardiac shadow.
- What is the diagnosis?
- What further investigation is indicated?

A81

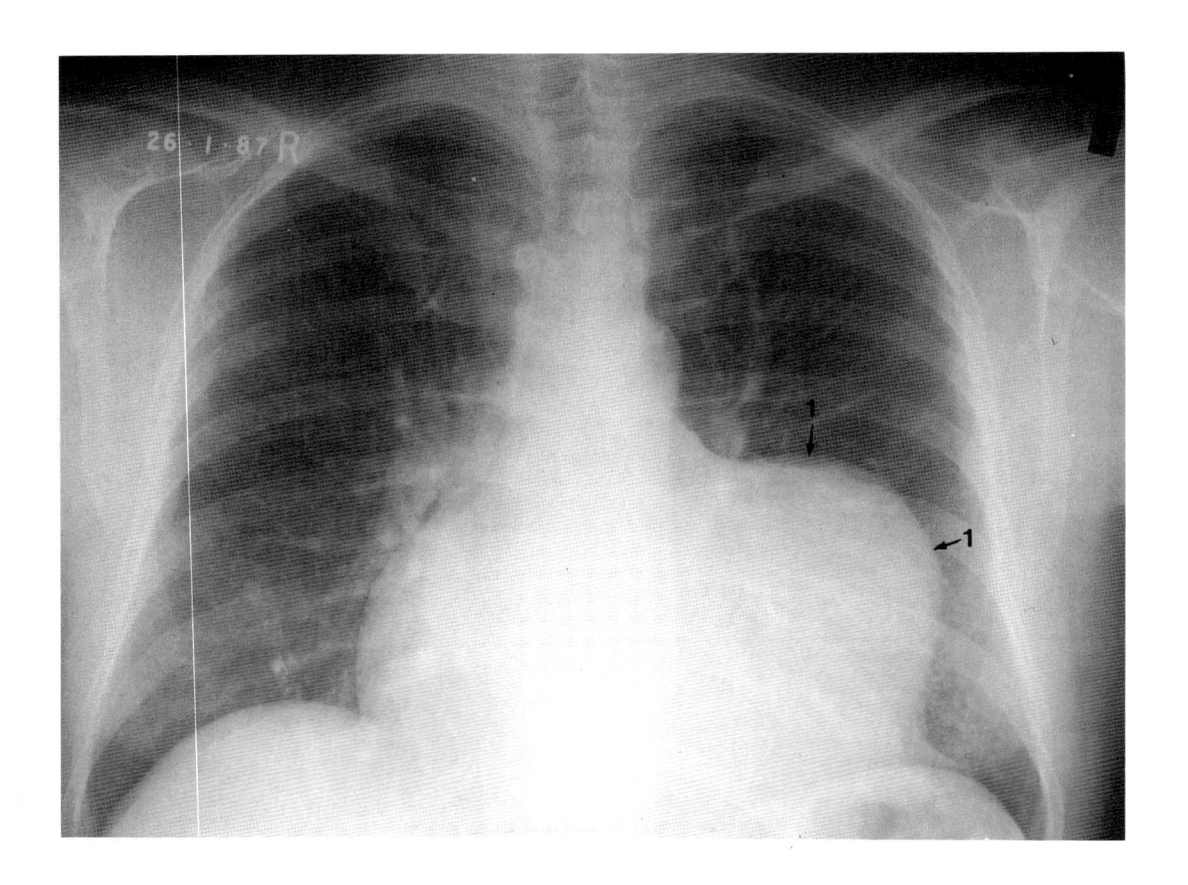

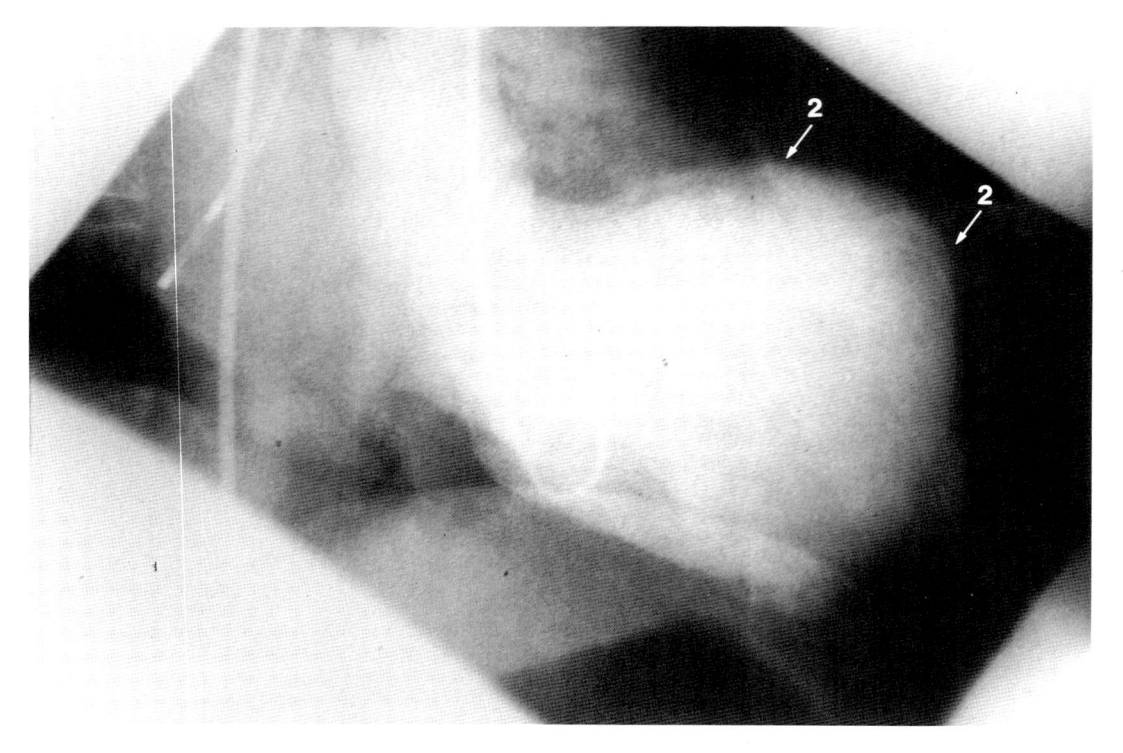

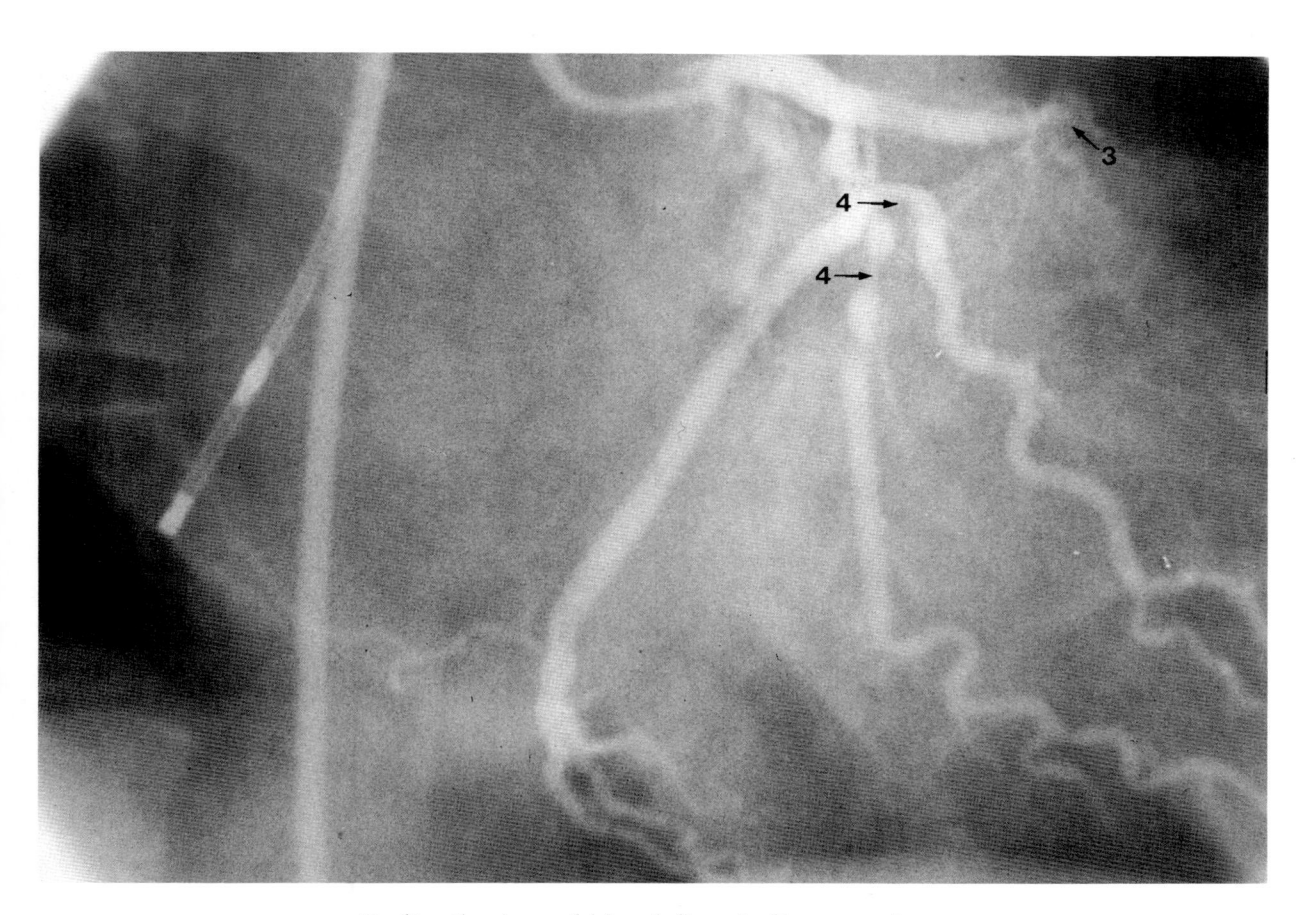

Redistribution of blood flow indicates pulmonary venous hypertension. The cardiac shadow shows a discrete bulge on the left heart border (1). The diagnosis is left ventricular aneurysm.

Cardiac catheterisation is now indicated to assess the state of the left ventricle and the coronary arteries with a view to aneurysmectomy and, possibly, coronary artery bypass surgery. The left ventriculogram demonstrates a large apical aneurysm (2). The left coronary arteriogram shows occlusion of the left anterior descending artery (3) and left circumflex artery strictures (4).

Q82

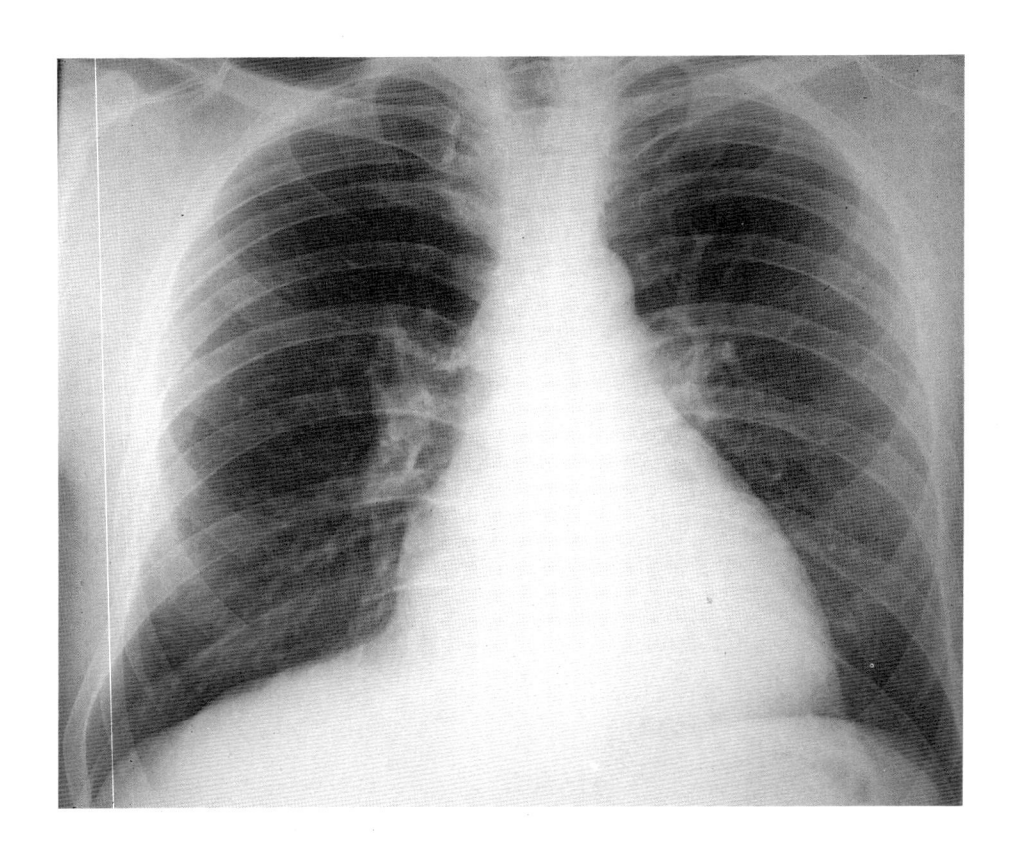

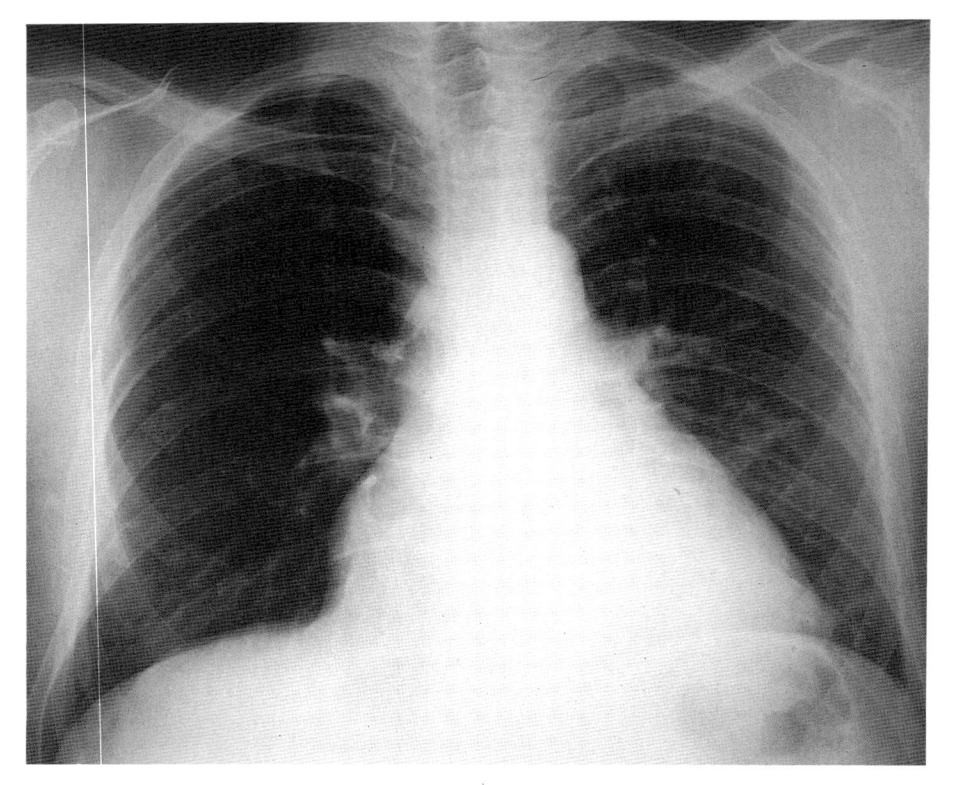

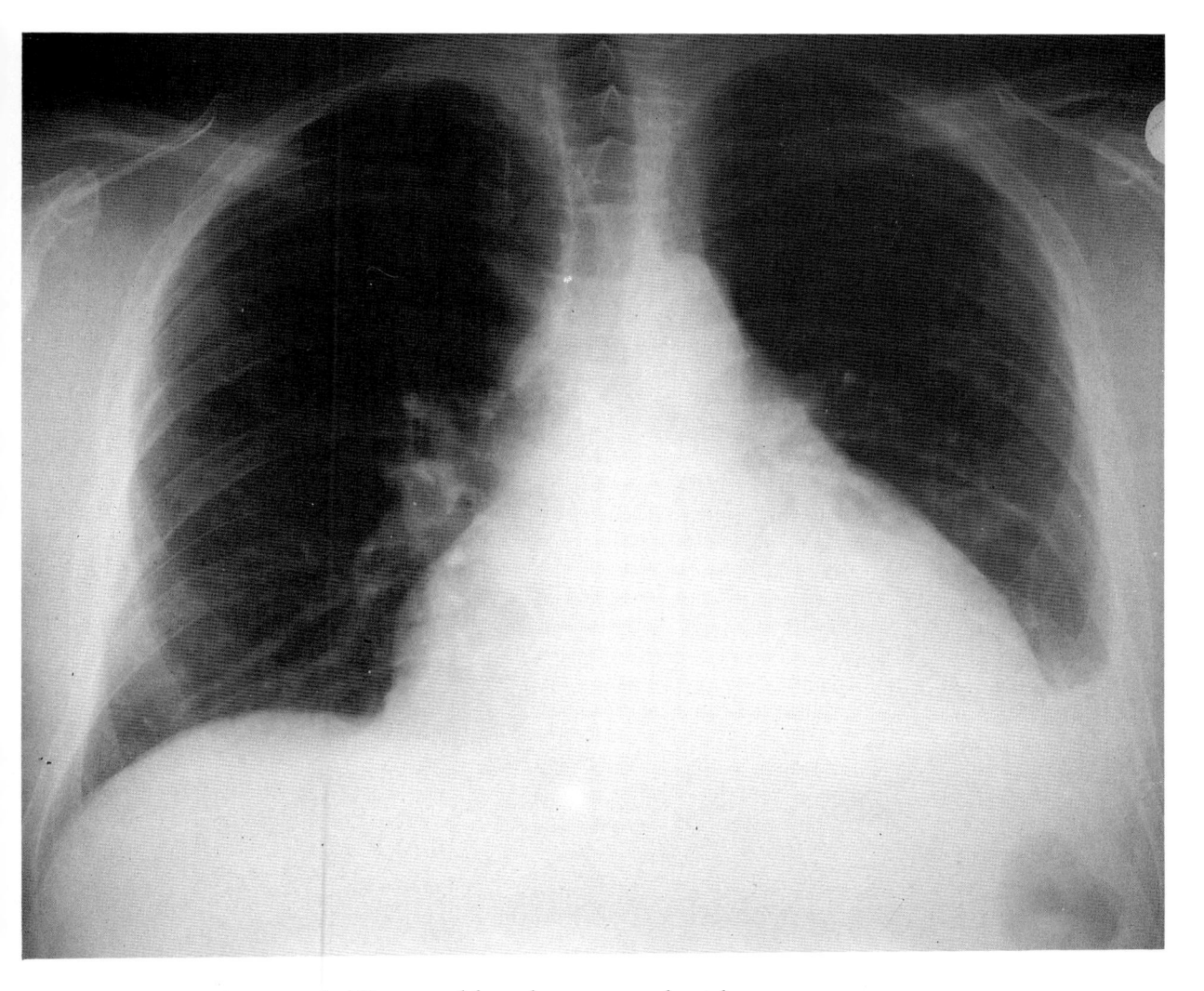

A 50-year-old male presented with acute myocardial infarction. The first CXR is on presentation. The patient was recovering well, but three weeks later developed chest pain and fever. The second CXR was taken at this time, and the third CXR six days later.

- What change has occurred between the first and second films?
- What further complication is seen on the last film?
- What other investigation would you do?
- What is the diagnosis?

A82

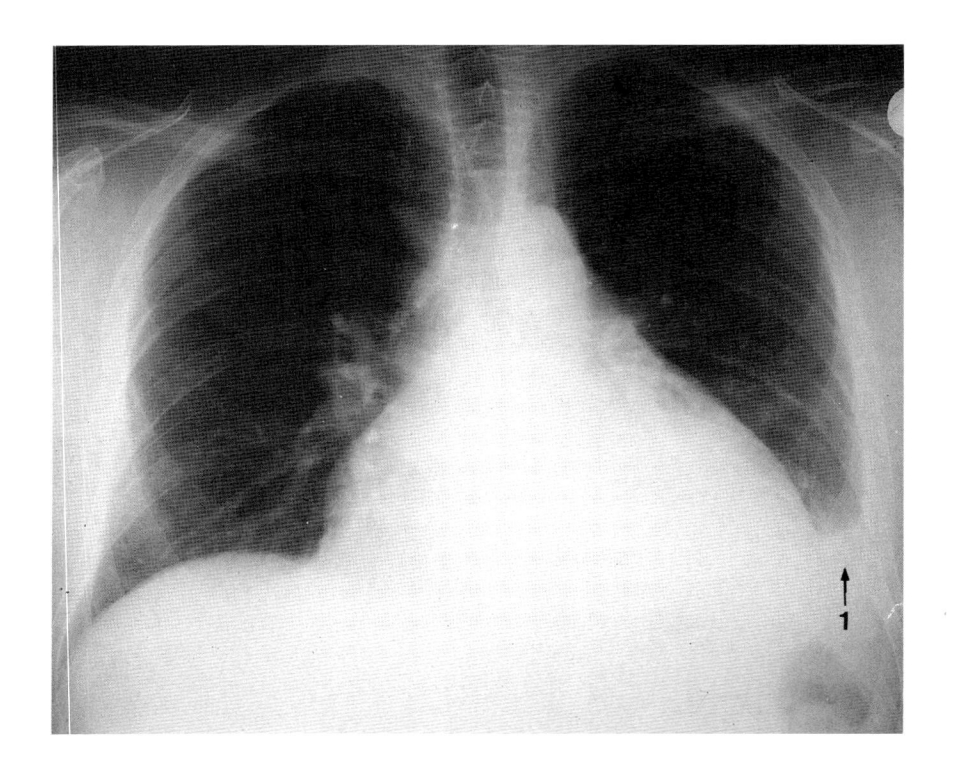

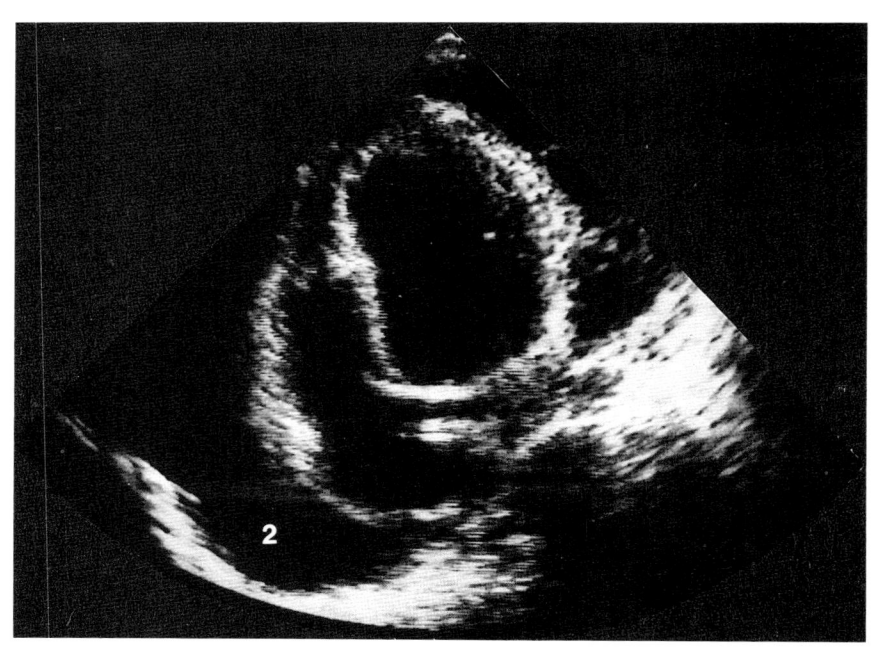

Between the first and second films the cardiac shadow has enlarged, but there are no signs of heart failure. The last film shows that a left pleural effusion has developed (1). A cardiac ultrasound should be undertaken. This demonstrates a pericardial effusion (2). The diagnosis is post-myocardial infarction or Dressler's syndrome.

Q83

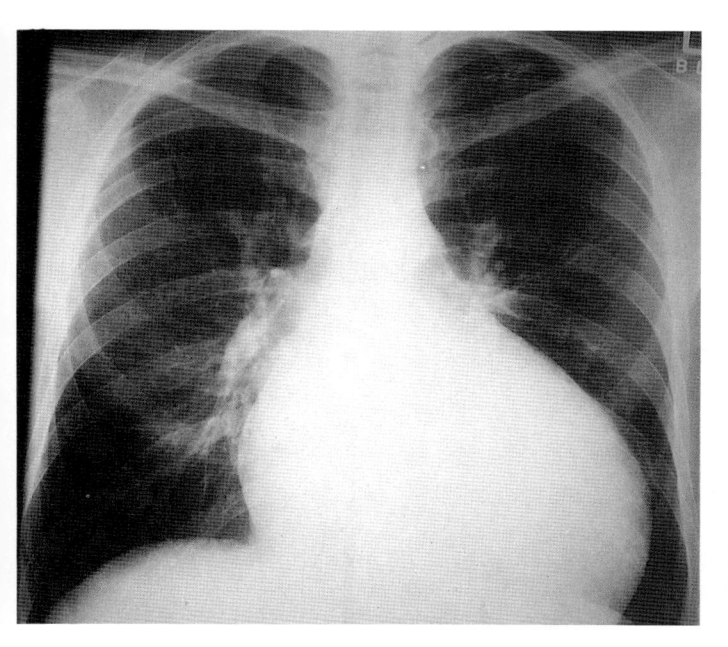

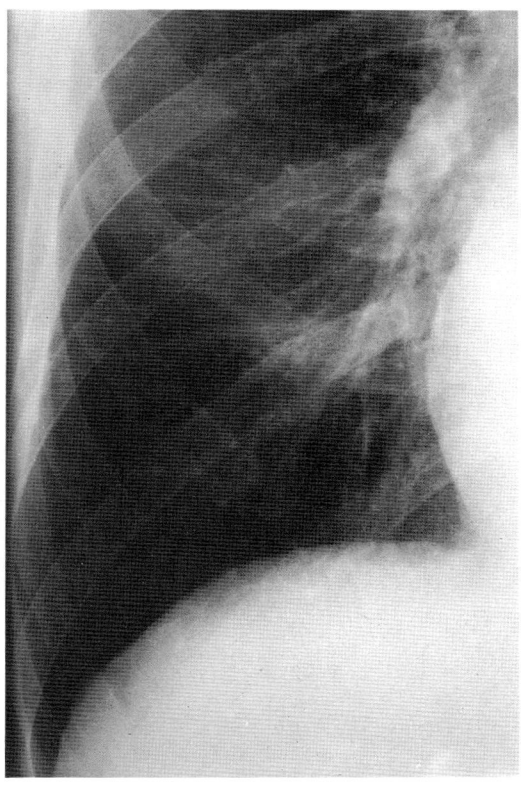

A 29-year-old man presented with dyspnoea at rest. The CXR shows a large globular heart shadow.

- Comment on the pulmonary vasculature.
- Is this a pericardial effusion?
- What is the diagnosis?

A83

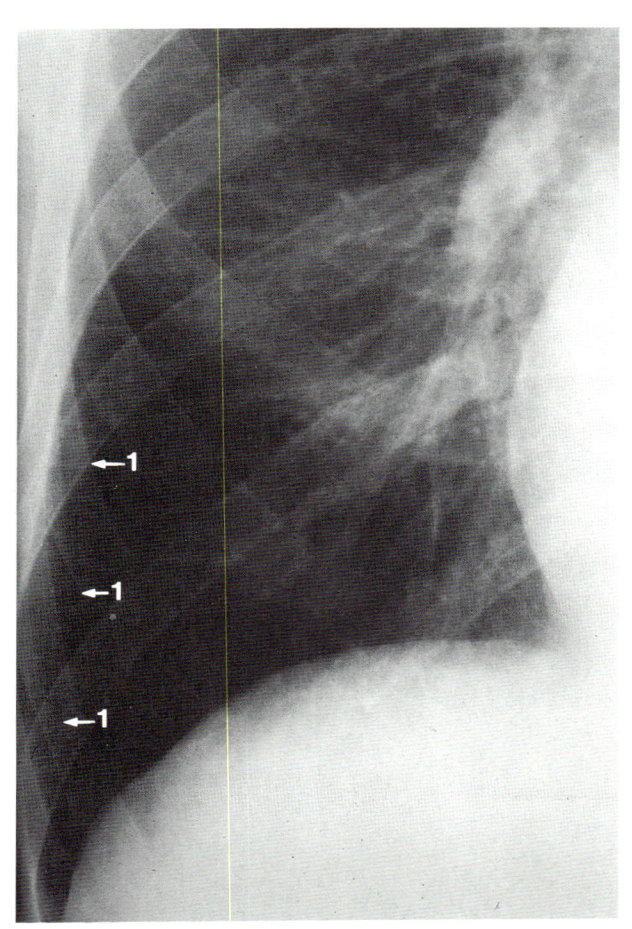

Redistribution of blood flow and interstitial lines (1) indicate pulmonary venous hypertension. This is not a pericardial effusion. A pericardial effusion does not cause pulmonary venous hypertension. This vasculature pattern with cardiomegaly indicates left heart failure. The diagnosis is congestive cardiomyopathy. The gated blood pool scan shows severe, generalised left ventricular hypokinesis, with virtually no change between systole and diastole.

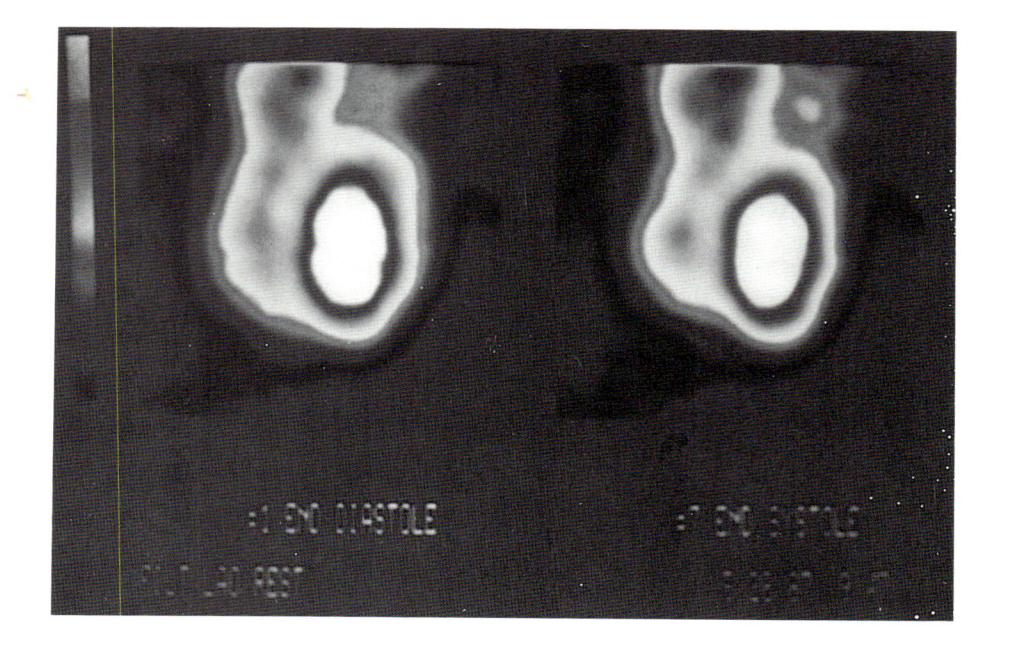

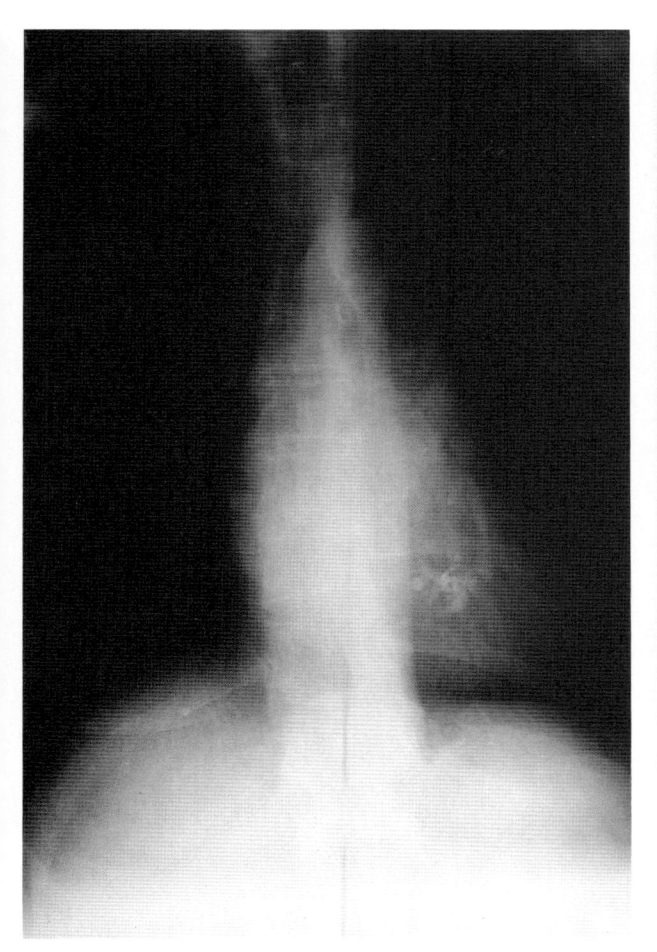

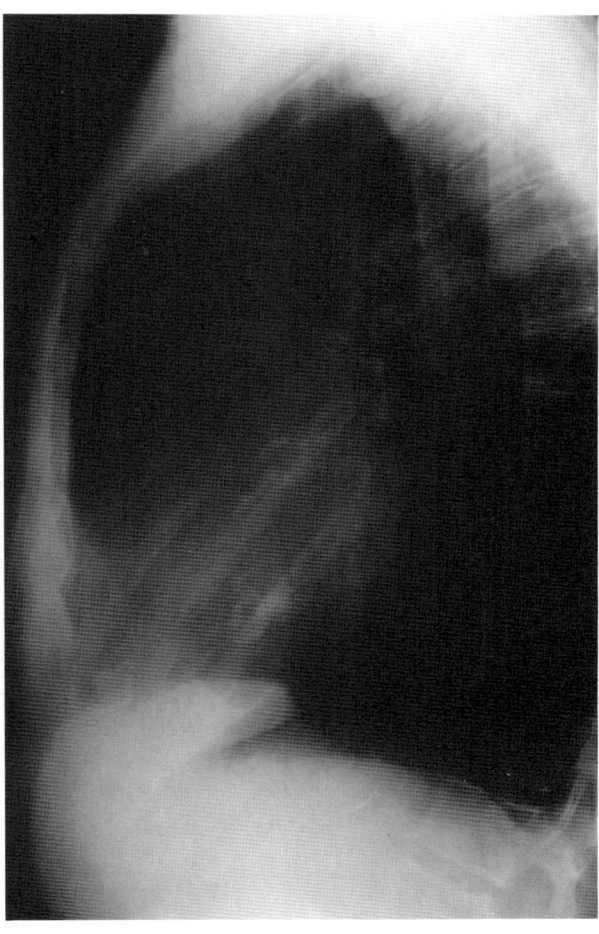

A 58-year-old female presented with orthopnoea.

- What structure is abnormally calcified?
- What is the diagnosis?

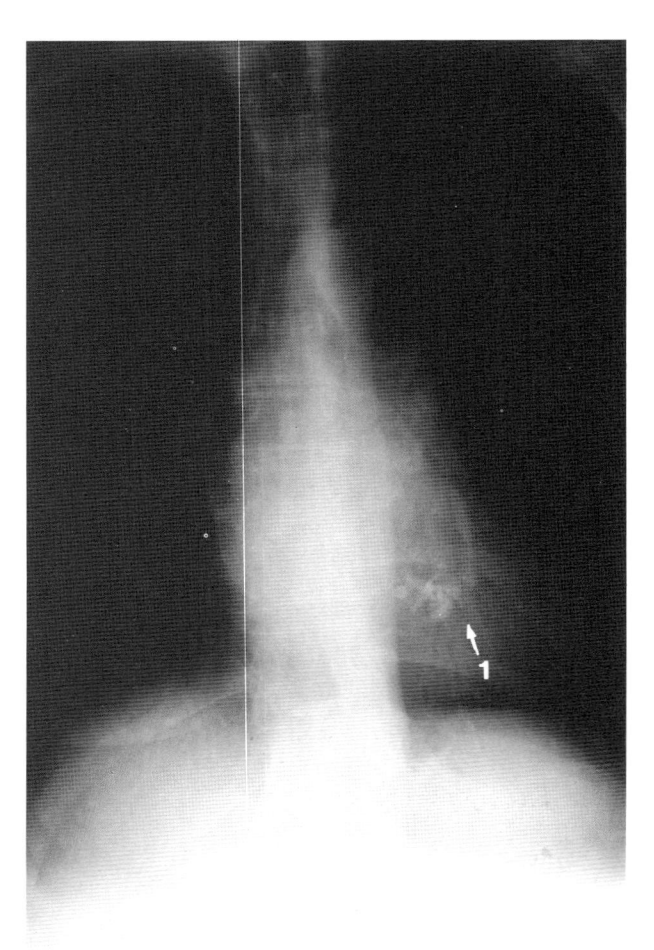

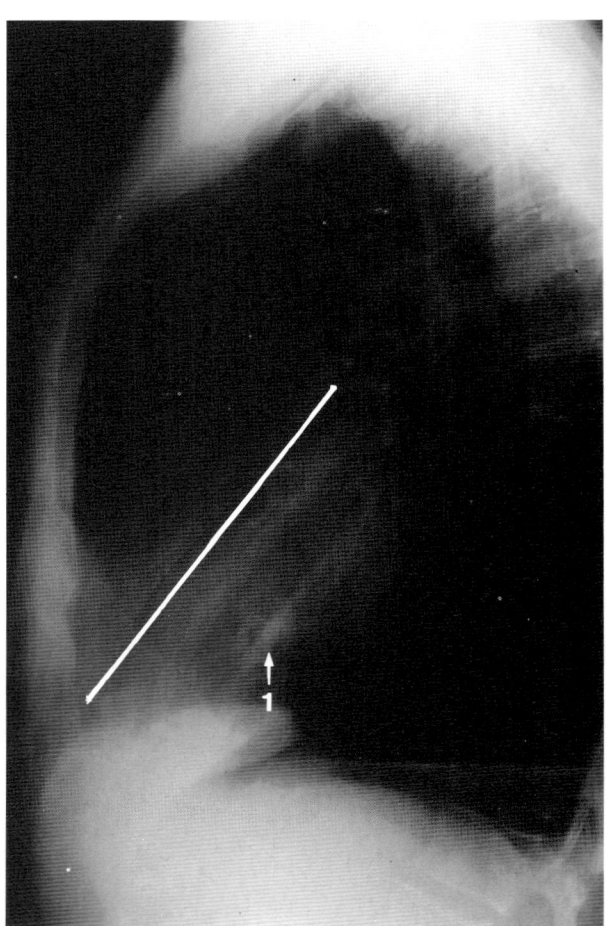

The mitral valve is abnormally calcified. The calcification (1) is situated posterior to a line drawn from the carina to the anterior costophrenic angle, and on the PA film it is to the left of the spine. The diagnosis is mitral stenosis.

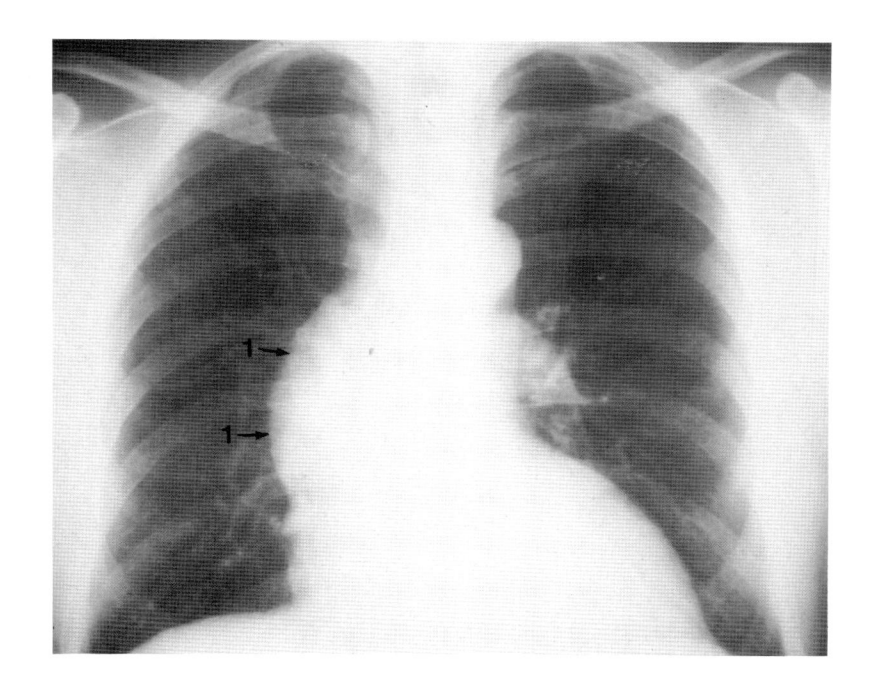

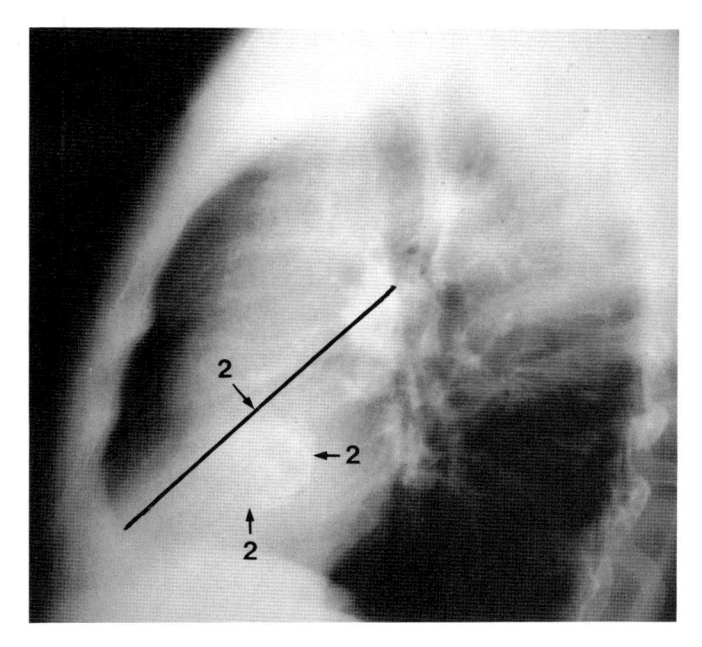

A 40-year-old man presented with chest pain and shortness of breath.

- What structure is abnormally calcified?
- What is this structure (1)?
- What is the diagnosis?

A85

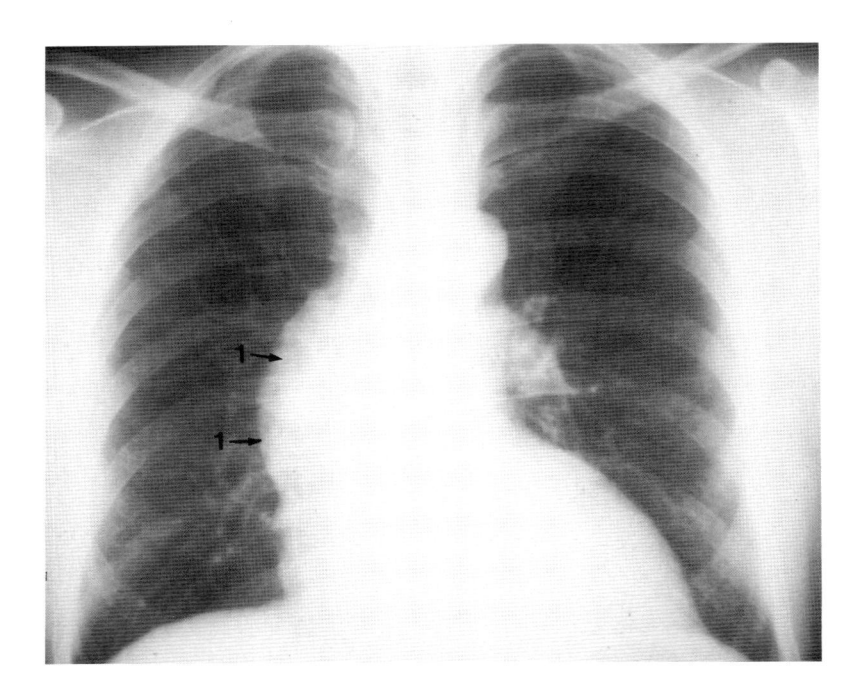

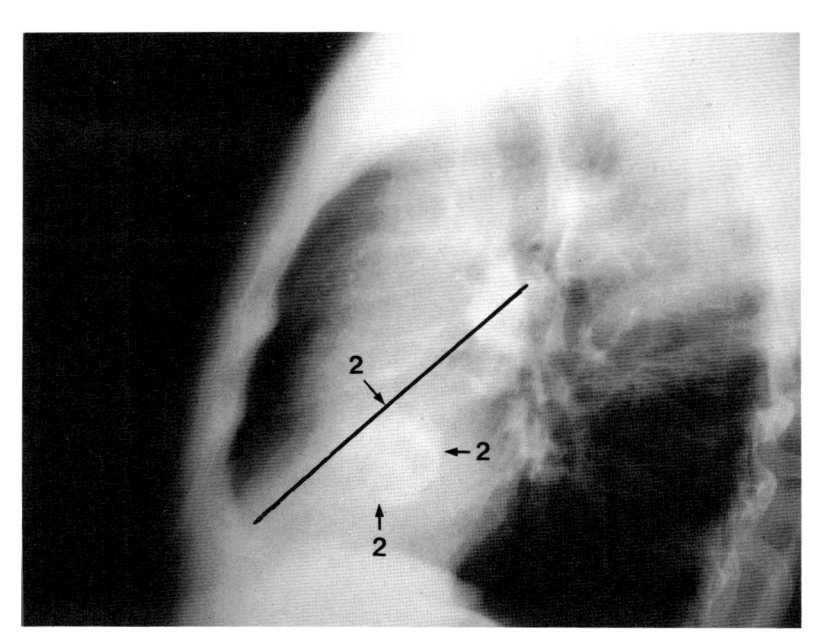

The aortic valve is abnormally calcified (2). The calcification is mostly anterior to a line drawn from the carina to the anterior costophrenic angle. It overlies the spine on the PA film and cannot be seen. (1) = the ascending aorta. It is prominent due to post-stenotic dilatation. The diagnosis is calcific aortic stenosis.

Q86

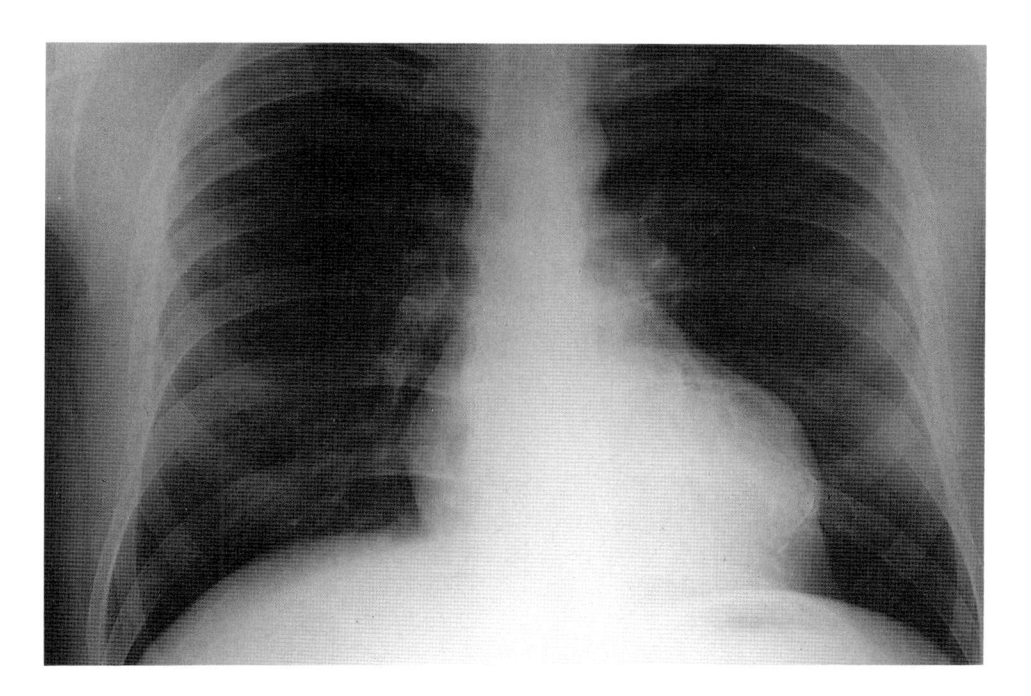

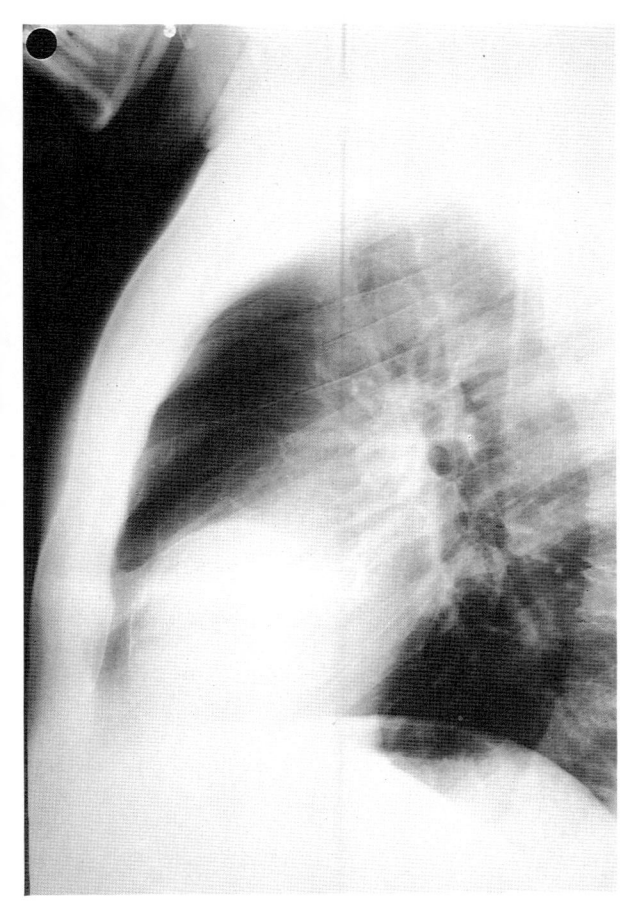

A 62-year-old man presented with a history of ischaemic heart disease.

- Comment on the cardiac shadow.
- What is the diagnosis?

A86

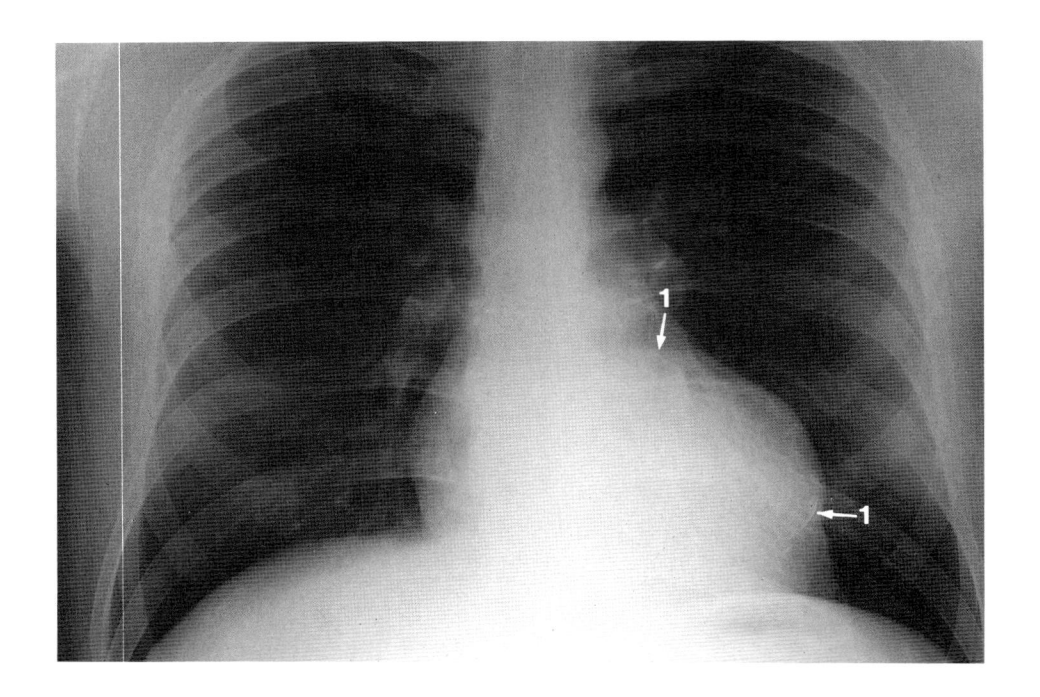

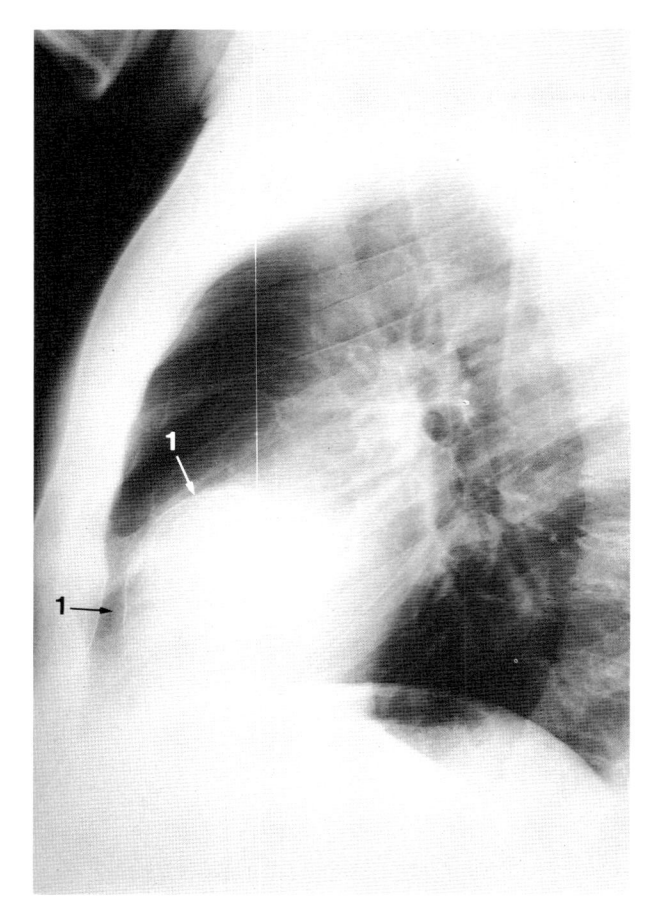

The heart is mildly enlarged. The left heart border and apex are more convex than usual, and a thin calcific density outlines the convexity (1). The diagnosis is calcified left ventricular aneurysm.

Q87

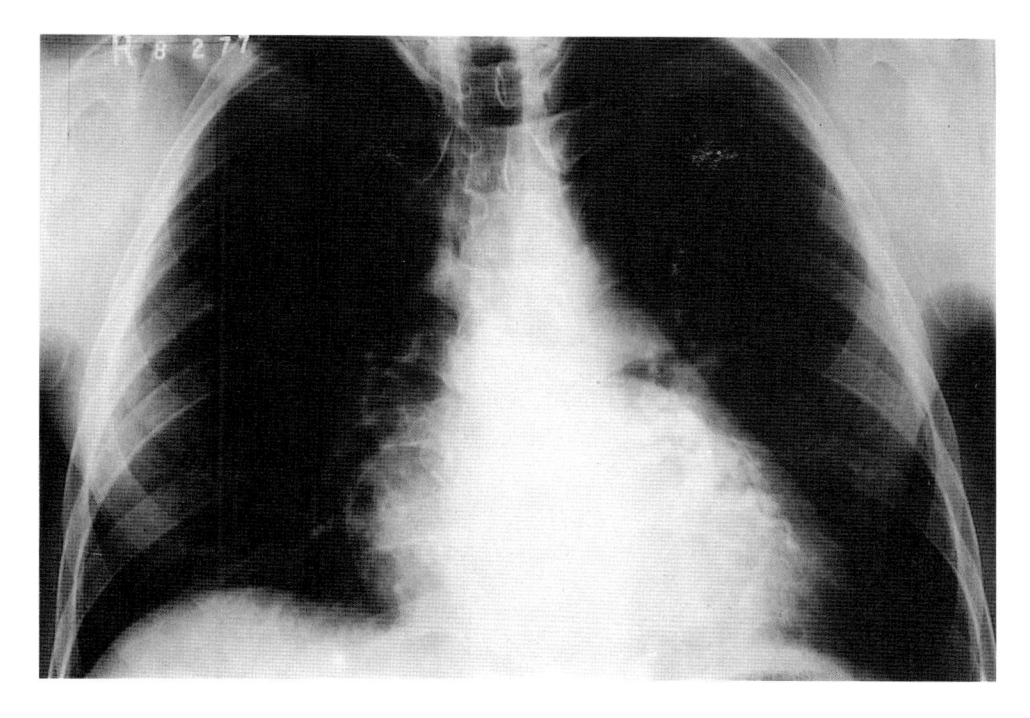

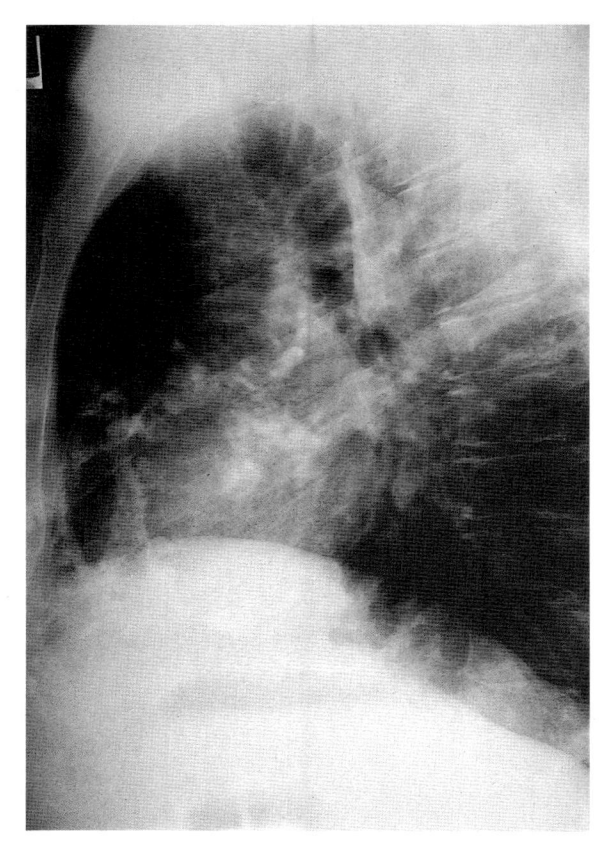

A 42-year-old man presented with exertional dyspnoea. On physical examination the pulse was paradoxical and the neck veins were distended.

- What does the CXR show?
- What is the diagnosis?

A87

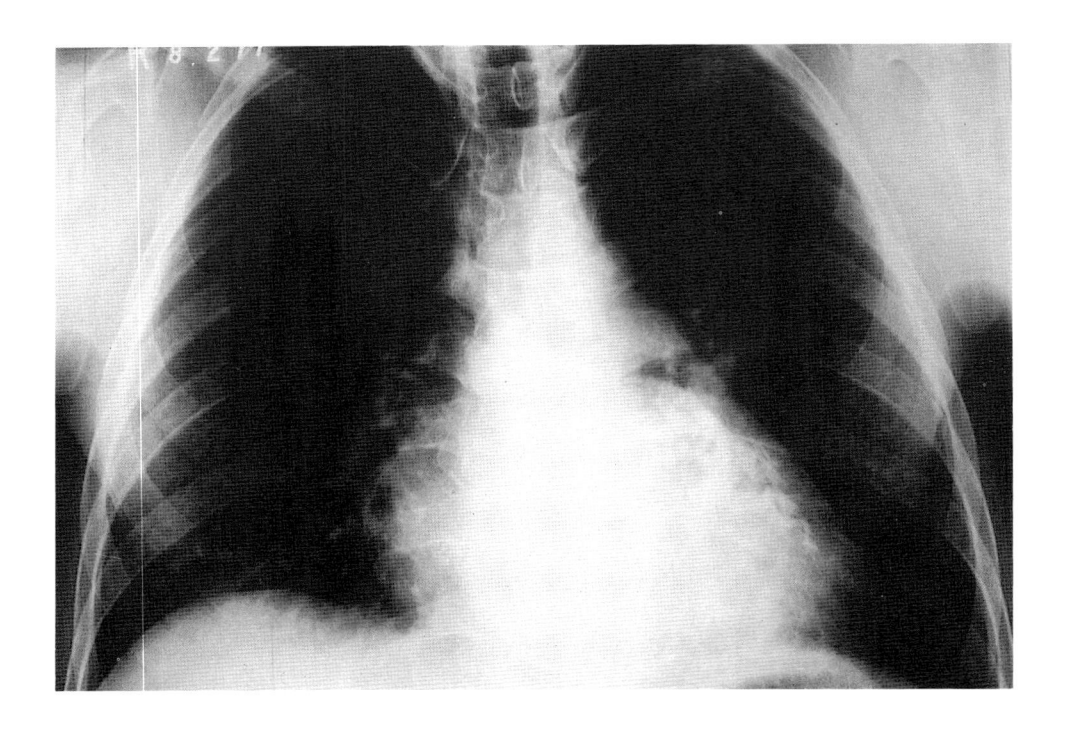

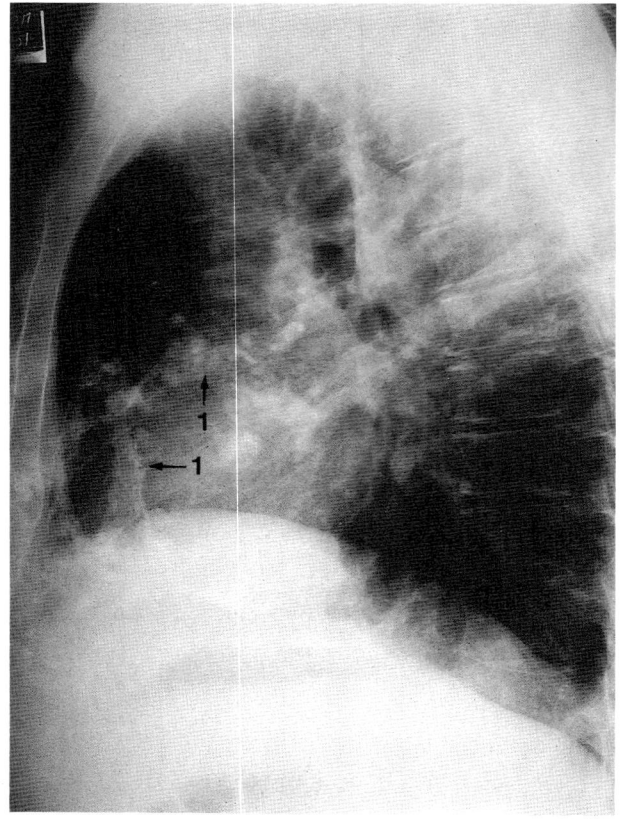

Extensive calcification is present over the heart. On the lateral film it is seen particularly densely in the atrioventricular and interventricular grooves (1). The diagnosis is constrictive pericarditis.

Q88

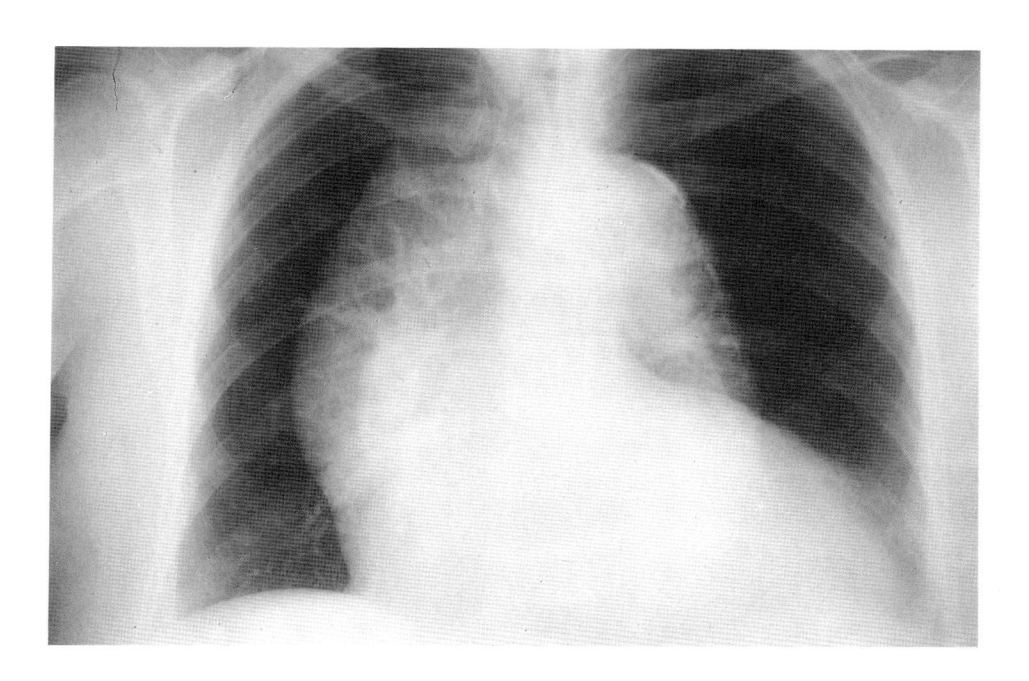

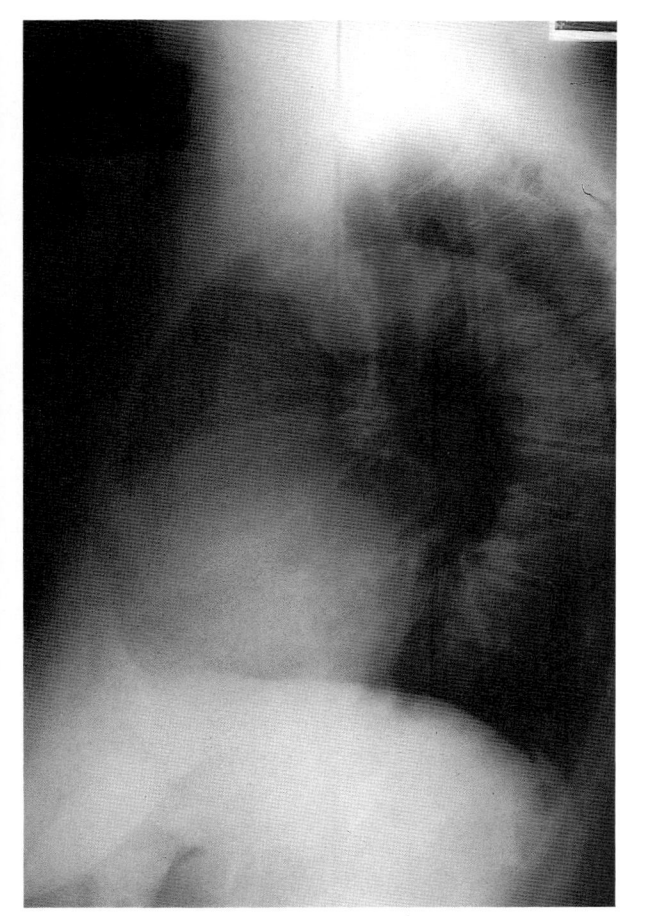

A 69-year-old female with systemic hypertension presented with chest pain and shortness of breath and an early diastolic murmur.

- Comment on the cardiac shadow.
- Comment on the aorta.
- What is the diagnosis, and what other investigation would you do?

A88

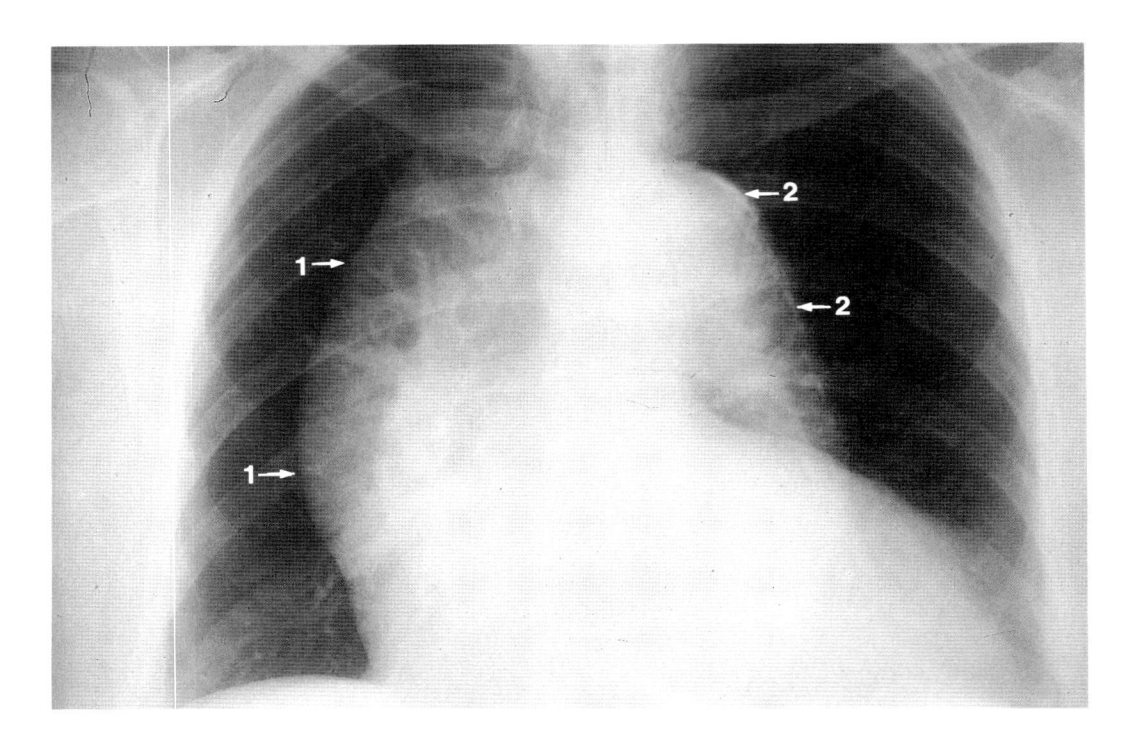

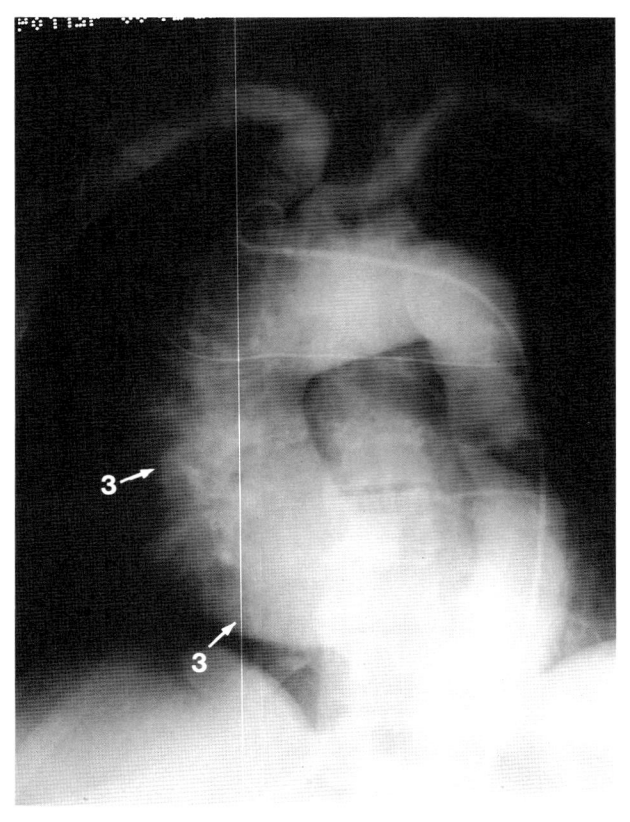

The heart is enlarged, the shape suggesting left ventricular enlargement. The aorta is unfolded. The ascending aorta is prominent (1). The descending aorta is not dilated, but is diffusely calcified (2). The diagnosis is aneurysm of the ascending aorta. The next investigation is an arch aortogram to assess the aorta and aortic valve. This demonstrates the aneurysm (3) confined to the ascending aorta. There was also mild aortic regurgitation.

Q89

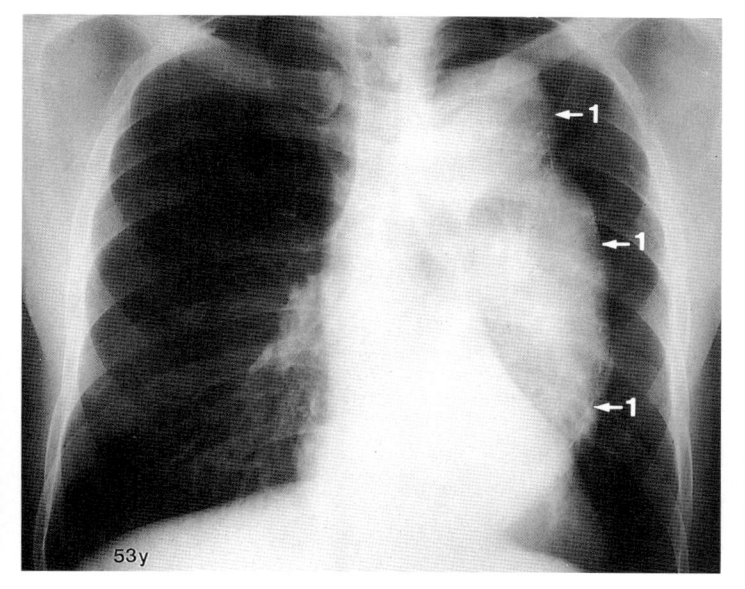

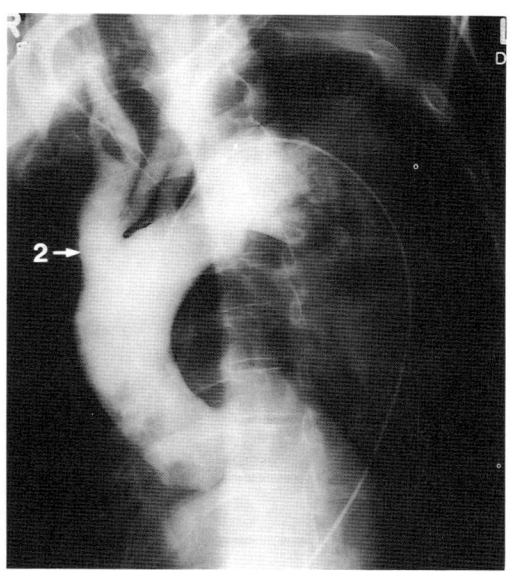

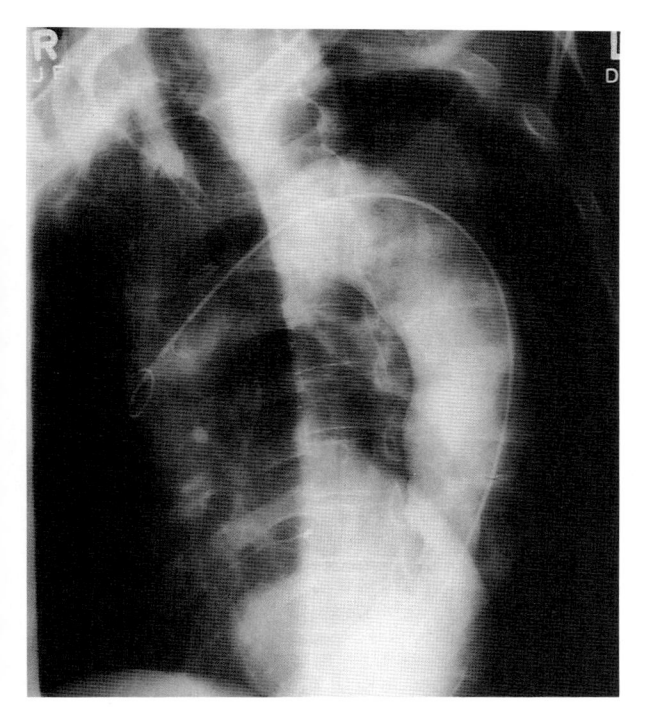

A 53-year-old male presented with systemic hypertension and vague chest pain.

- What is this structure (1)?
- Describe the angiogram.
- What is the diagnosis?
- Instead of the angiogram, what other investigation might have been done?

A89

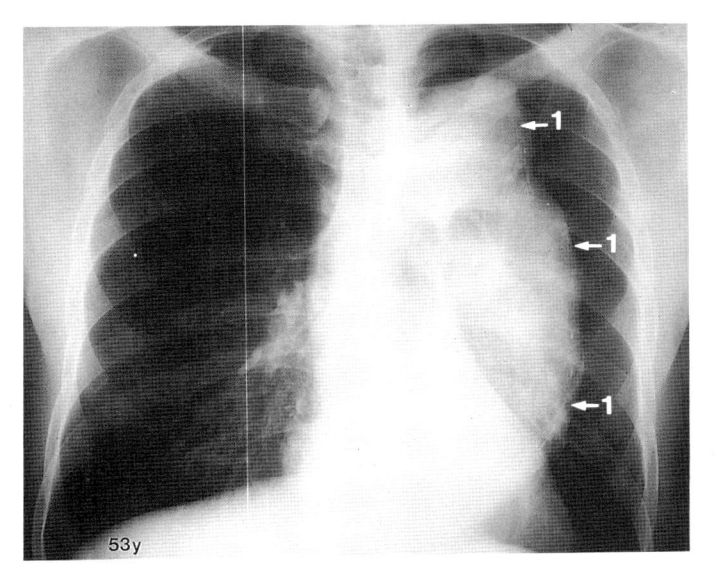

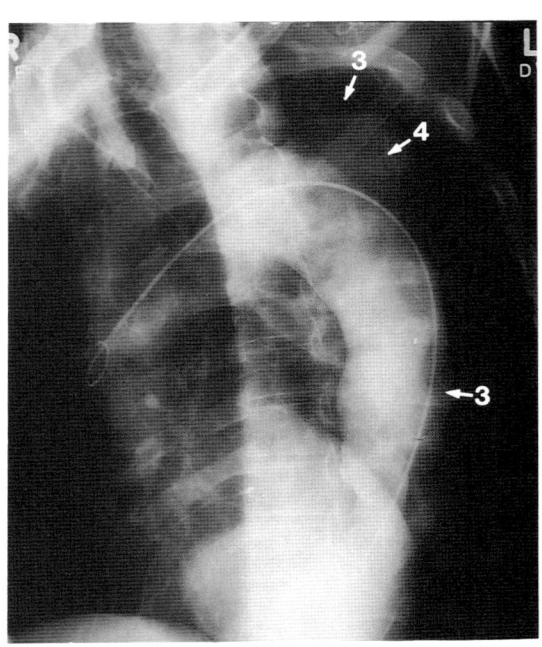

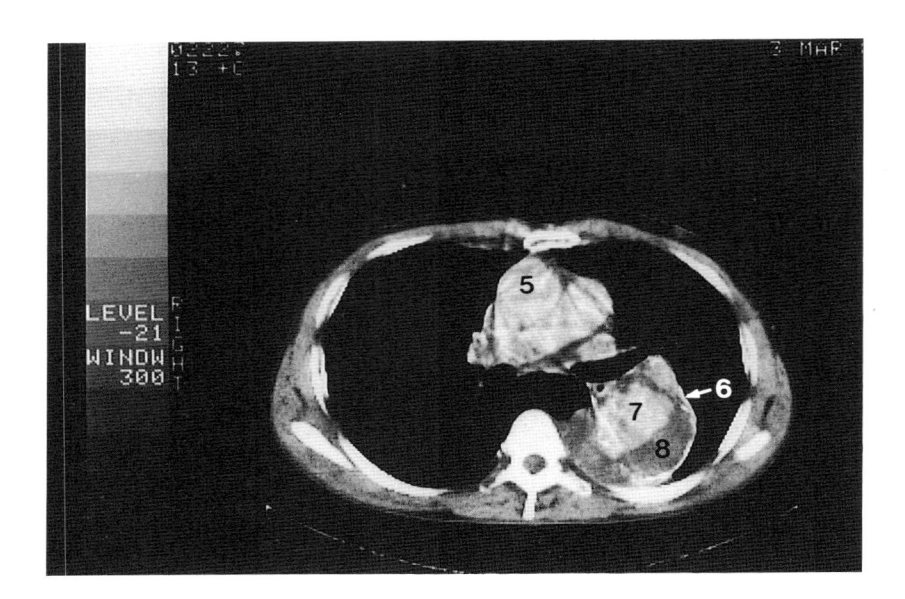

(1) = the descending aorta. It is dilated. The angiogram consists of two frames from an arch aortogram, left anterior oblique projection. There is: a normal ascending aorta; a common origin of innominate and left carotid arteries (2); and an aneurysm of the descending aorta, commencing immediately distal to the origin of the left subclavian artery (3). A false lumen does not opacify and is filled with blood clot (4). The diagnosis is dissecting aneurysm of descending aorta.

A contrast enhanced CT scan might have been performed. This shows normal ascending aorta (5), dilated descending aorta (6) with opacified true lumen (7) and clot-filled false lumen (8). Alternatively, an MRI scan would have given similar information.

Q90

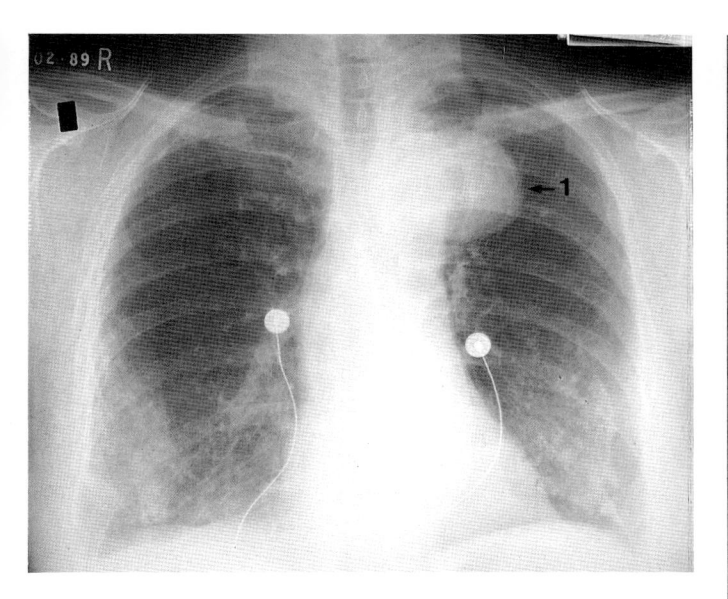

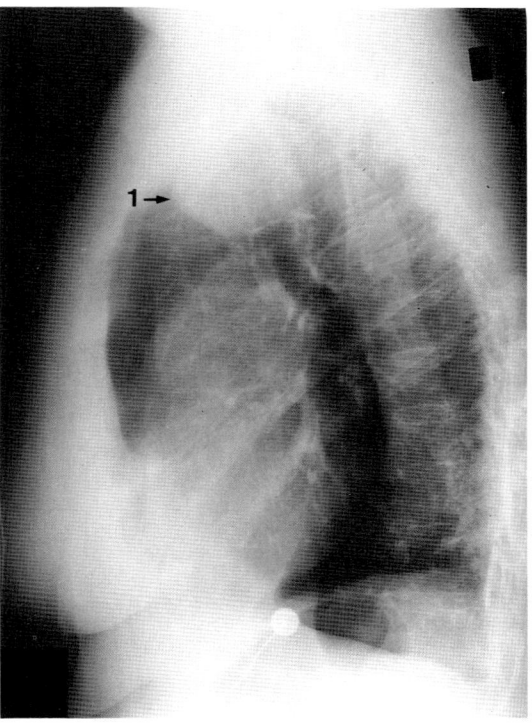

A 58-year-old female presented with mild central chest pain. She gave a history of chest infections many years earlier.

- Describe the abnormalities on the chest x-ray.
- What is the differential diagnosis of the opacity (1), and what further investigations would you do?

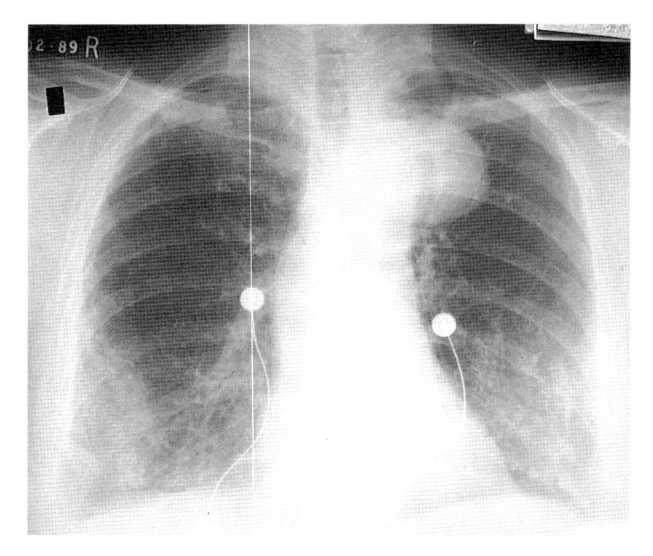

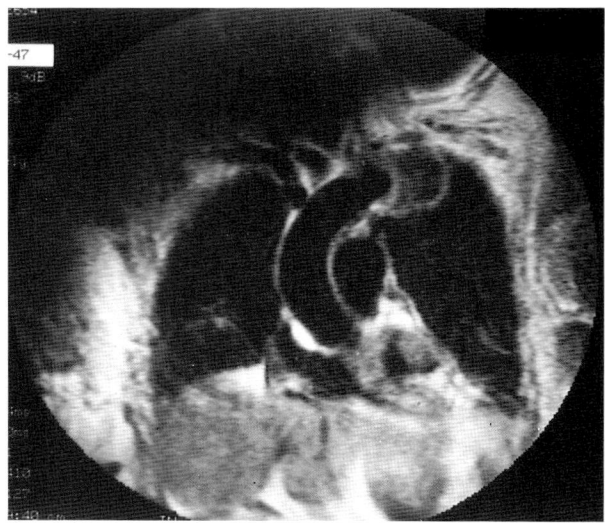

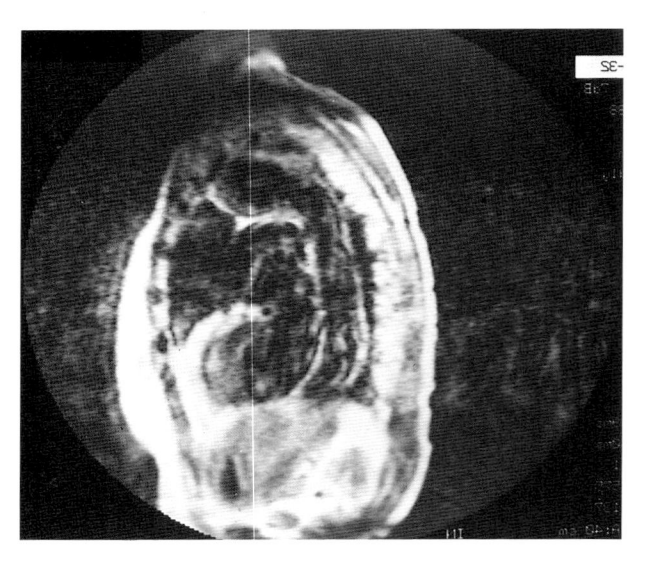

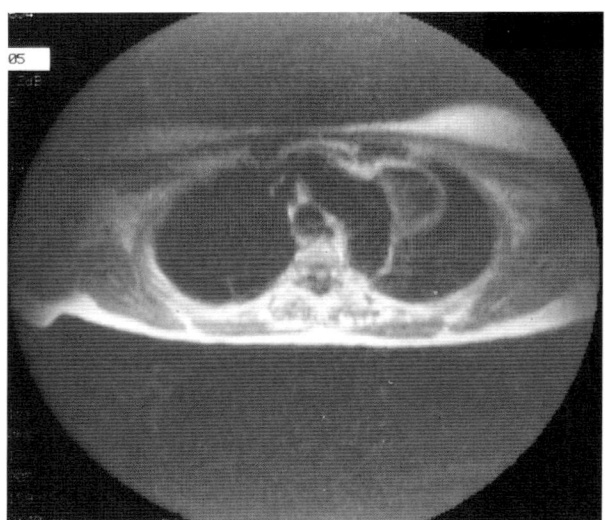

The chest x-ray shows extensive, bilateral lower zone pleural calcification and a round opacity (1) contiguous with the aortic knuckle. The pleural calcification is consistent with previous tuberculous pleurisy. The differential diagnosis of (1) lies between a mediastinal mass, a lung mass, and an aortic aneurysm.

Before considering a biopsy of some sort it is essential to exclude an aortic aneurysm. An MRI scan was performed, although a contrast enhanced CT scan or aortogram would also be appropriate. The scan shows the mass in coronal, sagittal, and transverse planes. It is an aneurysm of the aortic arch and contains thrombus.

Q91

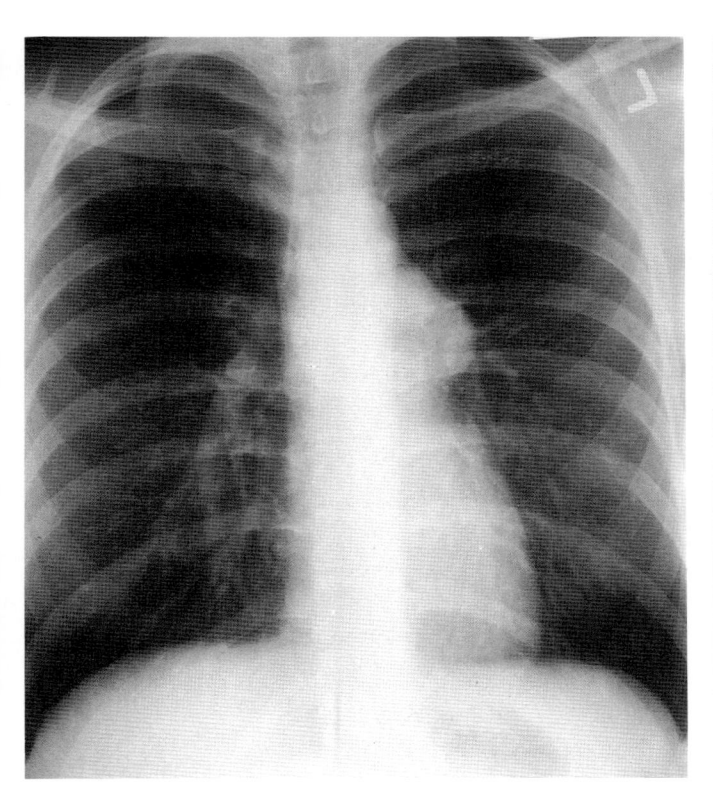

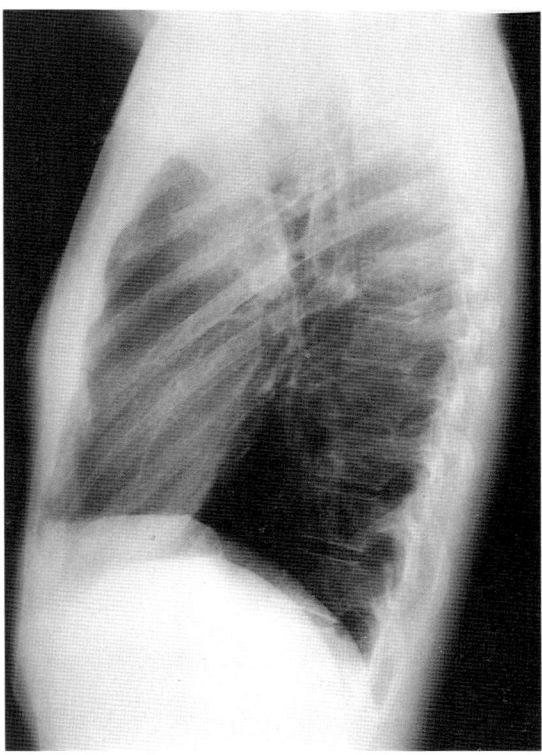

A 26-year-old female presented with generalised weakness, fatigue and double vision.

- What abnormality does the CXR show?
- What is the differential diagnosis?
- What is the diagnosis in this case?

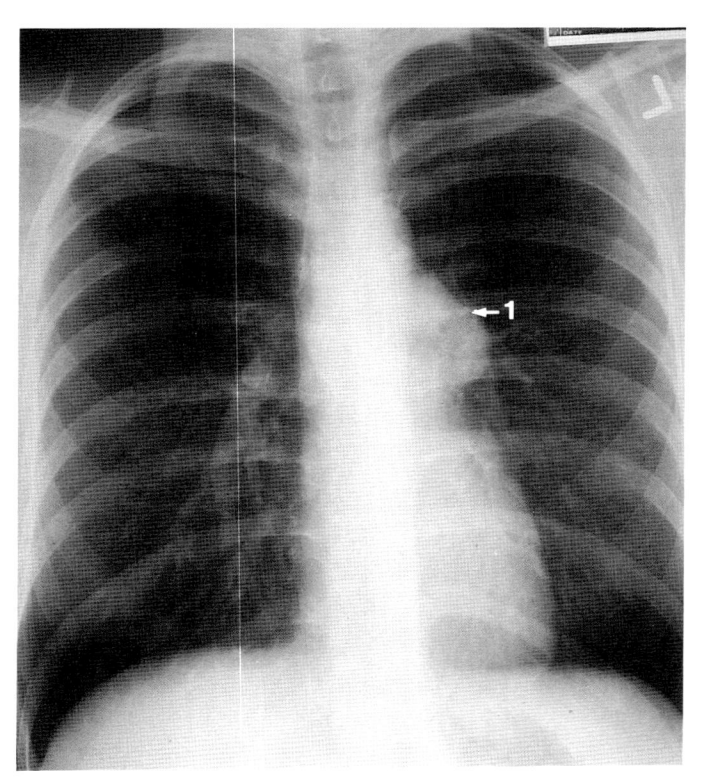

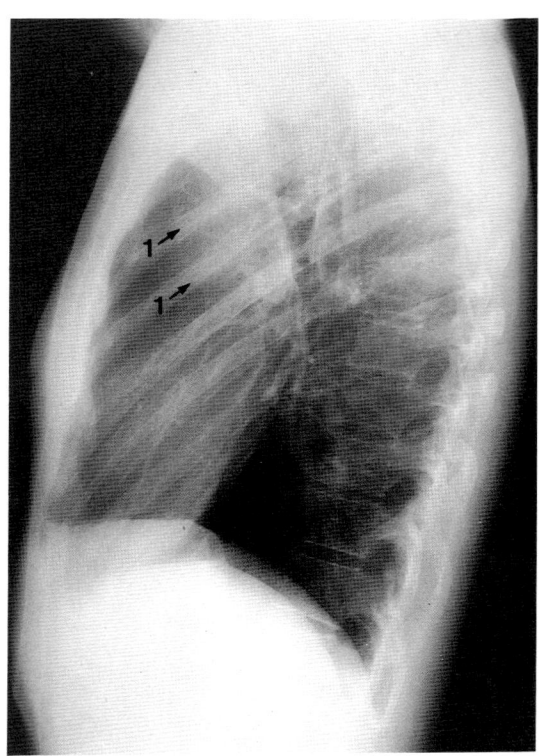

The CXR shows an anterior mediastinal mass (1). The differential diagnosis is:

a) Lymphadenopathy.
b) Retrosternal thyroid.
c) Thymoma.
d) Teratodermoid tumour.

The diagnosis in this case is thymoma, associated with myasthenia gravis.

Q92

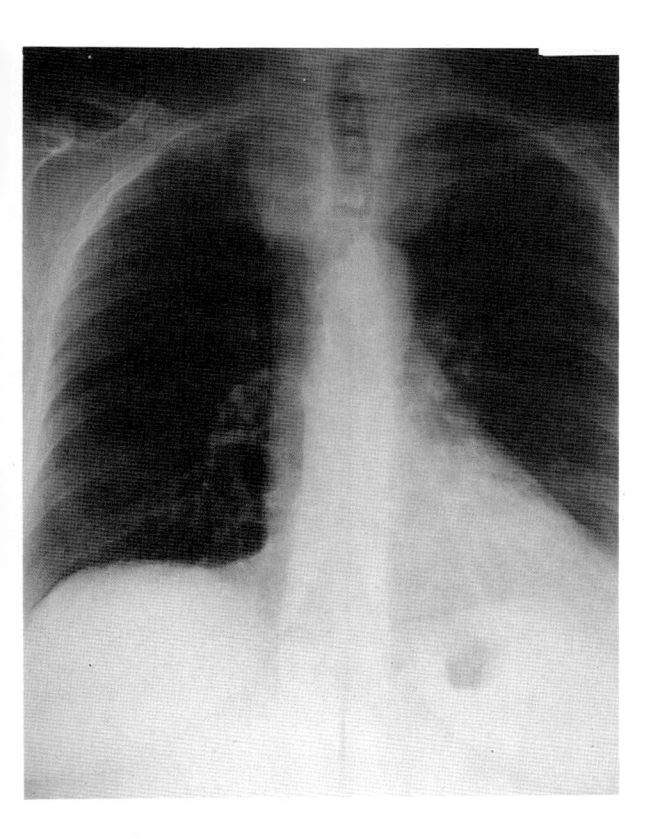

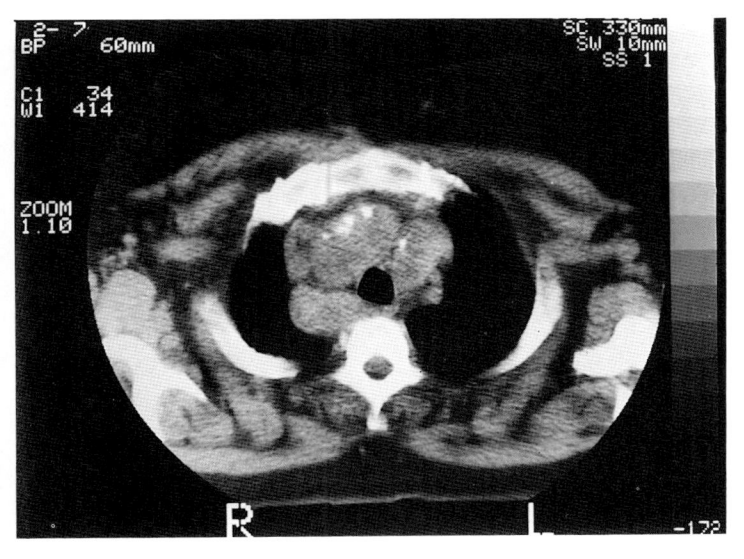

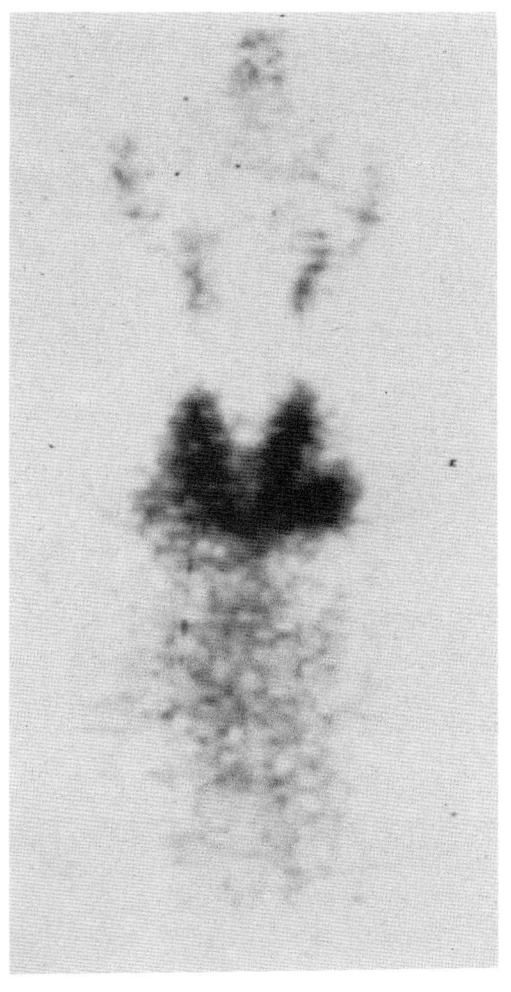

A 59-year-old female complained of a tight feeling in the neck.

- What abnormality is seen on the CXR?
- What does the radionuclide scan show?
- What abnormality is seen on the CT scan?
- What is the diagnosis?

A92

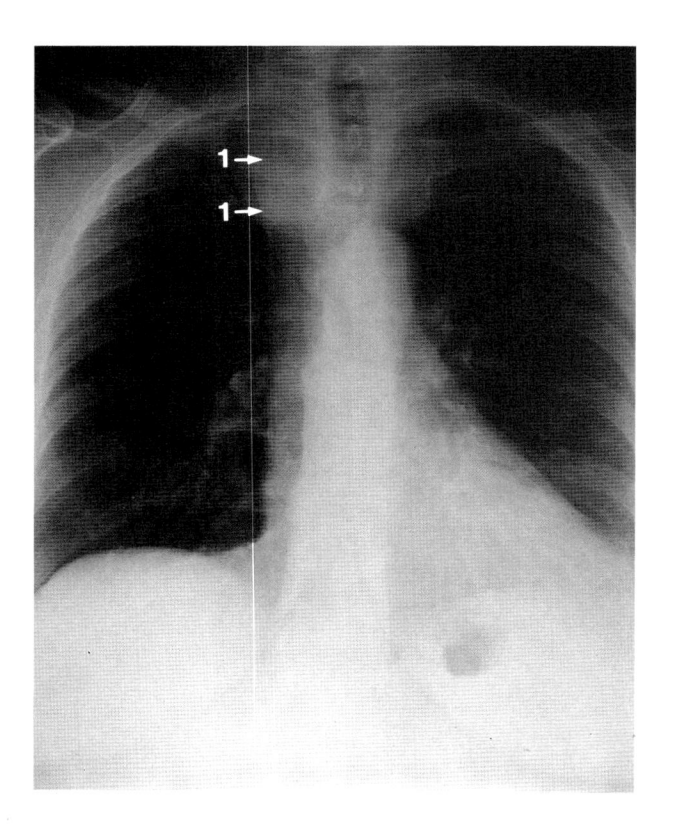

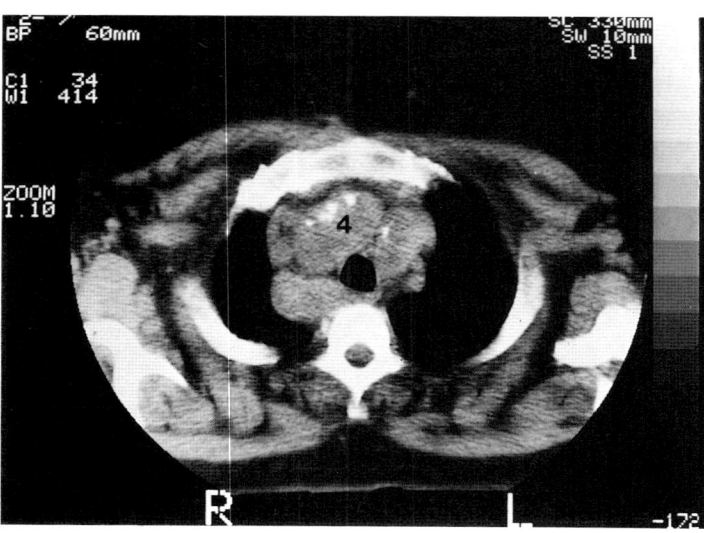

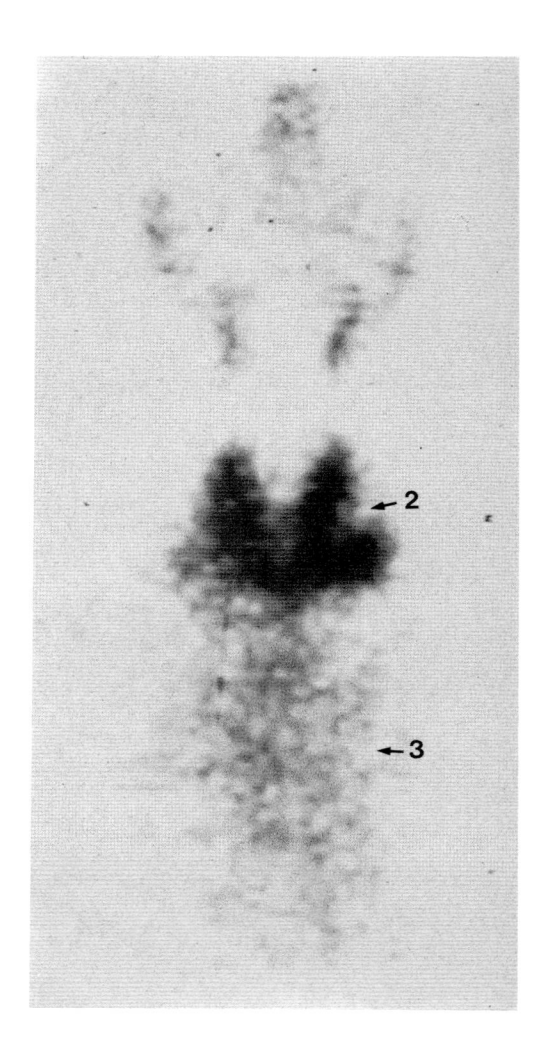

The CXR shows a superior mediastinal mass (1), which is causing mild deviation of the trachea to the left. The radionuclide scan shows uptake of isotope in the thyroid, with a small defect in the left lobe (2). There is also uptake of isotope extending into the thorax (3). A partly calcified soft tissue mass anterior to the trachea (4) is seen on the CT scan. The diagnosis is an intrathoracic, multinodular goitre.

Q93

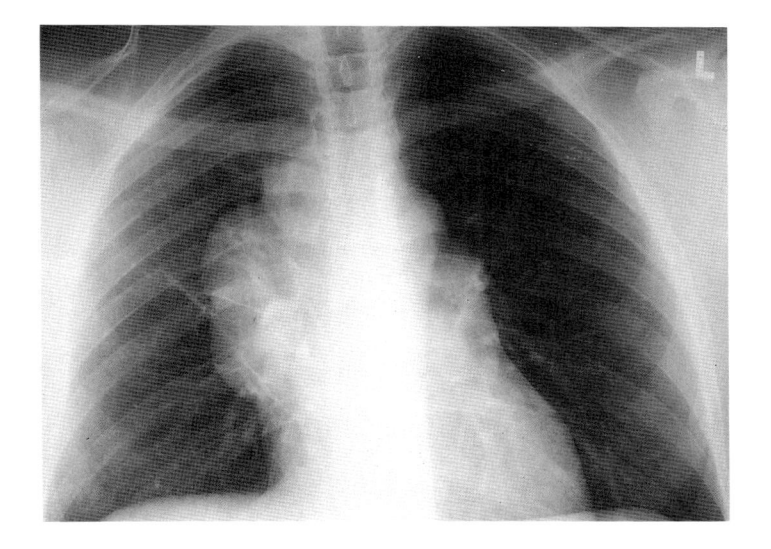

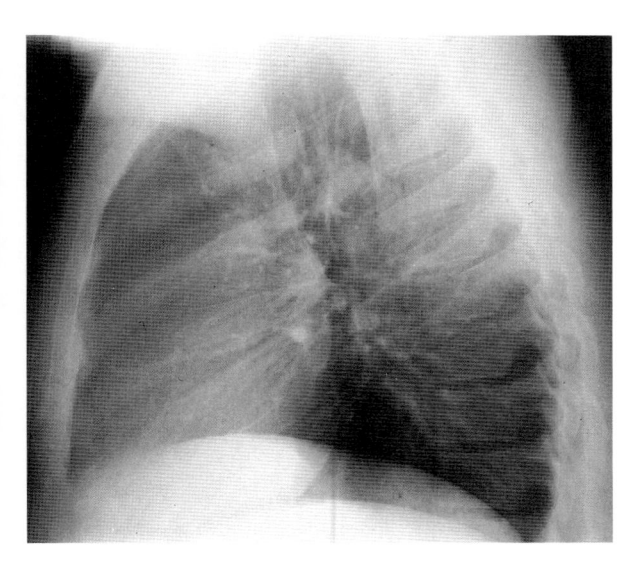

A 31-year-old male presented with chest discomfort and night sweats.

- What does the CXR show?
- What does the lateral CXR show?
- Does the CT scan add any information?
- What further investigation would you do?
- What is the diagnosis?

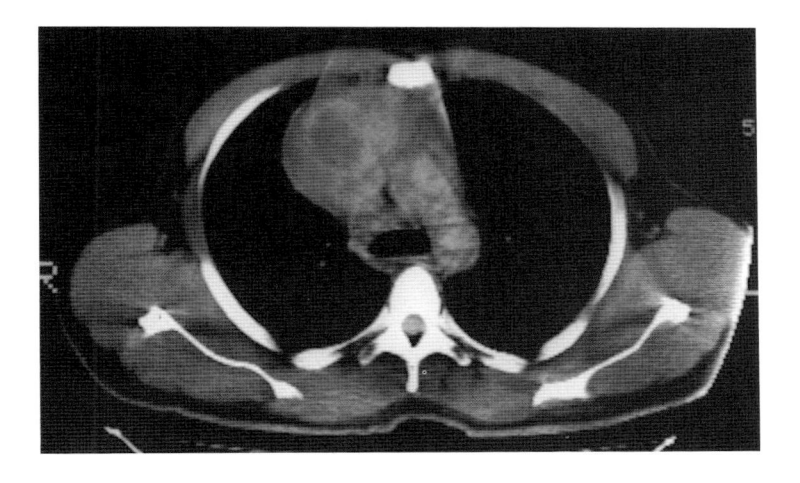

A93

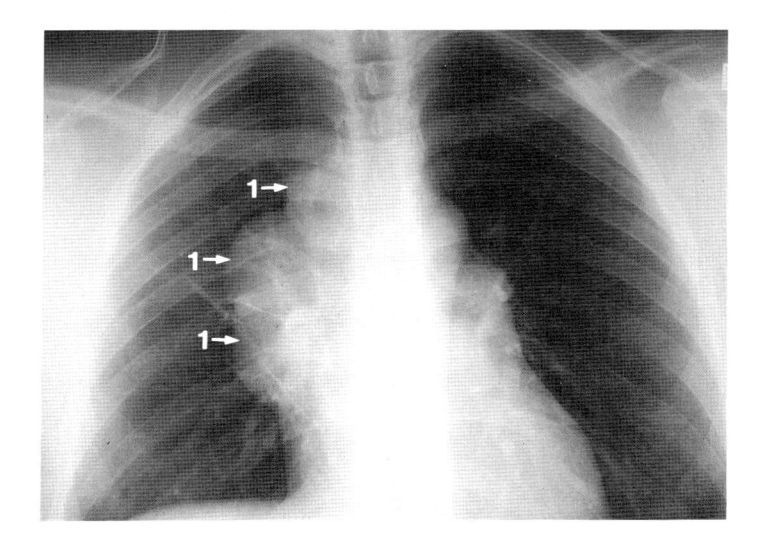

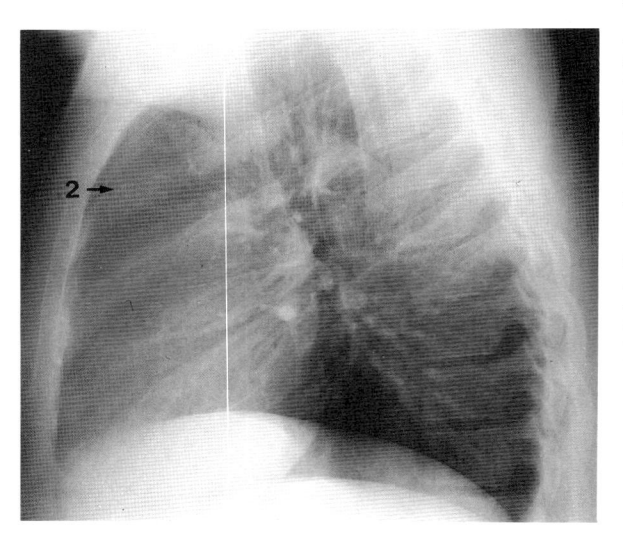

The CXR shows lobulated masses in the right paratracheal region and overlying the right hilum (1). The lateral CXR shows that the retrosternal space is occupied by soft tissue (2). This slice of the CT scan does not add any information. It does, however, confirm the retrosternal mass (3).

A histological diagnosis is necessary: mediastinoscopy was performed in this case, but a percutaneous needle biopsy could have been easily performed. The diagnosis is Hodgkin's lymphoma.

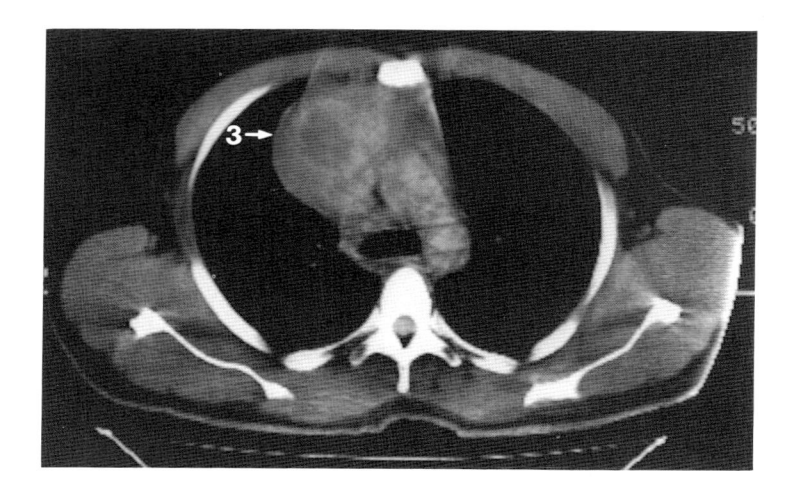

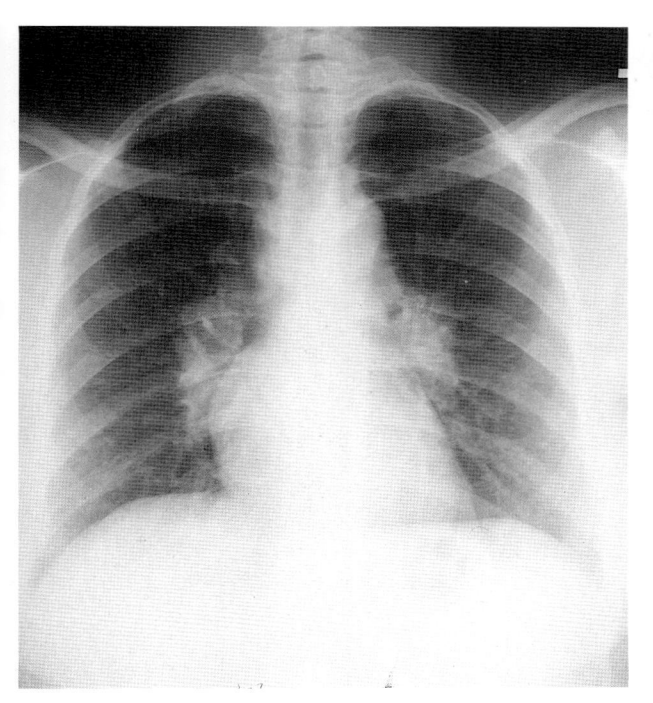

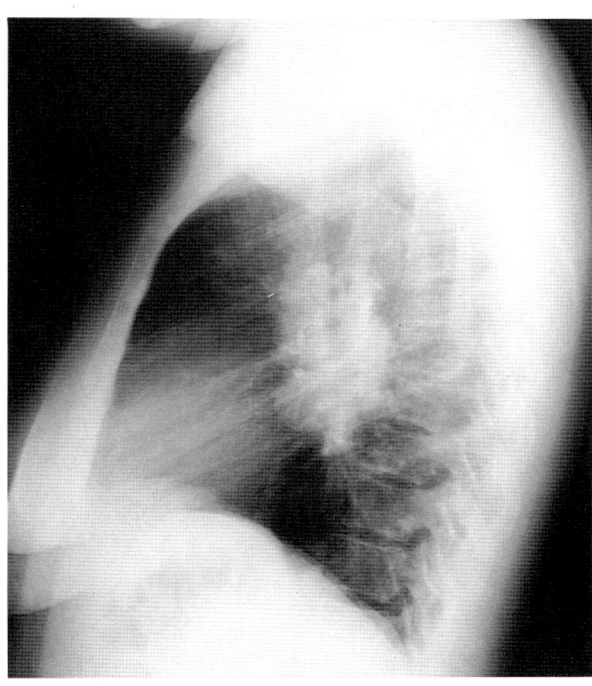

A 32-year-old asymptomatic female had this CXR taken for pre-employment purposes.

- Describe the CXR abnormalities.
- Is the retrosternal space clear?
- What is the diagnosis?

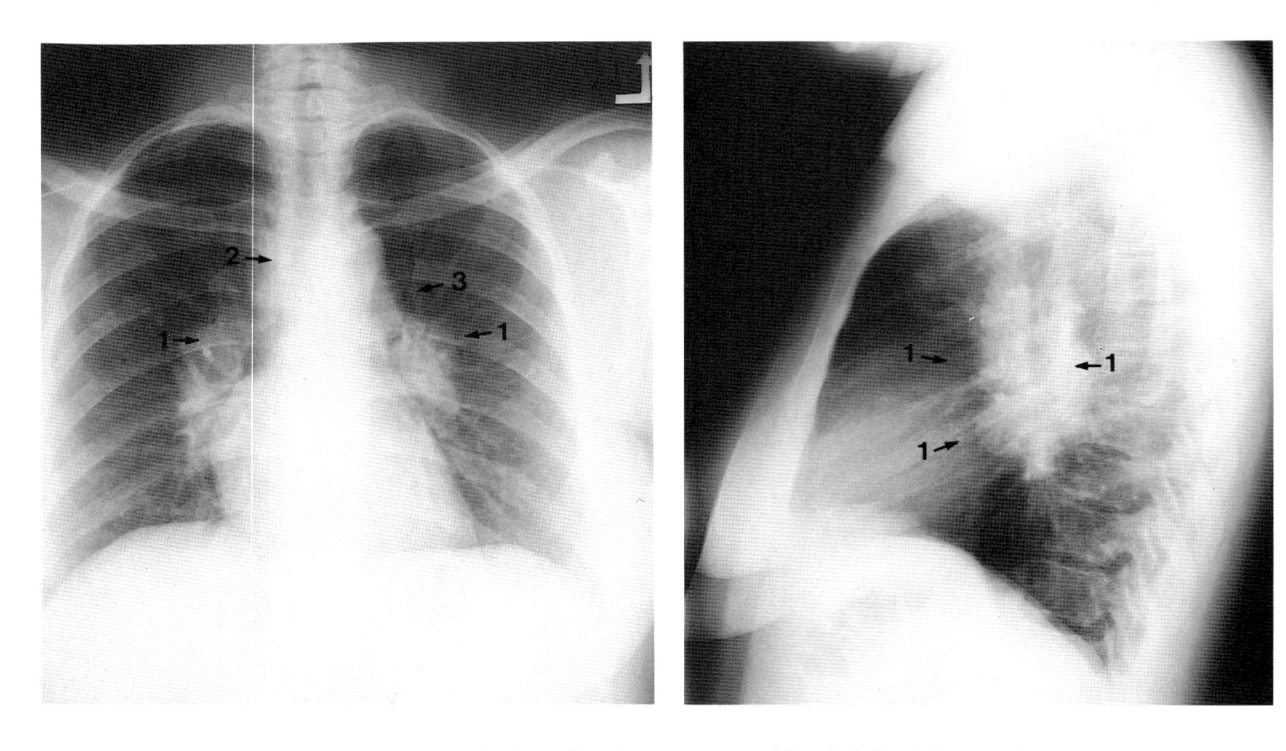

There is lobulated enlargement of both hila (1). Increased right paratracheal shadowing is present (2). Lymph node enlargement is also present in the aortico-pulmonary window (3). The retrosternal space is clear, unlike in case 93. The diagnosis is sarcoidosis.

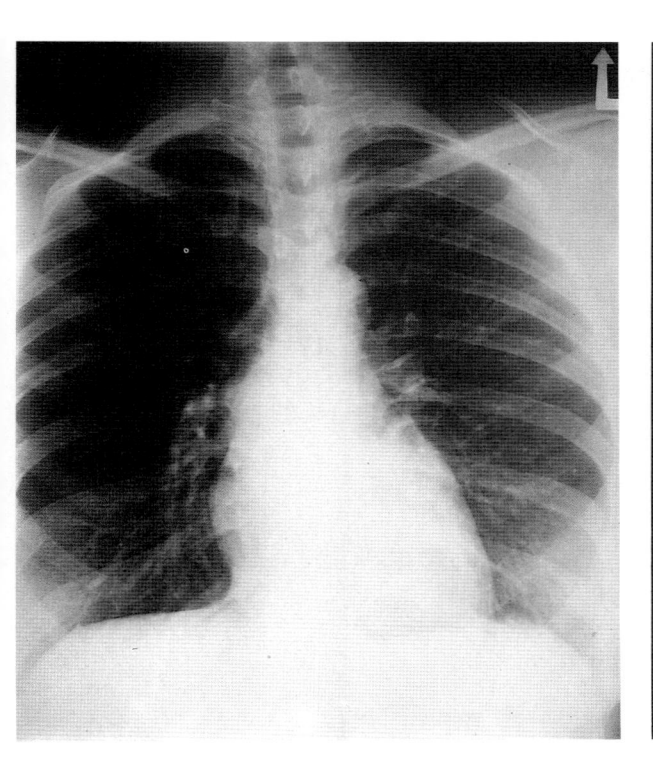

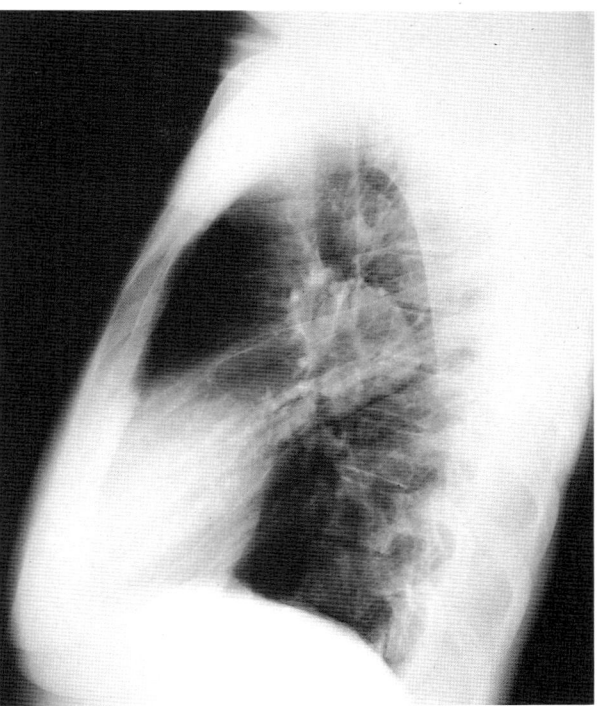

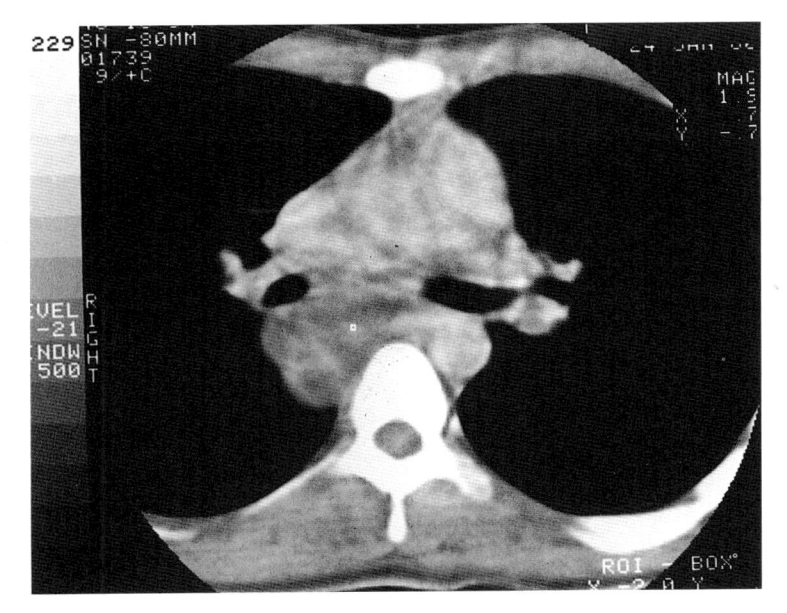

A 24-year-old female presented with a tooth abscess. A routine CXR was taken prior to general anaesthetic. There were no chest symptoms.

- What does the CXR show?
- What does the CT scan show?
- What is the differential diagnosis?

A95

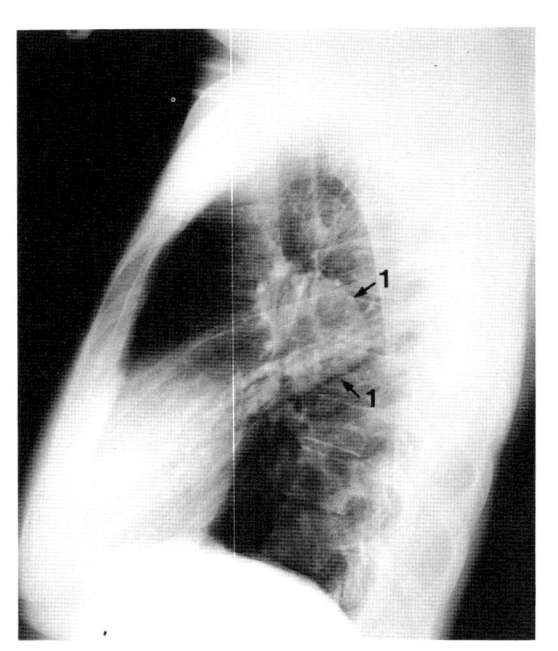

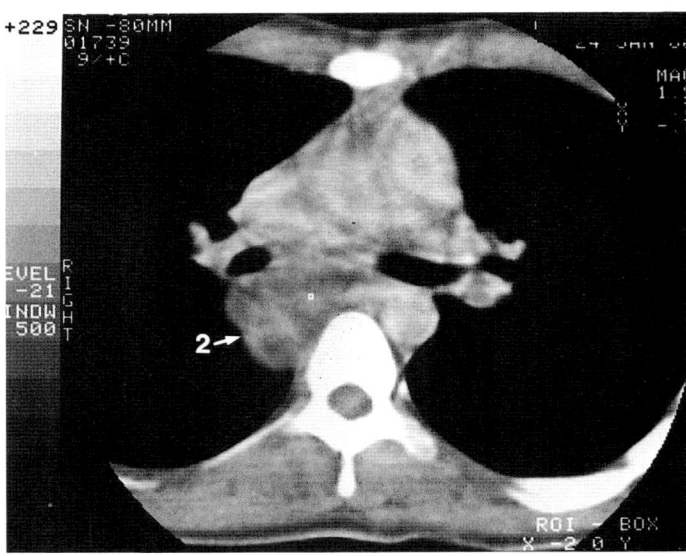

The PA film is normal, but on the lateral film a middle mediastinal mass is seen (1). The CT scan shows that the mass occupies the azygo-oesophageal recess (2). The differential diagnosis is lymphadenopathy or bronchogenic cyst. This patient had a bronchogenic cyst.

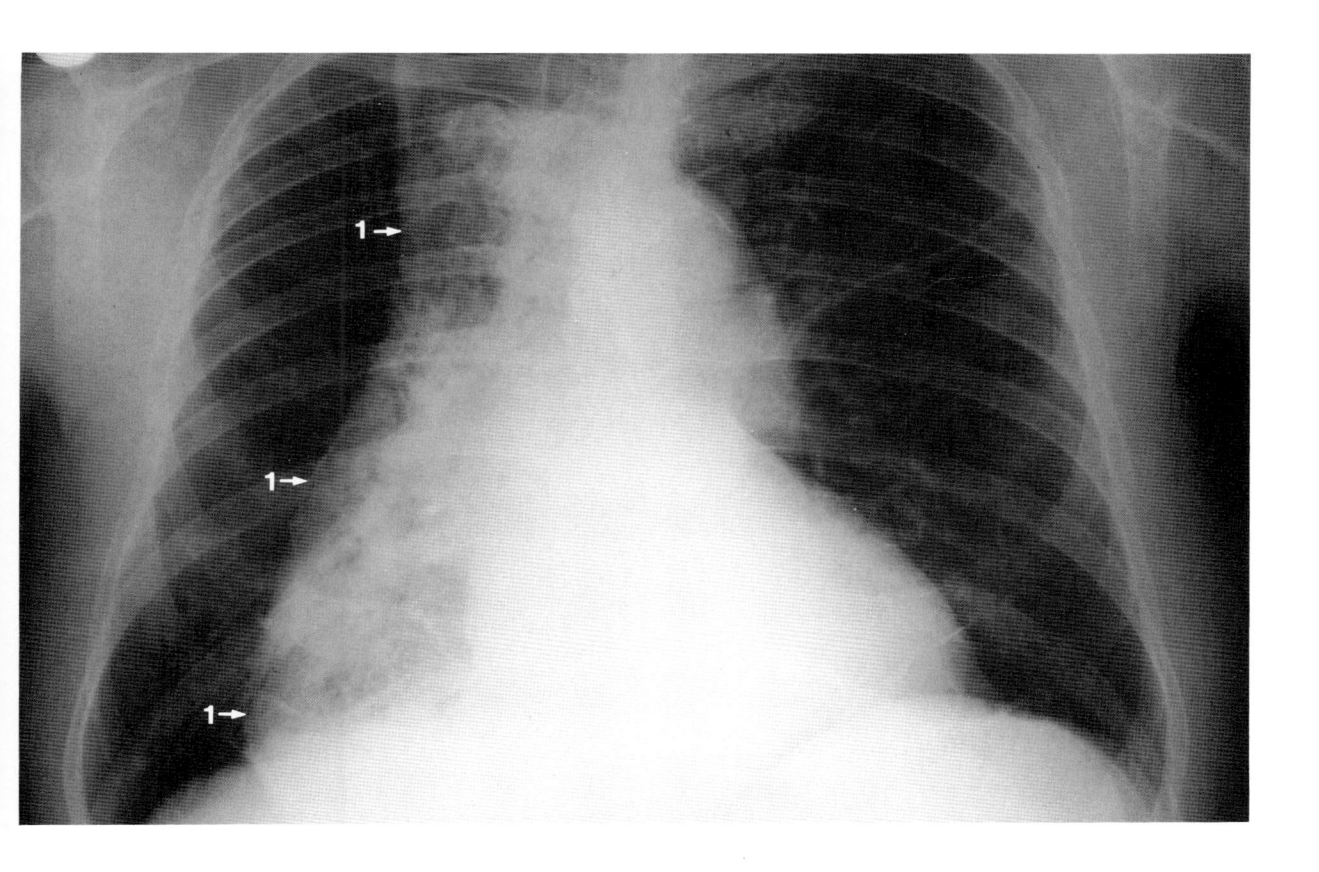

A 57-year-old man presented with persistent vomiting.

- What is the density (1) in the right hemithorax?
- What is the probable diagnosis?
- What further investigation would you do?

A96

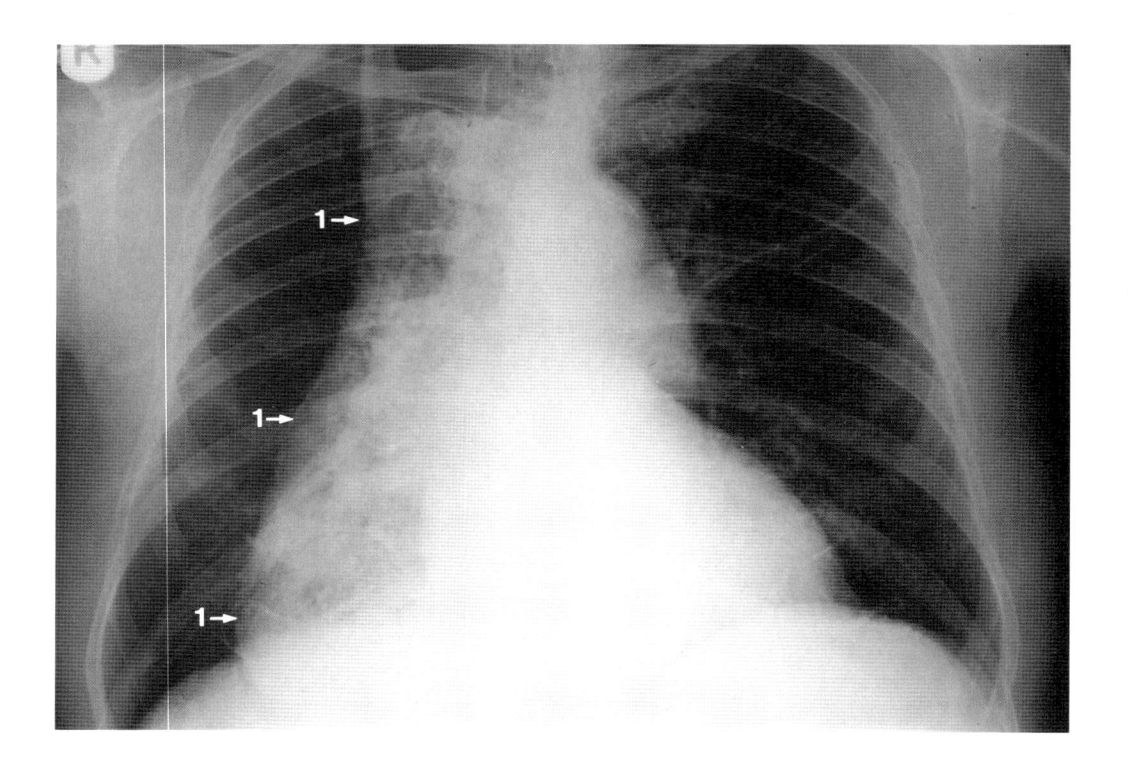

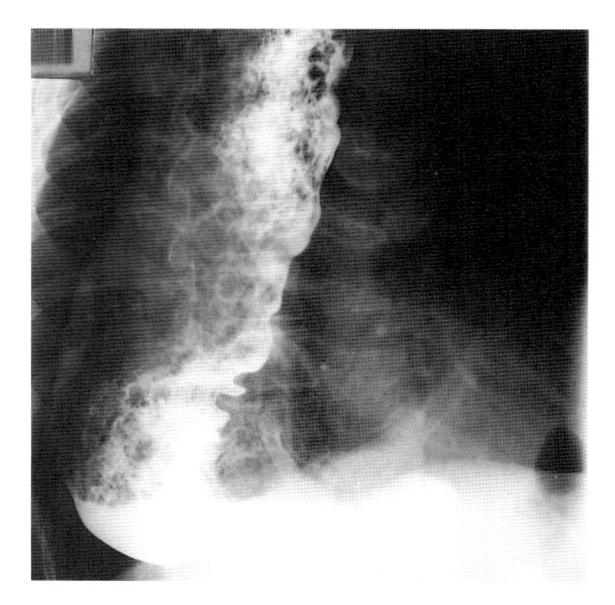

The density in the right hemi-thorax is a dilated oesophagus, full of food debris. The probable diagnosis is achalasia. The next investigation is a barium swallow. Note how the barium has passed through the food residue and settled at the lower end of the oesophagus.

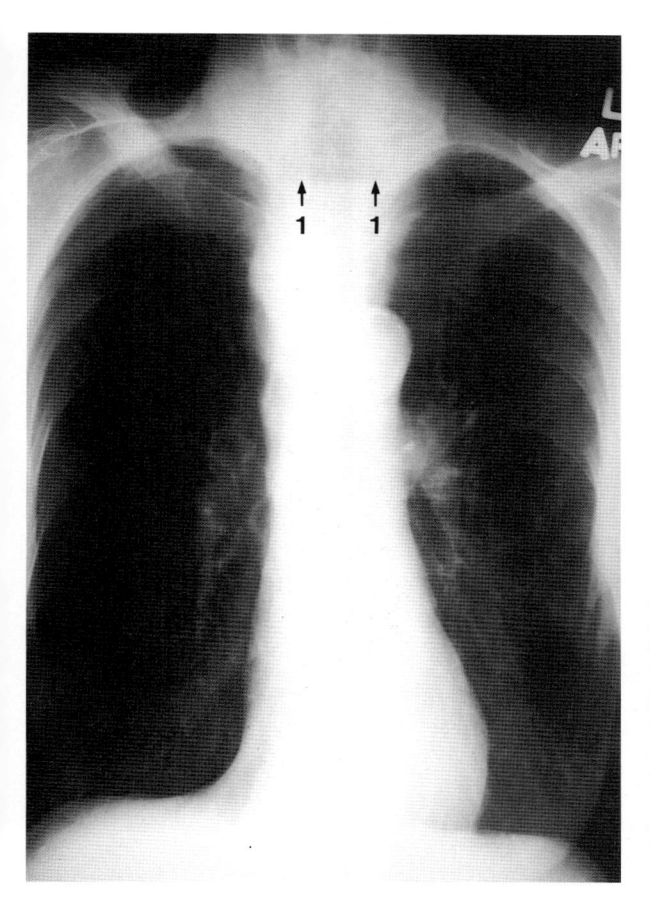

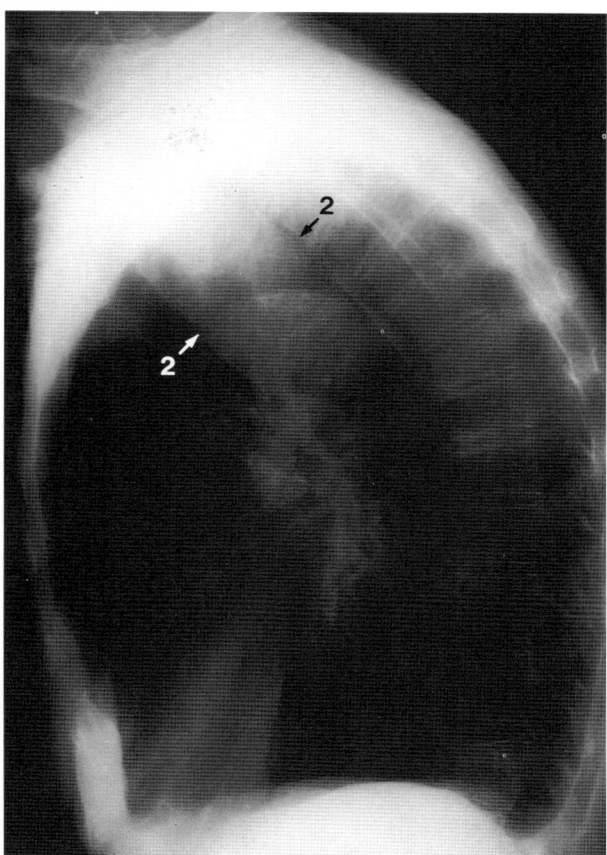

A 75-year-old female presented with dysphagia and vomiting.

- What is this density (1)?
- What is this density (2)?
- Why is the patient vomiting?
- What examination would you do next?

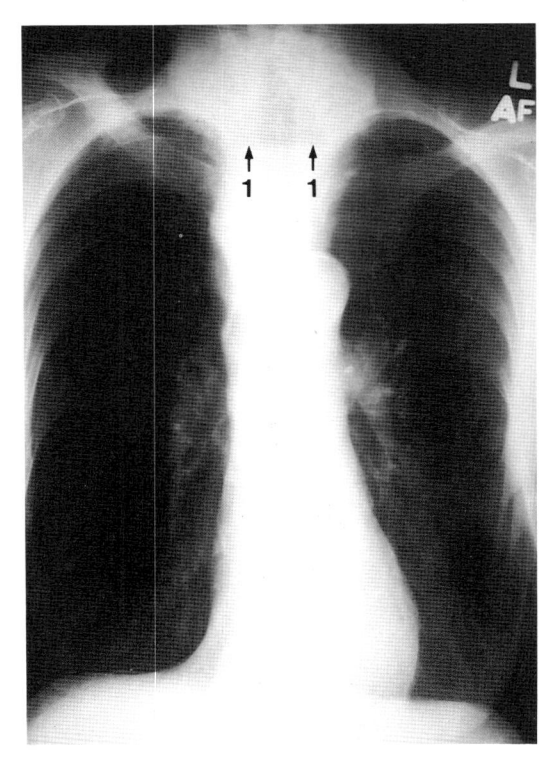

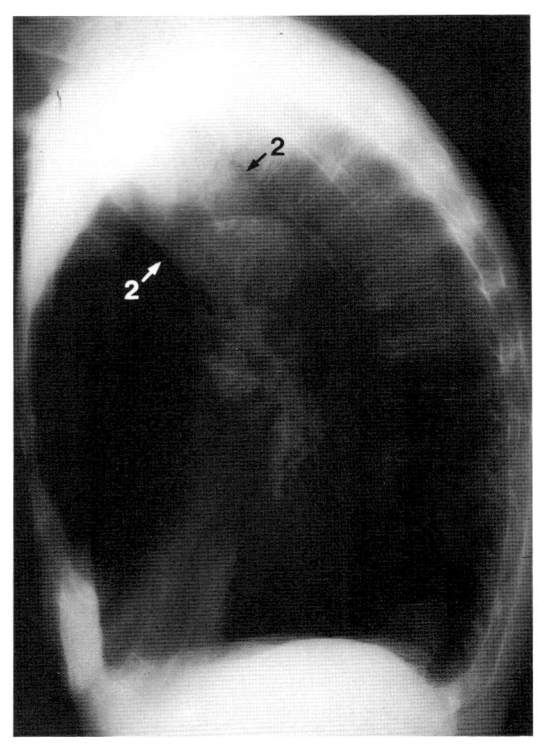

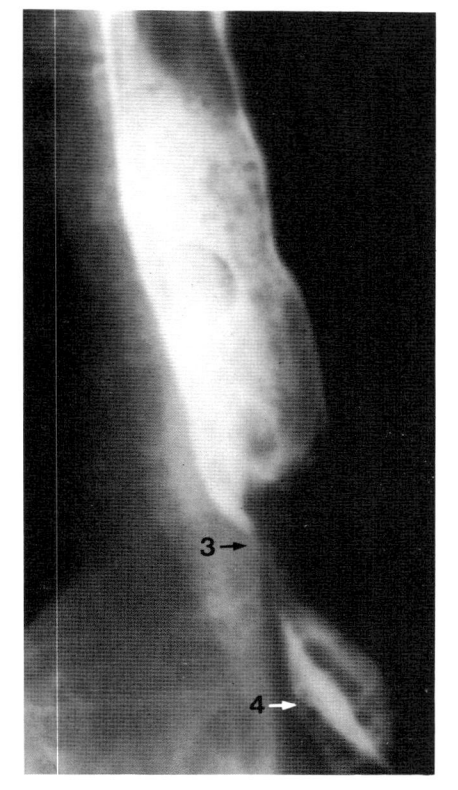

(1) = a fluid level. (2) = a dilated, fluid-filled oesophagus. The patient is vomiting because the oesophagus is obstructed. A barium swallow should be undertaken. It shows a tight, distal oesophageal stricture (3) secondary to a hiatus hernia (4). Oesophogoscopy was performed to exclude malignancy.

Q98

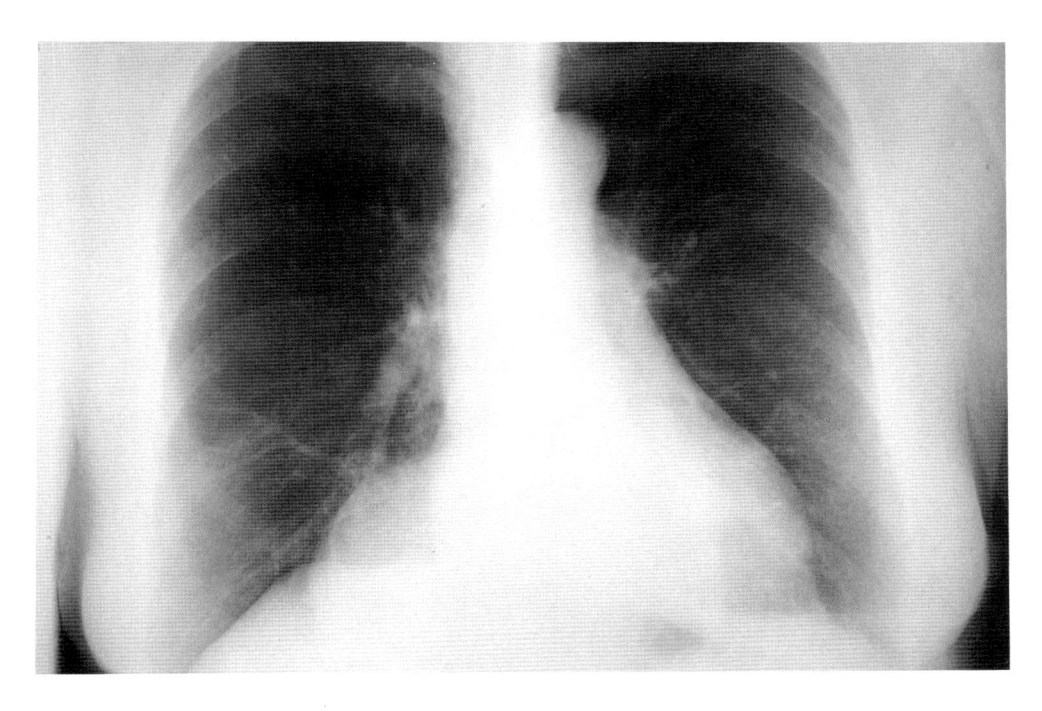

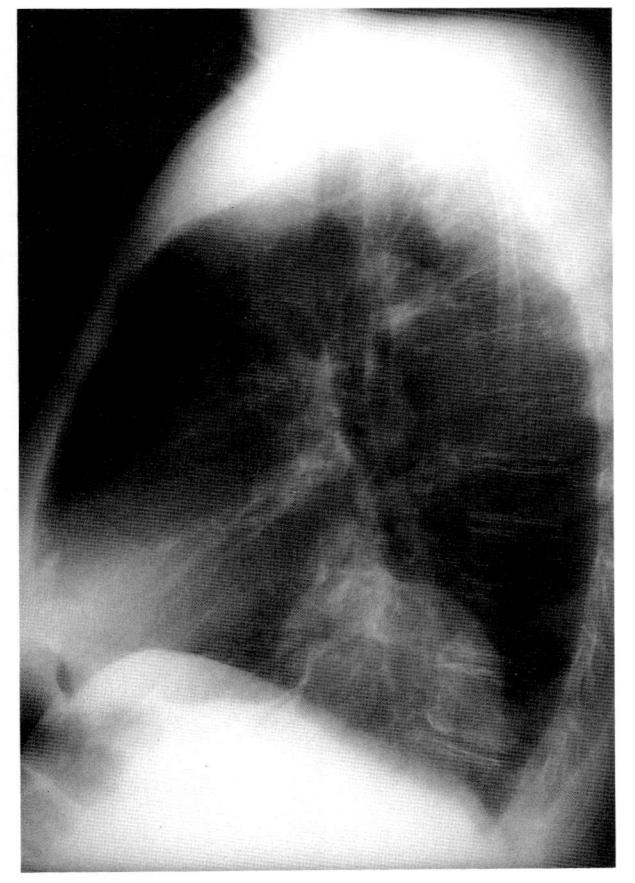

A 54-year-old female presented, complaining of "heartburn".

- What does the CXR show?
- What is the diagnosis?
- How would you prove it?

A98

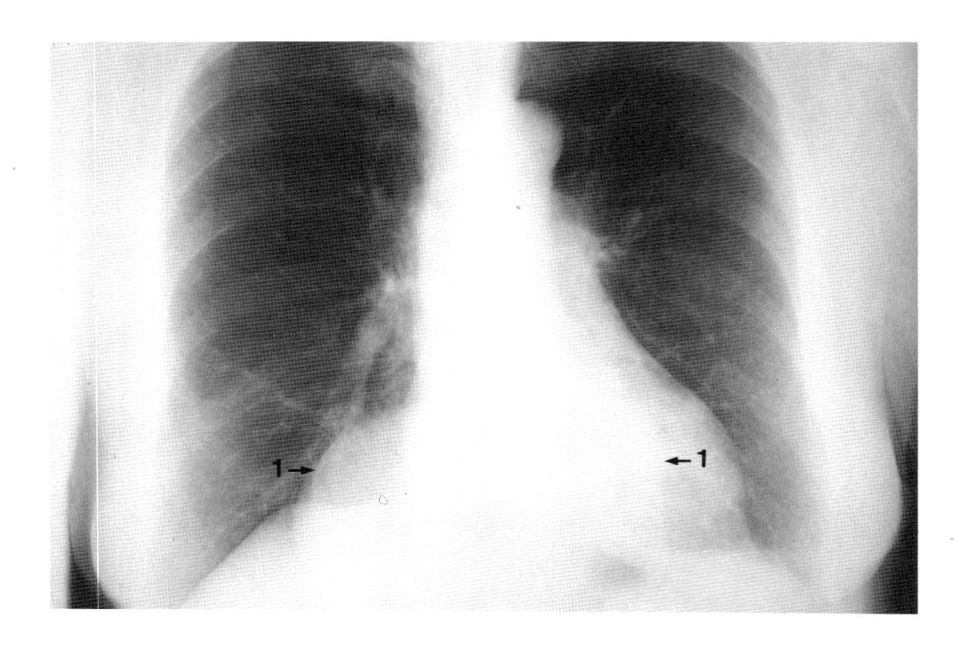

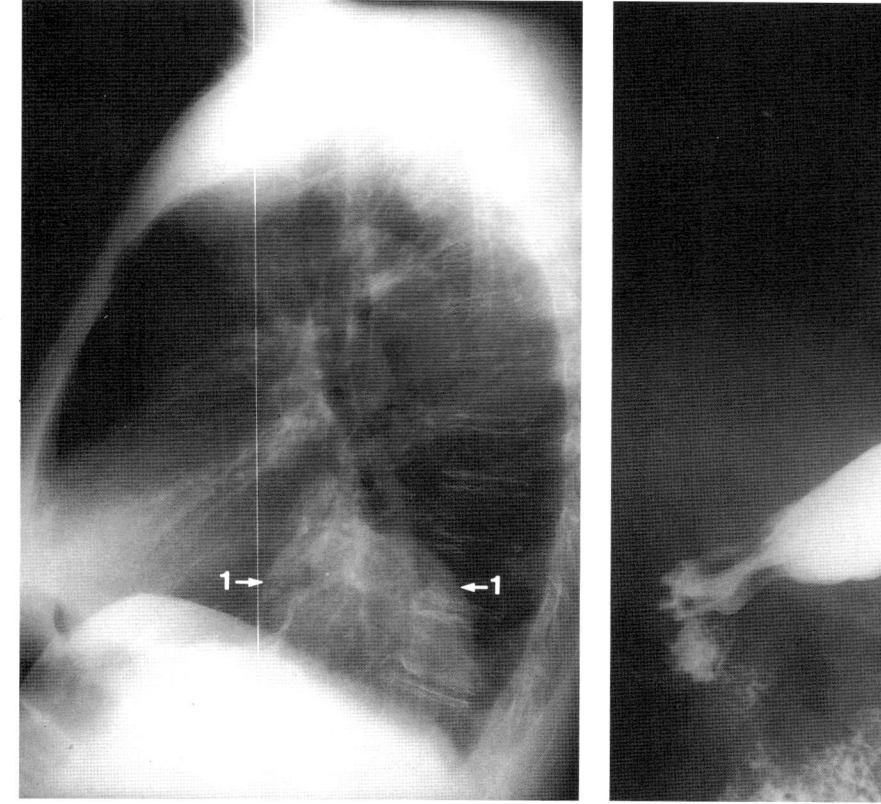

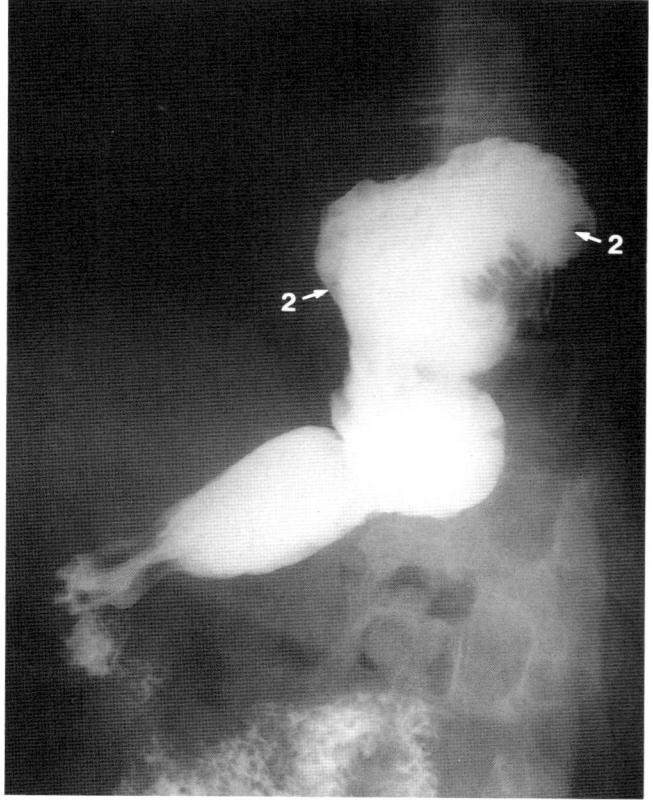

The CXR shows a retrocardiac opacity (1). The diagnosis is a hiatus hernia. It could be proved by a barium swallow and meal. The entire gastric fundus (2) is intrathoracic.

Q99

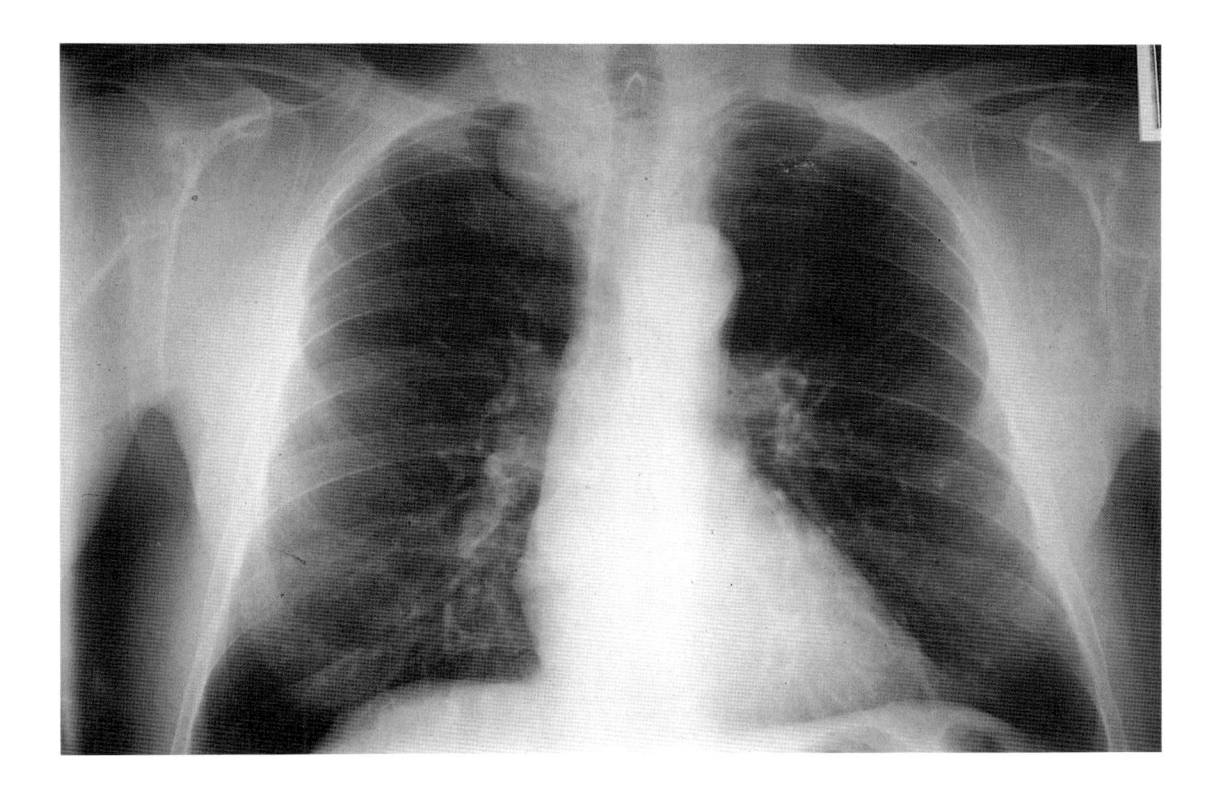

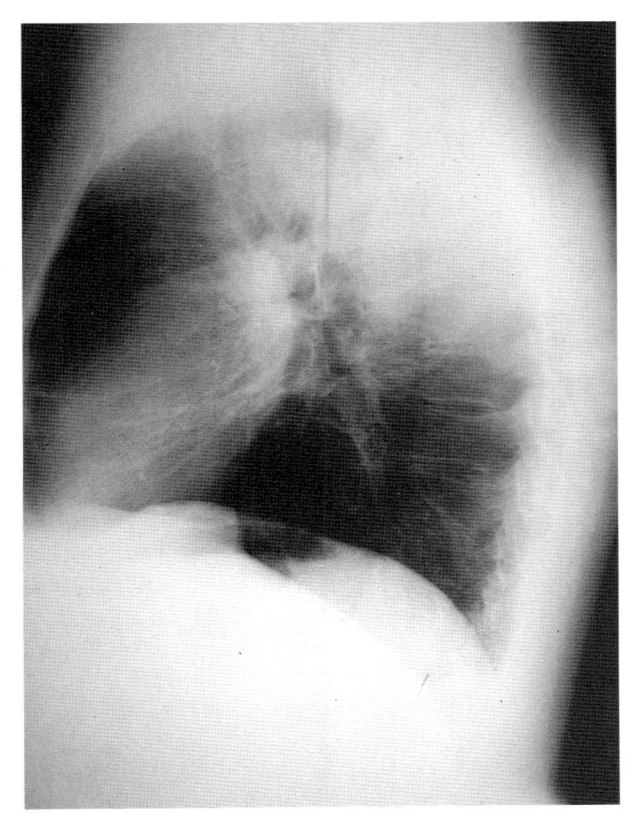

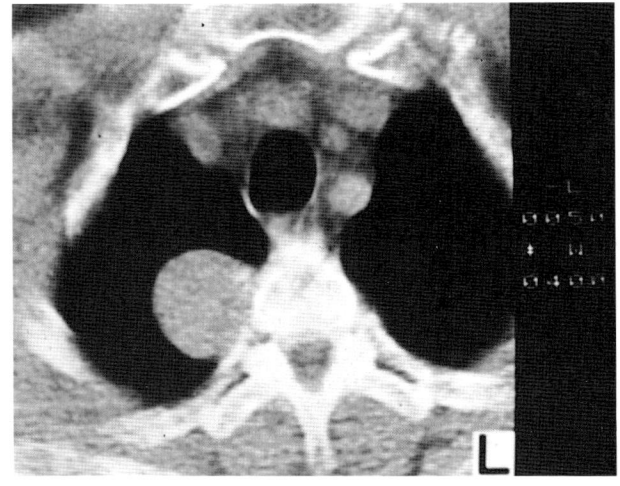

A 25-year-old male was asymptomatic when a routine CXR was undertaken.

- What abnormality do you see?
- What is the diagnosis?

A99

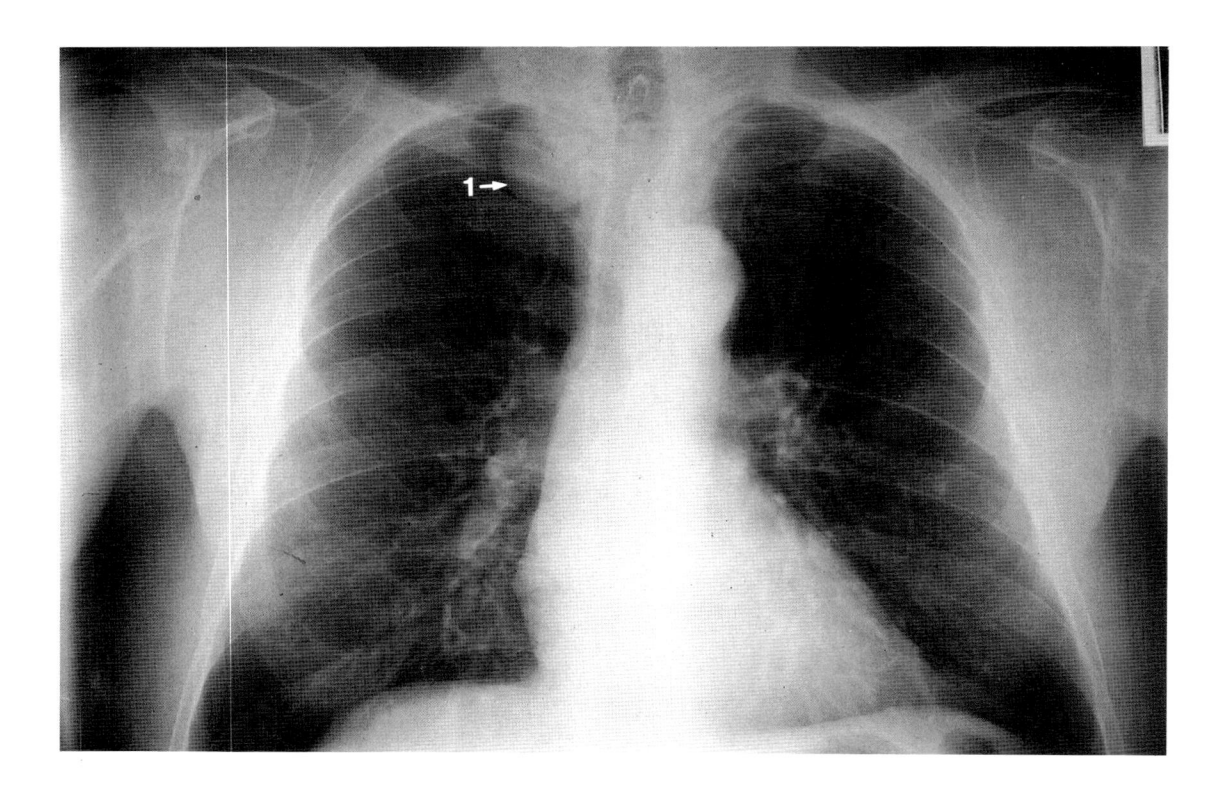

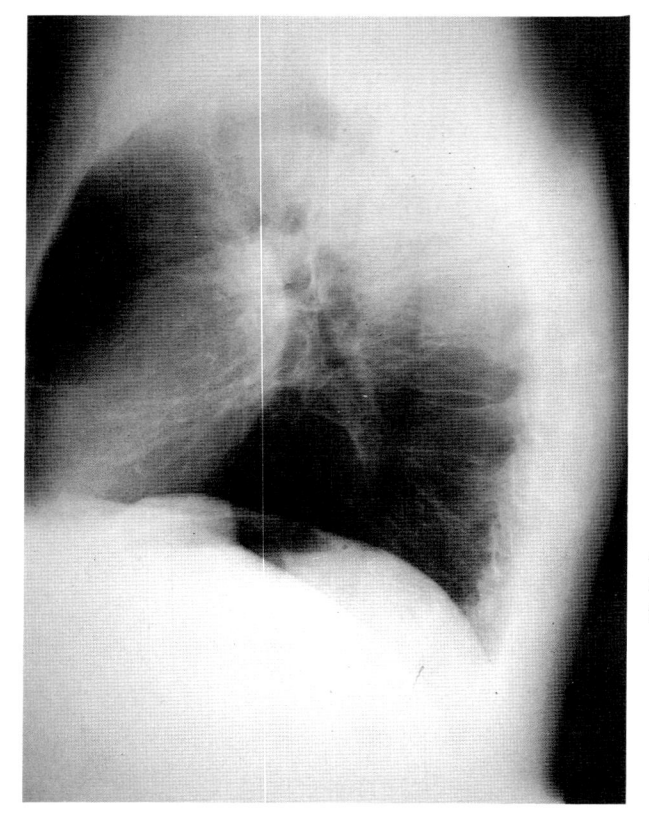

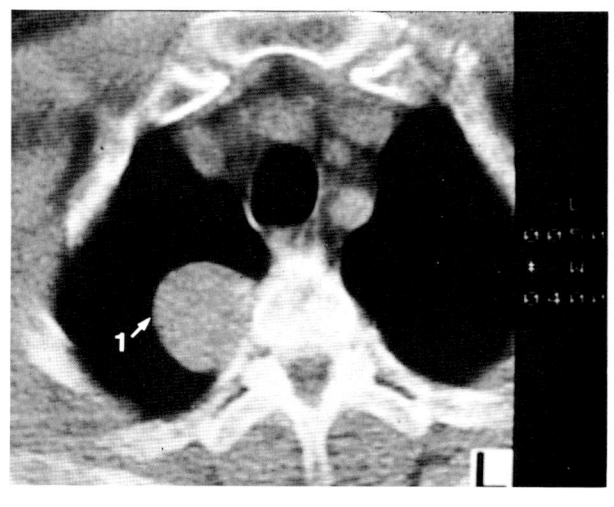

A round, well-circumscribed right paraspinal mass (1) is seen. The diagnosis is a neurogenic tumour. A neurofibroma was removed.

Index

References are to page numbers.

Abscess
— lung(s), 126
— subphrenic, 26
Achalasia, 198
Acquired immune deficiency syndrome (AIDS), 73, 74
Adenocarcinoma, 36, 112
AIDS, 73, 74
Air bronchogram, 65, 66, 72, 78
Air trapping, 102
Alveolar pulmonary oedema, 136
Alveolitis, cryptogenic fibrosing, 80
Aneurysm
— aortic arch, 186
— ascending aorta, 182
— calcified, ventricular, 178
— dissecting, of descending aorta, 184
— left ventricular, 167
Anterior mediastinal mass, 188, 192
Aorta
— ascending, aneurysm of, 182
— coarctation of, 12
— descending, dissecting aneurysm of, 184
Aortic
— aneurysm, MRI of, 186
— arch
 — aneurysm of, 186
 — right-sided, 147, 148, 156
— knuckle, 11, 12
— regurgitation, 164
— stenosis, 176
— valve, 12, 126
 — bicuspid, 12
 — calcification, 175, 176
 — replacement, 125
Aortogram, 12, 182, 184
Appendix, perforated, 26
Arteriogram, pulmonary, 122
Arterio-venous malformation (AVM), 122
Asbestos exposure, 42, 43, 44, 83
Asbestosis, 43, 44, 84
Ascending aorta
— aneurysm of, 182
— post-stenotic dilatation, 12
Aspergillus, 128
Atrial septal defect, 138
— Eisenmenger, 150
— ostium primum, 158
Atrioventricular septal defect, 158

Barium
— follow-through, 28
— meal, 30, 202
— swallow, 53, 54, 129, 130, 139, 140, 198, 200
Bone
— erosion, 13, 14, 18, 112
— sclerosis, 19, 20
Breast, carcinoma, 8
Bronchiectasis, 106
Bronchitis, chronic, 123
Bronchogenic cyst, 196
Bronchogram, 106
— air, 65, 66, 72, 78
Bronchopleural fistula, 46
Bronchoscopy, 46, 47, 48, 53, 116
Bronchus, carcinoma of, 14, 45, 48, 49, 50, 53, 54, 56, 58, 59, 60, 84, 110, 112, 114, 116, 124

Calcific aortic stenosis, 176
Calcification
— pleural, 43, 44
— popcorn, 120
— pulmonary, 22
Calcified nodular shadowing, 92
Calcified nodule, 118
Carcinoid tumour, 116
Carcinoma
— breast, 8
— bronchus, 14, 49, 50, 53, 54, 56, 58, 59, 60, 84, 110, 112, 114, 116, 124
— larynx, 96
— metastatic thyroid, 18, 86
— squamous cell, 53, 84, 124
Cardiac catheterisation, 141, 167
Cardiac outline, 5, 6
Cardiomyopathy, congestive, 39, 172
Cardiovascular silhouette, 5, 6
Cavitating, pulmonary mass, 87, 88
Cavitation, 76, 88, 96, 124, 126
Cavities
— multiple pulmonary, 96
— pulmonary, 128
Cavity, solitary pulmonary, 124, 126
Chest
— injuries, 15
— pain, 17, 31, 41, 69, 111, 135, 183, 185
— x-ray, 185, 186
 — expiration, 32, 101, 102
 — normal, 5
 — oblique, 44
Chronic obstructive airways disease, 98, 99, 100, 127, 128
Coarctation of aorta, 12
Collapse
— left lower lobe, 58
— left upper lobe, 56
— right lower lobe, 54
— right middle lobe, 52
— right upper lobe, 50
Collapsed lung, 47, 48
Congestive cardiomyopathy, 39, 172

Consolidation
— left lower lobe, 70
— left upper lobe, 65, 66
— lingular, 68
— right lower lobe, 64
— right middle lobe, 62
— right upper lobe, 60
Constrictive pericarditis, 180
Coronary arteriogram, left, 167
Cryptogenic fibrosing alveolitis, 80
CT
— of dissecting aneurysm of aorta, 184
— of lung, 14
— of mediastinum, 59, 60, 189, 190, 191, 192, 195, 196, 203, 204
— of pleura, 41, 42
— of thyroid, 189, 190
Cyanosis, 143, 145, 147, 149, 159, 160
Cyst
— bronchogenic, 196
— emphysematous, 104
— lung, 104
— testicular, 119
Cystic fibrosis, 108

Diaphragm, 24, 108
— hemi-, 26, 58, 108
— rupture of, 30
Diaphragmatic hernia, congenital, 28
Dilated oesophagus, 198, 200
Dissecting aneurysm of aorta, 184
— CT of, 184
Down's syndrome, 157, 158
Dysphagia, 53

Ebstein's anomaly of the tricuspid valve, 160
Echocardiogram, 162, 170
Effusion
— encysted, 40
— lamellar, 40
— pleural, 26, 36, 37, 38, 110, 136, 170
Eisenmenger atrial septal defect, 150
Emboli, recurrent pulmonary, 152
Emphysema
— pulmonary, 98, 128
— surgical, 72
— unilateral, 102
Emphysematous cyst, 104

Fallot, tetralogy of, 156
Fibrosis
— bilateral, upper lobe, 100
— cryptogenic fibrosing, 80
— cystic, 108
— progressive massive (PMF), 87, 88
— pulmonary, 22, 82
— radiation, 78
— upper lobe, 100, 128
Film
— lateral CXR, 5
— PA, 5
Fistula, bronchopleural, 44
Fungus balls/mycetomas, 128

Gated blood pool scan, 172
Goitre, intrathoracic, multinodular, 190
Granuloma, pulmonary, 118
Great arteries, transposition of, 144

Haemoptysis, 47, 49, 55, 83, 121, 123, 127
Hamartoma, pulmonary, 120
Heart, 10, 48, 178, 180
— border, 51, 52
— enlarged, 138, 182
— failure, 39, 129
— size, normal, 136
Hemi-diaphragm, 26, 58, 108
— rupture of, 30
Hemithrorax, 29, 37, 47, 48
Hernia, 30
— congenital diaphragmatic, 28
— hiatus, 200, 202
Hilar
— elevation, 99, 100, 128
— enlargement, 108
— lymphadenopathy, 194
— mass, 50, 60, 114, 116
Histiocytic lymphoma, 77
Histoplasmosis, 90, 92
Hodgkin's lymphoma, 77
Hydropneumothorax, 16
Hypertension
— pulmonary arterial, 98, 128, 150, 152
— pulmonary venous, 129, 130, 131, 132, 134, 167, 172
Hypertransradiant lung, 8, 102

Interstitial lines, 132, 133
Interstitial lung disease, 34, 79, 80, 81, 82, 83, 84
Interstitial pulmonary oedema, 132
Irradiation, 178

Kerley B lines, 132, 133
Klebsiella aeruginosa, 64, 126

Larynx, carcinoma of, 96
Left atrial
— appendage, enlarged, 132
— enlargement, 130, 140, 161, 162
Left ventricular
— aneurysm, 167
— calcified, 178
— enlargement, 167
Left ventriculogram, 167
Ligature, broken, 46
Lingular consolidation, 68
Lung(s), 79, 80, 97
— abnormal, 65, 107

— abscess, 126
— aerated, 54
— changes in, 81, 83
— collapsed, 16, 37, 47, 48, 72
— compressed, 104
— CT of, 14
— cyst, 104
— density, 7, 42, 43, 101
— opacities, 94
— parenchyma, 33, 34
— shadowing in, 74, 79, 107
Lymph node, 54, 60, 108
Lymphadenopathy
— paratracheal, 191, 192, 194
— pre-tracheal, 60
— hilar, 194
— sub-carinal, 54
Lymphoma, histiocytic, 77

Macleod's syndrome, 102
Malignant mesothelioma, 142
Mass
— anterior mediastinal, 188, 192
— apical, 13, 14
— hilar, 50, 60, 114, 116
— pleural, 36, 42
— posterior mediastinal, 204
— pulmonary, 83, 84
— cavitating, 87, 88
— solitary, 110, 111, 112
— retrocardiac, 202
Mastectomy, 8
Mediastinal mass
— anterior, 188, 192
— posterior, 204
— superior, 190
Mediastinum, 27, 28, 38, 46, 47, 57, 58
— CT of, 59, 60, 189, 190, 191, 192, 195, 196, 203, 204
Mesothelioma, 42
Metastases
— military pulmonary, 86
— multiple pulmonary, 94, 96
— pulmonary, 8, 114
Metastatic thyroid carcinoma, 18, 86
Metastasis
— pleural, 35, 36
— rib, 18, 114
Miliary
— pulmonary metastases, 86
— shadowing, 90
— tuberculosis, 90
Mitral
— regurgitation, 162
— stenosis, 131, 132, 174
— valve
— calcification, 174
— disease, 130
MRI of aortic aneurysm, 186

Myasthenia gravis, 188
Mycetomas / fungus balls, 128
Myocardial infarction, 117, 165
— acute, 133, 136, 169

Neurofibroma, 204
Neurogenic tumours, 204
Nodular shadowing, calcified, 92
Nodule, calcified, 118

Oedema, pulmonary
— alveolar, 136
— interstitial, 132
Oesophageal stricture, 200
Oesophagoscopy, 200
Oesophagus, 82, 198, 200
— dilated, 82
Oligaemia, pulmonary, 156

Pancoast tumour, 14
Patent ductus arteriosus, 142, 144
Peptic ulcer, 24
Pericardial
— calcification, 180
— effusion, 170
Pericarditis, constrictive, 180
Pleura
— CT of, 41, 42
— ultrasound of, 35, 38
Pleural
— calcification, 43, 44
— effusion, 26, 34, 36, 37, 38, 47, 110, 136, 170
— encysted, 40
— lamellar, 40
— infection, 22
— mass, 36, 42
— plaques, 42, 44
— shadowing, apical, 14
Pneumoconiosis, coal miner's, 87, 88
Pneumocystis carinii, 74
Pneumomediastinum, 72
Pneumonectomy, 45, 46
Pneumonia, 68
— acute, 62
— lobar, 62, 64
— right-sided, 115
— staphylococcal, 76
— varicella, 92
— viral, 71, 72
Pneumonitis, radiation, 78
Pneumoperitoneum, 24
Pneumothorax
— spontaneous, 32
— tension, 72
Popcorn calcification, 120
Post-myocardial infarction syndrome, 170
Post-stenotic dilatation
— ascending aorta, 12, 176
— pulmonary trunk, 153, 154

Posterior mediastinal mass, 204
Pulmonary
— arterial hypertension, 98, 128, 150, 152
— arteriogram, 122, 146
— arterio-venous malformation (AVM), 122
— artery, enlargement of, 108
— calcification, 22
— cavities, 128
  — multiple, 96
— cavity, solitary, 124, 126
— emboli, recurrent, 152
— emphysema, 98, 128
— fibrosis, 22
— granuloma, 118
— hamartoma, 120
— mass, 83, 84
  — cavitating, 87, 88
  — solitary, 110, 111, 112
— metastases, 8
  — miliary, 86
  — multiple, 94, 96
— metastasis, 114
— nodule, solitary, 118, 120
— oedema
  — alveolar, 133, 134, 136
  — interstitial, 132
— oligaemia, 156, 160
— plethora, 138, 140, 144, 146, 148, 158
— trunk
  — enlargement of, 149, 150, 151, 152, 153, 154
  — post-stenotic dilatation, 153, 154
— tuberculosis, 21, 22, 65, 66, 76, 100
— valve stenosis, 154
— venous hypertension, 129, 130, 131, 132, 134, 167, 172
— venous return, 146

Radiation
— fibrosis, 78
— pneumonitis, 78
Redistribution of blood flow, 129, 130, 133, 134, 167
Reticulo-nodular shadowing, 79, 80, 82, 84
Retrocardiac mass, 202
Rheumatic fever, 131
Rheumatic mitral valve disease, 130
Rheumatoid disease, 34
Rib
— fracture, 16
— metastasis, 18, 114
— notching, 12
Right atrial enlargement, 158, 159, 160
Right ventriculogram, 144, 156

Sarcoidosis, 90, 194
Sarcomas, 96

Scan, gated blood pool, 172
Scan of thyroid, isotope, 190
Scleroderma, 82
Sclerosis, bony, 19, 20
Shadowing
— nodular, 85, 86
  — calcified, 92
— reticulo-nodular, 79, 80, 82, 84
Sickle cell disease, 20
Spine, 19, 77
Squamous cell carcinoma, 53, 84, 124
Staphylococcal pneumonia, 76
Streptococcus pneumoniae, 68
Sternum, depressed (pectus excavatum), 10
Stomach, herniation of, 30
Subphrenic abscess, 26
Superior mediastinal mass, 190
Surgical emphysema, 72
Swyer-James' syndrome, 102
Syndromes
— Down's, 157, 158
— Macleod's, 102
— Post-myocardial infarction, 170
— Swyer-James', 102

Tetralogy of Fallot, 155, 156
Thoracoplasty, 21, 22
Thymoma, 188
Thyroid
— CT of, 189, 190
— isotope scan of, 190
— metastatic carcinoma, 18
Tomography, 117, 118, 119, 120, 121, 127, 128
Total anomalous pulmonary venous return, 146
Trachea, 46, 48, 55, 56, 82
Transposition of the grest arteries, 144
Truncus arteriosus, 148
Tuberculosis, 66, 92
— miliary, 90
— pulmonary, 21, 22, 65, 66, 76, 100

Ulcer, peptic, 24
Ultrasound of pleura, 35, 38
Unilateral emphysema, 102

Valve stenosis, pulmonary, 154
Varicella, pneumonia, 92
Ventilation Perfusion (VP) lung scan, 152
Ventricular
— aneurysm, 167
  — calcified, 178
— hypertrophy, 153
— hypokinesis, 172
— septal defect, 140
Ventriculogram
— left, 167
— right, 144, 156